NURSING CASE STUDIES ON IMPROVING HEALTH-RELATED QUALITY OF LIFE IN OLDER ADULTS

Meredith Wallace Kazer, PhD, APRN, AGPCNP-BC, FAAN, completed her BSN degree magna cum laude at Boston University. Following this, she earned an MSN in medical–surgical nursing with a specialty in geriatrics from Yale University and a PhD in nursing research and theory development at New York University. During her time at NYU, she was awarded a predoctoral fellowship at the Hartford Institute for Geriatric Nursing. In this capacity, she became the original author and editor of the series *Try This: Best Practices in Geriatric Nursing*. She was the managing editor and research brief editor for the *Journal of Applied Nursing Research*. Dr. Kazer is an award-winning researcher and an adult and gerontological primary care nurse practitioner. She currently maintains a practice in Connecticut with a focus on chronic illness in older adults, clinical experience that informs her scholarly work. Her work has been disseminated in 10 books, over 70 peer-reviewed journal publications, 26 book chapters, and over 100 research and invited presentations. She is the recipient of the Connecticut Nurse Association Virginia Henderson Award for Outstanding Contributions to Nursing Research, the Springer Publishing Company Award for Applied Nursing Research, and four *American Journal of Nursing* Book of the Year Awards. In addition, she is the recipient of the Eastern Nursing Research Society/John A. Hartford Foundation Junior Investigator Award, and in 2011 she was inducted as a fellow into the American Academy of Nursing, an appointment reserved for nurse leaders at the forefront of the profession nationwide.

Kathy Murphy, PhD, MSc, BA, RGN, RNT, Dip Nur, Dip Nur Ed, is a registered general nurse and has held clinical manager posts in older people's services and emergency department nursing. For the past 20 years, she has worked in nursing education, first at Oxford Brookes University, UK, and then at the National University of Ireland, Galway, and is currently a professor of nursing at NUI, Galway. Her research interests are in quality of life of older people, dementia, and chronic disease management, and she has been involved in a number of national research studies, all utilizing mixed methods.

NURSING CASE STUDIES ON IMPROVING HEALTH-RELATED QUALITY OF LIFE IN OLDER ADULTS

Meredith Wallace Kazer, PhD, APRN, AGPCNP-BC, FAAN

Kathy Murphy, PhD, MSc, BA, RGN, RNT, Dip Nur, Dip Nur Ed

Editors

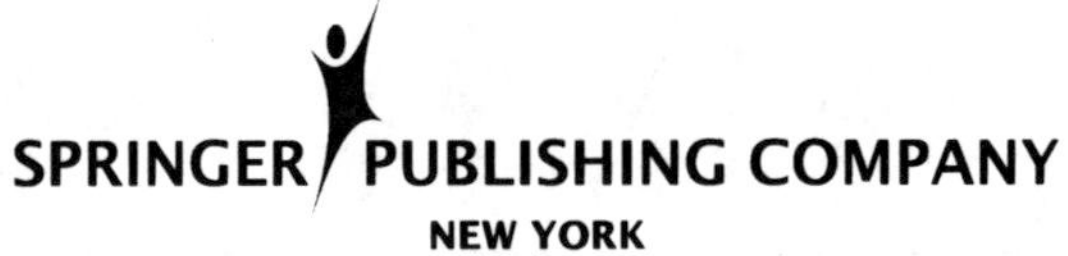

Springer Publishing Company, LLC
11 West 42nd Street
New York, NY 10036
www.springerpub.com

Acquisitions Editor: Elizabeth Nieginski
Production Editor: Kris Parrish
Composition: S4Carlisle Publishing Services

ISBN: 978-0-8261-2703-7
e-book ISBN: 978-0-8261-2704-4

15 16 17 18 / 5 4 3 2 1

Library of Congress Cataloging-in-Publication Data

Nursing case studies on improving health-related quality of life in older adults / [edited by] Meredith Wallace Kazer, Kathy Murphy.
p. ; cm.
Includes bibliographical references and index.
ISBN 978-0-8261-2703-7—ISBN 978-0-8261-2704-4 (e-book)
I. Kazer, Meredith Wallace, editor. II. Murphy, Kathy, 1953- , editor.
[DNLM: 1. Geriatric Nursing—methods. 2. Case Reports. 3. Quality of Life. WY 152]
RC954
618.97'0231—dc23 2014047655

Printed in the United States of America by Gasch Printing.

CONTENTS

CONTRIBUTORS

Helen Bartlett, PhD, MSc, BA
Monash University
Subang Jaya, Selangor, Malaysia

Simon Burrow, MA (Social Work), BA (Hons; Social Policy)
The University of Manchester
Manchester, United Kingdom

Matthew Carroll, PhD, BA (Hons)
School of Rural Health
Monash University, Gippsland Campus
Churchill, Victoria, Australia

Dympna Casey, PhD, MA, BA, RGN
School of Nursing and Midwifery
National University of Ireland, Galway
Galway, Ireland

Christine Cauffield, PsyD, MS, BS
Cauffield and Associates—Integrated Behavioral Healthcare
Sarasota, Florida

Glenda Cook, PhD, MA (Medical Ethics), BSc (PSCH), RNT, RGN
Northumbria University
Newcastle Upon Tyne, United Kingdom

Adeline Cooney, PhD, MMSc, BSc, RGN
National University of Ireland, Galway
Galway, Ireland

Mary Courtney, PhD, RN
School of Nursing, Midwifery & Paramedicine
Australian Catholic University
Victoria, Australia

Ann Coyle, PhD, OT
Ann Coyle Health Service Executive
Dundalk County, Louth, Ireland

Colleen Doyle, PhD
School of Nursing, Midwifery & Paramedicine
Australian Catholic University
Victoria, Australia

Jenneke Footitt, PhD, RN
School of Nursing, Midwifery & Paramedicine
Australian Catholic University
Victoria, Australia

Rosemary Ford, PhD, MSc, BSc, DipPH, RN, RM
School of Nursing, Midwifery & Paramedicine
Australian Catholic University
Victoria, Australia

Mary Gannon, PgDip Nursing (Gerontology), MHSc, RGN
School of Nursing and Midwifery
National University of Ireland, Galway
Nursing & Midwifery Planning Development Unit
Galway, Ireland

Catherine Houghton, PhD, MSc, RGN, RPN
School of Nursing and Midwifery
National University of Ireland, Galway
Galway, Ireland

Andrew Hunter, MSc, BA, RMN
School of Nursing and Midwifery
National University of Ireland, Galway
Galway, Ireland

Cecily Hunter, PhD
School of Nursing, Midwifery & Paramedicine
Australian Catholic University
Victoria, Australia

Cynthia S. Jacelon, PhD, RN, CRRN, FAAN
School of Nursing
University of Massachusetts
Amherst, Massachusetts

David Jackson, RN
School of Nursing, Midwifery & Paramedicine
Australian Catholic University
Victoria, Australia

Anna Ramió Jofre, PhD, RN
Campus Docent Sant Joan de Déu
University of Barcelona
Barcelona, Spain

Meredith Wallace Kazer, PhD, APRN, AGPCNP-BC, FAAN
Fairfield University
School of Nursing
Fairfield, Connecticut

John Keady, PhD, RMN, RNT
The University of Manchester
Manchester, United Kingdom

Marcella Kelly, MSc, RGN, RM, PHN
School of Nursing and Midwifery
National University of Ireland, Galway
Galway, Ireland

Mary Kjorven, MSN, BSN, GNC
Interior Health
Kelowna, British Columbia, Canada

Alison E. Kris, PhD, RN
Fairfield University
School of Nursing
Fairfield, Connecticut

Kimberly O. Lacey, DNSc, MSN, CNS, CNE
Department of Nursing
Southern Connecticut State University
New Haven, Connecticut

Kathleen Lovanio, MSN, ANP-BC
School of Nursing
Fairfield University
Fairfield, Connecticut

Bernadette Madara, EdD, APRN-BC
Department of Nursing
Southern Connecticut State University
New Haven, Connecticut

Diana R. Mager, DNP, RN-BC
School of Nursing
Fairfield University
Fairfield, Connecticut

Pauline Meskell, PhD, MSc, BSc, PGC-TLHE, Dip AP, RGN
School of Nursing & Midwifery
National University of Ireland, Galway
Galway, Ireland

Teresa Moore, MSc (Primary Care), H Dip (Primary Care), Dip (Management), RNID, RGN
Education Centre
St. Brendan Campus
Loughrea, County Galway, Ireland

Stephanie B. Mostone, RN, BSN, OCN
Fairfield University
School of Nursing
Fairfield, Connecticut

Kathy Murphy, PhD, MSc, DipN, BA, RN, RNT
School of Nursing and Midwifery
National University of Ireland, Galway
Galway, Ireland

Jean M. O'Connor, DNP, MPH, MS, FNP, ARNP-C
Cauffield and Associates—Integrated Behavioral Healthcare
Sarasota, Florida

Kathleen O'Neil-Meyers, MSN, BC
U.S. Department of Veterans Affairs
West Haven, Connecticut

Eamon O'Shea, PhD, MA, MSc, BA
School of Business, Public Policy and Law
National University of Ireland, Galway
Galway, Ireland

Claire O'Tuathail, PGCTLHE, MSc, PGDip Gerontology, RGN
School of Nursing and Midwifery
National University of Ireland, Galway
Galway, Ireland

Theresa Tavella Quell, PhD, MSN, RN
School of Nursing
Fairfield University
Fairfield, Connecticut

Laura Martínez Rodríguez, PhD, RN
Campus Docent Sant Joan de Déu
University of Barcelona
Barcelona, Spain

Kathy L. Rush, PhD, RN
University of British Columbia—Okanagan Campus
School of Nursing
Kelowna, British Columbia, Canada

Assumpta Ryan, PhD, MEd, BSc (Hons), RMN, RGN, RNT, PGCTHE
School of Nursing
University of Ulster
Londonderry, Northern Ireland

Catherine Sweeney, H.Dip Nursing, BA, RGN, ENB 998
Director of Nursing
Mowlam Healthcare
Limerick, Ireland

Juliana Thompson, MA, BSc, BA, RN
Northumbria University
Newcastle Upon Tyne, United Kingdom

Claire Welford, PhD, MSc, DipNS, BNS–Hons, RGN, PGCTLHE
Practice Development Facilitator
Mowlam Healthcare
Limerick, Ireland

Vanessa M. White, BBSc (Hons)
Australian Institute of Primary Care & Aging
La Trobe University
Victoria, Australia

Min-Lin Wu, PhD, RN, MN
Australian Catholic University
Victoria, Australia

Toyoaki Yamauchi, PhD, MD, ND, FNP
Graduate School of Medicine
Nagoya University
Nagoya, Japan

PREFACE

This book fulfills a substantial need among the gerontological nursing literature. While quality of life (QOL) is often discussed in relation to the care of older adults, there is a substantial gap between patient and family wishes and clinical practice implementation. This gap can be filled only through knowledge and communication. Through the development of this book we aim to advance education for nurses in clinical practice in an attempt to resolve gaps in the care of older adults. Gerontological nursing care has made substantial advances over the past several decades; however, we continue to support efforts toward further improvement. We are hopeful that this book will lead gerontological nurses toward a higher level of care. Nurses caring for older adults are poised and ready for this advancement. The strength of this book is the ability to link real patient cases with the evidence and provide practical strategies for improving this care.

In this book, we have chosen to highlight a number of commonly occurring issues among older adults. The first section examines global issues that are important to QOL. As in the entire book, each chapter opens with a case study, reviews the literature, and provides specific strategies for improving QOL for individuals and families. The cases showcase the experiences of older people as they struggle to maintain autonomy, dignity, and a sense of self amid the aging process and declining health. The chapters provide a lens through which to examine challenges of aging and strategies that may be implemented to promote QOL. The middle section of the book is organized around 15 chapters that direct the lens toward a number of environmental issues that impact the QOL of older adults. The cases contained in this section explore the experiences of older adults at home and in assisted living and nursing home environments. Evidence-based literature reviews enhance the discussion of care issues that impact older adults and their families. The authors of these chapters use clinical experience and the evidence to improve understanding of issues that impact the QOL of older adults across these multiple care environments. The final section of this book is organized around 12 chapters that may function as a clinical resource guide for clinicians. Cases are presented to improve clinical reasoning and improve understanding of issues that older adults encounter in preventing and managing acute and chronic disease states.

Some of the chapters focus on commonly occurring medical issues; others explore less common health care conditions.

As we prepared this book, we selected contributors who are on the front lines of health care for the aged and have been involved in both clinical practice and research. In this way, the cases are realistic and moving. In addition, the literature selected is up to date and comprehensive. We understand that these cases are not the beginning and end of all knowledge on the topic areas presented, but we are confident that they will inspire the necessary dialogue. As readers journey through these cases and the supporting literature, it is our hope that they will increase their understanding of issues that impact older adults across environments of care and stimulate effective assessment and management strategies.

We are hopeful that this book stimulates discussion, knowledge development, and improved care for the rapidly increasing population of older adults worldwide. However, we understand that it is only a small contribution. We are indebted to our contributors for sharing in our desire to increase the care of older adults and to Springer Publishing Company for investing in this care. However, we also look forward to a future when the care proposed within this volume becomes standard and an improved QOL for older adults is realized. It is only with such contributions that this goal may be attained.

Meredith Wallace Kazer
Kathy Murphy

ACKNOWLEDGMENT

The authors wish to gratefully acknowledge the contributions of Reverend Michael Fahey, S.J., Scholar in Residence at Fairfield University, who devoted his time and attention to the thoughtful and comprehensive editing of this book. We remain forever in his debt.

I

FOUNDATIONS OF QUALITY IN OLDER ADULT CARE

KATHY MURPHY

Maintaining quality of life (QOL) into older age is one of the important challenges facing the growing aging population and governments across the world. While QOL is a useful and widely used expression, its apparent simplicity masks the complexity and ambiguity surrounding the actual meaning of the concept. QOL is difficult to define and to measure as it is made up of interacting objective and subjective dimensions, which may change over time in response to life and health events and experiences (Bowling, 2003). What is really important, therefore, is to ensure that health care is focused on the components of QOL that matter to older people and have in place strategies for maximizing QOL into older age.

The opening section of the book is devoted to an exploration of the issues that are important to QOL of older people. In most of the chapters of this section, QOL is divided into specific domains. Each chapter contains a case study, supporting literature, and specific strategies for improving QOL within that domain. The cases reveal the experiences of older adults in a variety of environments as they struggle to maintain their quality, autonomy, or dignity within the context of aging and deteriorating health. The chapters provide insights into some of the challenges that occur in QOL issues across living environments and strategies that can be used by nurses to promote quality of life.

Each chapter presents a case study and supporting literature; the case study gives both the objective and the subjective appraisal of the issues described. Consideration of the material in the chapters will enable nurses to increase their understanding of issues that extend across environments of care and strategies they can use to maximize good assessment and management. The cases in this section describe some of the QOL concepts that underpin the foundations of care for older people. Using the case study framework, nurses can develop enhanced clinical knowledge regarding how the ethos of care can impact on the QOL of older adults and how some of these issues can be addressed.

This section of the book is organized around eight chapters that focus attention on a number of environmental and theoretical issues that impact the QOL of older adults. The first chapter explores the case of an older woman who lives alone following the death of her husband. Now, while physically well, she is finding life a struggle, is feeling low, and finds it increasingly difficult to do the work of maintaining her home. Through the review of literature, Drs. Murphy and Kazer explore the overall concept of QOL and strategies to enhance QOL. In the second chapter, Dr. Coyle explores the impact of person-centered care on the QOL of older adults living in nursing home environments. She describes the concept of person-centered care and identifies solutions and strategies to enable care to become more person centered.

In Chapter 3 of this section, Dr. Welford and Ms. Sweeney consider the issues impacting on the autonomy of an older man recently admitted to nursing home care. Relevant exploration of the literature into the concept of autonomy is provided in this chapter. Care planning strategies and the use of a core daily life plan are explored in this chapter. The ability to make choices in the way you live your life in nursing home environments is explored in the next chapter of this book. In Chapter 5, Dr. Murphy challenges caregivers to find ways to promote independence amid institutional climates that often engender dependency. In Chapter 6, Dr. Jacelon explores the challenge of maintaining dignity across care environments and describes how this concept is increasingly important as people age.

Chapter 7 explores the complex issues of risk, what this means, and the tools that can be used to help nurses make risk assessments balanced alongside consequences. The need for risk avoidance to be balanced with older adults' needs, values, and overall QOL is identified. In the last chapter in this section, Dr. Kazer explores the complex issues of sexuality and aging through a case study of an older woman who is experiencing some difficulties with intercourse.

The many case studies and evidence-based literature reviews contained within this section expand the discussion of meaningful QOL substantially. The authors of these chapters use clinical experience and sources to enhance understanding of issues that impact the QOL of older adults. The solutions and strategies contained herein are, in many cases, easily implementable and can significantly impact the QOL of older adults and their families. Each chapter presents a unique QOL issue and uses the case study approach to broaden understanding of nurses and, consequently, to promote QOL for older adults.

Reference

Bowling, A. (2003). Current state of the art in quality of life measurement. In A. J. Carr, I. J. Higginson, & P. Robinson (Eds.), *Quality of life* (pp. 1–8). London, England: BMJ Books.

1 QUALITY OF LIFE

KATHY MURPHY AND MEREDITH WALLACE KAZER

Subjective

"I am just so alone now."

Objective

Mrs. Abigail Ames is a 72-year-old woman who lives alone in a small town on the west coast of Ireland. Her husband died last year. He had a massive myocardial infarction while gardening and died instantly. Mrs. Ames has three grown-up children who are all living abroad. Mrs. Ames visited her family practitioner last week because she was feeling down. She said she has found life on her own quite lonely—her husband had been her main companion. She has one sister who is living in Northern Ireland and, while they get on well, they rarely see each other because both are widowed and neither can drive. After the death of her husband, there was a lot to do, and the children had been over a few times in the first year, but, she says, "They have their lives to get on with now." The children bought her a new dog, her beloved dog Toto, as they were concerned about her being in the house alone, and she said she still feels nervous about nights on her own. Mrs. Ames has a good work pension; she was a university administrator, owns her own house, and says she has no financial concerns. Her house is a bungalow, well equipped and cared for. She is a very organized person who has a personal computer and laptop and what she describes as reasonable IT skills. She is finding the garden a burden, especially as she cannot get the lawnmower to start, so recently she has stopped cutting the grass and has the young boy across the road do it for her. Mrs. Ames used to enjoy golf and reading, but lately her eyesight has deteriorated, and she is finding reading difficult, especially at night. Mrs. Ames is a Catholic, but has found herself less interested lately in the organized church. Mrs. Ames says that her life is lonely and difficult, and she finds it hard to pass the day. She misses her children and her husband, and has lost interest in going out.

On examination, Mrs. Ames is 156 cm (61 in.) in height and weighs 190 lbs. (86 kg). Her blood pressure (BP) is 170/90; her pulse (P) is 120 respirations, 22 per minute; she is overweight with a BMI of 29; her waist circumference is 88 cm (35 in.). She says she has put on a bit of weight since giving up her daily walk that she used to do with her husband, and has recently stopped cutting the grass also. Overall, her physical health has been good; she has recently been prescribed BP medication, but otherwise describes herself as physically well. Recently, she has been feeling low in mood, which she attributes to her husband's death. Her current medications are Lisinopril 20 mg po daily. She is not a member of any local groups at present.

Literature Review

Populations across the world are aging; the World Health Organization (2012) predicts that the proportion of the population over 60 will double, rising from 11% in 2000 to 22% by 2050. The number of people over 80—the older old age group—is predicted to rise even more markedly, quadrupling between 2000 and 2050 and reaching 395 million. Currently, it is estimated that, in the United States, 10,000 individuals a day are turning 65 years old; this trend is expected to continue for over the next two decades, and by 2030, 20% of the population, or 72.1 million people, will be older adults (Administration on Ageing, 2010). In this context, it is important to think about the quality of life of older people and the strategies that nurses can use to enable older people to live well.

Quality of life (QOL) has gained increased attention as a significant factor in the care and management of many nursing problems over the past several decades. In the past, physical problems generally led to more rapid mortality and subsequently less suffering. Little attention was paid to the impact that those physical problems had on other aspects of life. Today, previously incurable diseases are now treated and sometimes eradicated, leading to the prolongation of human life. The end result is a population of older adults previously nonexistent in recent history. The challenge this newly evolved population presents is in designing health care systems that seek not only to prolong the quantity of life, but also to improve the QOL. In fact, Senator Charles McMathias Jr. in 1979 showed early insight into the challenges of the growing older population when he stated:

> I simply cannot believe that we, who accomplished the miracle of prolonging life, are willing now to watch that miracle turn into a Frankenstein monster. We cannot let longer lives mean only more suffering and greater loneliness. We must make those extra years shine for our elderly. I believe we will. (McMathias, 1979, p. 386)

George and Bearon (1980) tell us that QOL had its origins in the concept of "the good life" as described by the philosopher Aristotle; both concepts are fundamentally about the QOL. Aristotle proposed that "the good life" was a life that was worthwhile, fulfilling, virtuous, and lived in a way that enabled the capacity for rational action to be realized (Smith, 2000). Traditional Chinese philosophy also made reference to QOL, suggesting that a good QOL was achievable if there was harmony between yin and yang (Zhan, 1992). John Seth, a Scottish philosopher writing in the 19th century (Seth, 1889, p. 43), proposed that longevity and QOL should be seen as equally important and viewed enhancing QOL as a moral end toward which mankind should aspire (Smith, 2000).

The term QOL did not appear in the *International Encyclopedia of Social Sciences* until 1968. Bond and Corner (2004) suggest that research interest in QOL was ignited around this time within the context of expanding economies and increasing affluence. It was not until the late 1970s, however, that entries regarding QOL began to appear in health care literature, and research into the impact of care on QOL has expanded exponentially in the past three decades (Bowling, Banister, Sutton, Evans, & Windsor, 2002; Bowling et al., 2003; Fry, 2000; Gurland & Katz, 1991). QOL has become an important outcome measure for many care interventions, so it is important to understand what it is.

QOL is difficult to define and measure precisely. QOL is comprised of both objective and subjective elements, which may change over time and are impacted by life, deteriorating health, and overall experiences (Bowling, 2003; Murphy, O'Shea, & Cooney 2007a). Some researchers have attempted to understand QOL by examining what life is, what quality is, and how they intersect. *Taber's Cyclopedic Medical Dictionary* (2005) defines *life* as the "state of being alive; quality manifested by metabolism, growth, reproduction, and adaptation to environment; state in which the organs of an animal or plant are capable of performing all or any of their functions." Webster defines life as "the quality that distinguishes a vital and functional being from a dead body; a principle or force that is considered to underlie the distinctive quality of animate beings." Interestingly, the word *quality* is seen in both definitions of life. This reveals that the two words that form the concept are closely related and well understood by both health care professionals and lay people. In addition, the listing of the manifestation of the qualities of metabolism, growth, reproduction, and adaptation empowers the construct of multidimensionality.

Human needs may also provide part of the foundation for QOL, and this can be an important influence on the theory and practice of measurement (Bowling & Gabriel, 2004; Browne, O'Boyle, McGee, McDonald, & Joyce, 1997). Maslow's (1970) *A Theory of Human Motivation and Personality* outlines a needs-based approach to measuring QOL that adopts a hierarchical stance. At the bottom of the hierarchy are the basic needs, which are the physiological needs, followed by the safety and security needs. These needs are deemed to be essential for human survival, and it is not until they have been fully satisfied that an individual will seek to fulfill higher level needs. When the physiological and safety needs have been gratified, then love and affection and belongingness needs will emerge. These include the need for affectionate relationships; for example, with family and friends. When this need is satisfied, the individual will strive to fulfill the esteem needs that include a feeling of self-respect and self-confidence and the gaining of the respect of others. Finally, Maslow maintains that even if all of the aforementioned desires are met, an individual will not be at peace until he or she has fulfilled the need for self-actualization, that is, that "the individual is doing what he/she, individually, is fitted for" (Maslow, 1970). In other words, the individual must be able to realize and express his or her full potential, whatever the circumstances, what Sen (1993) might describe as maximizing capabilities.

In an attempt to isolate the concerns relevant to individual QOL values, researchers have attempted to define QOL by evaluating the needs and values of individuals within different population groups or environments of care. There has therefore been a focus on QOL of older people (Bond & Corner, 2004; Bowling et al., 2003; Grewal et al., 2006), QOL of older people living in long-stay care (Ball et al., 2000; Berglund & Ericsson, 2003; Cooney, Murphy, & O'Shea, 2009; Hubbard, Downs, & Tester, 2003; Kane et al., 2003; Leung, Wu, Lue, & Tang, 2004; Murphy et al., 2007a; Tester, Hubbard, Downs, MacDonald, & Murphy, 2004), and QOL and disability (Bowling, 2007; Bowling et al., 2003; Farquhar, 1995; Grewal et al., 2006), resulting in a wide spectrum of opinion and perspectives. QOL also has relevancy across disciplines and has been explored within economics, sociology, psychology, philosophy, medicine, nursing, social history, and geography (Bowling & Brazier, 1995; Farquhar, 1995). Bringing together all these diverse perspectives is important in order to really understand what QOL is. However, because disciplines examine QOL through different disciplinary lenses and older people experiencing different circumstances and living environments may emphasize different components of QOL, this exploration has given rise to a variety of interpretations (Anderson & Burckhardt, 1999).

Measurement of QOL has therefore been problematic. Initially, QOL scales designed to capture QOL focused on objective indicators such as finances and assets. However, it quickly became evident that these elements were not sufficient for fully understanding QOL. Therefore, researchers started to include subjective measures within QOL scales such as well-being, happiness, and life satisfaction (Farquhar, 1995; Murphy, O'Shea, Cooney, & Casey 2007b; Smith, 2000). These subjective measures are important to ensure that QOL studies focus on what is important to people, but their inclusion gives rise to a more complex and individualized definition of QOL that in turn makes comparison complex and stakeholder consensus difficult to achieve. QOL, however, is now regularly used as an outcome measure in evaluation of health care interventions and in economic analysis (Bond & Corner, 2004; Smith, 2000). Issues of cost-effectiveness and Medicare revisions inspired exploration into the substantial expenditures to keep people alive for years on respirators and other life-sustaining equipment, only to have such people die or return to a life considered undesirable.

Gurland and Katz (1991) conducted an extensive review of QOL literature in the context of older people. Through a process of content analysis, they developed a list of 19 domains in which QOL should be evaluated. These domains include: mobility, four areas of activities of daily living, organizational skills, orientational skills, receptive communication, expressive communication, health and perceived health, mood and symptoms, social and interpersonal relations, autonomy, financial management, environmental fit, gratification, future image, general well-being, and effective coordination. The validity of this model has not yet been tested in the area of QOL assessment.

It is also clear that although full consensus in relation to the determining components of QOL of older people remains elusive, there are some important domains of QOL that are emerging across research studies. These are health; psychological well-being, including spirituality, social relationships, activities, home, and neighborhood; and financial circumstances (Bond & Corner, 2004; Bowling et al., 2003; Farquhar, 1995; Grewal et al., 2006).

Researchers often identify physical health as an important influence on QOL. However, there are some important differences in the value placed on physical health; people who are generally healthy are more likely to stress the importance of good health, whereas people with significant disabilities often emphasize the importance of abilities rather than physical health (Murphy et al., 2007b). Psychological well-being is also frequently identified as an important factor for good QOL because it can shape how you perceive your experiences and life in general. Spirituality has been identified as important, with many older people identifying this as central to their QOL.

According to Bond and Corner (2004), family and kinship, good social relationships (Bowling et al., 2003), and close bonds with others (Borglin et al. 2005) are critical to QOL. The quality of relationships has been found to be an influencing factor in the engagement that people have with their communities, families, and friends. Various studies have also found a positive correlation between engagement in meaningful activities and QOL for older people (Farquhar, 1995; Grewal et al., 2006), and involvement in social activities, local community, and voluntary organizations also contributes to a good QOL (Bowling et al., 2003).

Home and neighborhood have also been identified as important to QOL (Bowling et al., 2003) as the physical environment can help or hinder independence, provide material comforts, or hinder or facilitate outdoor activities. Material circumstances and income have been identified as important to QOL (Bowling et al., 2003; Murphy et al., 2007b). Income allows older people more opportunities to participate in economic, social, and cultural life.

Role and Cultural Considerations

Providers caring for Mrs. Ames must consider the multiple QOL dimensions within a cultural context in order to improve health outcomes for this client. From a physical perspective, she is accustomed to visiting her provider and has a strong relationship, illustrated by her ability to share her concerns. Little is known about her spiritual practices. However, she has been a practicing Catholic until recently. Thus, conducting a spiritual assessment and referral to clergy may be within the role of the provider. From the economic perspective, Mrs. Ames seems comfortable enough and may consider traveling in the future. The loss of her role as a wife appears to be among her biggest challenges. Referral to support services for grief counseling may be appropriate within the early months following her husband's death. Then reconnecting with social avenues, through social clubs, senior services, the church, and volunteer activities, may be instrumental in helping Mrs. Ames to connect with others. Her social life was strong prior to her husband's death, and this projects strong possibilities for the future. From a cultural perspective, she may be less inclined to ask for help. Thus, a consistent assessment regarding QOL issues at each appointment will help to keep these multiple dimensions of the concept a top priority from the provider perspective.

Strategies to Enhance QOL

Relationships and connection to others have been described as determining of QOL. Mrs. Ames said she was feeling low in mood, was lonely, and missed her children and husband. Therefore, considering strategies to reconnect Mrs. Ames to her sister, family, and friends is important to overall QOL. Mrs. Ames was a university administrator, and because she has good computer skills, Skype could be one technology that could help her connect to her family. Group Skype could give her the capacity to talk to her children together; raising this with her may help facilitate her connectedness. Her family also needs to understand that she is lonely, and discussing the importance of telling them with Mrs. Ames may help her to ask the family for more support. Connections to the local community are also important, particularly as so many people withdraw rather than engage as they get older. Mrs. Ames used to walk daily. There is a walking group that meets twice a week in the town where she lives, and joining this group may help Mrs. Ames to reduce weight and increase her overall fitness and connect her to some of the community activities. There is also a local book club, and although Mrs. Ames is finding reading more difficult because of her eyesight, an e-reader with adjustable fonts may help her with her reading issues and give her the confidence to join the group.

Purposeful activity is also a key QOL issue, and doing activities that are meaningful and fulfilling matters. Mrs. Ames has many skills that could be of great value to the local community; the local active retirement group has been struggling to find someone to do their accounts, and Mrs. Ames may be able to use her skills to benefit the group. Community nurses have a wealth of knowledge about what is happening at a local level and may be able to identify opportunities for engagement. Getting Mrs. Ames involved and engaged in community activities may impact positively on her mood and psychological well-being.

Mrs. Ames stopped cutting the grass when she found it difficult to start the lawnmower. Many older people reduce the level of physical activity they do as they age; however, this may impact negatively on their overall levels of fitness and physical health. Therefore, identifying ways of continuing to undertake physical activity is important. It may be that spreading the activity over a longer time and getting help to undertake the activity is a better strategy than stopping engagement in the activity altogether. Mrs. Ames could get the young boy to start the lawnmower for her or she could replace the lawnmower with one that starts more easily. This may all help to keep Mrs. Ames active and fit for longer.

There are many domains that are relevant to the QOL of older people, and as populations age across the world, it is important to ask how the care given by nurses impacts on the QOL of the older people they care for and what strategies can be used to improve QOL. To date, there are few books that provide evidence-based analysis of QOL among older adults and across environments of care, and none that focus on strategies that can improve QOL. This book identifies how nurses can contribute to improving the QOL of the older people for whom they care.

Clinical Reasoning Questions

1. Considering the multiple dimensions of QOL, what interventions would you recommend for Mrs. Ames?
2. To whom would you refer her and in what priority? How can shared decision-making systems be developed?
3. Mrs. Ames's health status is stable. However, what if she were ill and homebound? How would this change the plan of care?

4. Have you ever worked with clients such as Mrs. Ames before? If so, what strategies did you find most effective in improving their QOL?

References

Administration on Ageing. (2010). *Ageing statistics.* Retrieved from http://www.aoa.acl.gov/Aging_Statistics/Census_Population/census2010/Index.aspx

Anderson, K. L., & Burckhardt, C. S. (1999). Conceptualization and measurement of quality of life as an outcome variable for health care intervention and research. *Journal of Advanced Nursing, 29*, 298–306.

Ball, M. M., Whittington, F. J., Perkins, M. M., Patterson, V. L., Hollingsworth, C., King, S. V., & Combs, B. L. (2000). Quality of life in assisted living facilities: Viewpoints of residents. *Journal of Applied Gerontology, 19*(3), 304–325.

Berglund, A. L., & Ericsson, K. (2003). Different meanings of quality of life: A comparison between what elderly persons and geriatric staff believe is of importance. *International Journal of Nursing Practice, 9*(2), 112–119.

Bond, J., & Corner, L. (2004). *Quality of life and older people.* Berkshire, England: Open University Press.

Borglin, G., Jakobsson, U., Edberg, A., & Hallberg, I. (2005). The experience of quality of life among older people. *Journal of Aging Studies, 19*(2), 201–220.

Bowling, A. (2003). Current state of the art in quality of life measurement. In A. J. Carr, I. J. Higginson, & P. Robinson (Eds.), *Quality of life* (pp. 1–8). London, England: BMJ Books.

Bowling, A. (2007). Quality of life in older age: What older people say. In H. Mollenkopf & A. Walker (Eds.), *Quality of life in old age: International and multi-disciplinary perspectives* (pp. 15–30). Dordrecht, The Netherlands: Springer.

Bowling, A., Banister, D., Sutton, S., Evans, O., & Windsor, J. (2002). A multidimensional model of the quality of life in older age. *Aging of Mental Health, 6*(4), 355–371.

Bowling, A., & Brazier, J. (1995). Introduction. *Social Science & Medicine, 41*, 1337–1338.

Bowling, A., & Gabriel, Z. (2004). An integrational model of quality of life in older age: Results from the ESRC/MRC HSRC Quality of Life Survey in Britain. *Social Indicators Research, 69*, 1–36.

Bowling, A., Gabriel, Z., Dykes, L. M., Marriott-Dowding, L., Evans, O., Fleissig, A., . . . Sutton, S. (2003). Let's ask them: A national survey of definitions of quality of life and its enhancement among people aged 65 and over. *International Journal of Aging and Human Development, 56*(4), 269–306.

Browne, J. P., O'Boyle, C. A., McGee, H. M., McDonald, N. J., & Joyce, C. R. B. (1997). Development of a direct weighting procedure for quality of life domains. *Quality of Life Research, 6*, 301–309.

Cooney, A., Murphy, K., & O'Shea, E. (2009). Resident perspectives of the determinants of quality of life in residential care in Ireland. *Journal of Advance Nursing, 65*(5), 1029–1038.

Farquhar, M. (1995). Elderly people's definitions of quality of life. *Social Science & Medicine, 41*(10), 1439–1446.

Fry, P. S. (2000). Whose quality of life is it anyway? Why not ask seniors to tell us about it? *The International Journal of Aging and Human Development, 50*(4), 361–383.

George, L. K., & Bearon, L. B. (1980). *Quality of life in older persons: Meaning and measurement*. New York, NY: Human Sciences Press.

Grewal, I., Lewis, J., Flynn, T., Brown, J., Bond, J., & Coast, J. (2006). Developing attributes for a generic quality of life measure for older people: Preferences or capabilities? *Social Science & Medicine, 62*, 1891–1901.

Gurland, B. J., & Katz, S. (1991). Science of quality of life of elders: Challenges and opportunities. In J. E. Birren, J. E. Lubben, J. C. Rowe, & D. E. Deutchman (Eds.), *The concept and measurement of quality of life in the frail elderly* (pp. 335–343). London, UK: Academic Press.

Hubbard, G., Downs, M. G., & Tester, S. (2003). Including older people with dementia in research: Challenges and strategies. *Aging & Mental Health, 7*(5), 351–362.

Kane, R. A., Kling, K. C., Bershadsky, B., Kane, R. L., Giles, K., Degenholtz, H. B., . . . Cutler, L. J. (2003). Quality of life measures for nursing home residents. *Journal of Gerontology Series A Biological Sciences and Medical Sciences, 58*(3), 240–248.

Leung, K. K., Wu, E. C., Lue, B. H., & Tang, L. Y. (2004). The use of focus groups in evaluating quality of life components among elderly Chinese people. *Quality of Life Research, 13*(1), 179–190.

Maslow, A. H. (1970). *A theory of human motivation and personality* (2nd ed.). New York, NY: Harper & Row.

McMathias, C. (1979). Improving the quality of life for the elderly. *Journal of the American Geriatrics Society, 28*(9), 385–388.

Murphy, K., O'Shea, E., & Cooney, A. (2007a). The quality of life for older people living in long-stay settings in Ireland. *Journal of Clinical Nursing, 16*(11), 2167–2177.

Murphy, K., O'Shea, E., Cooney, A., & Casey, D. (2007b). *Quality of life of older people with a disability in Ireland*. Dublin, Ireland: National Council on Ageing and Older People.

Sen, A. (1993). Capability and well-being. In M. Nussbaum and A. Sen (Eds.), *The Quality of Life* (pp. 30–53). Oxford, UK: Clarendon Press.

Seth, J. (1889). The evolution of morality in normative ethics. *Mind, 14*(53), 27–49.

Smith, A. (2000). *Researching quality of life of older people: Concepts, measures and findings* (Centre for Social Gerontology Working Paper No. 7). Keele, UK: Keele University.

Taber's Cyclopedic Medical Dictionary. (2005; 20th ed.). Philadelphia, PA: F.A. Davis.

Tester, S., Hubbard, G., Downs, M., MacDonald, C., & Murphy, J. (2004). Frailty and institutional life. In A. Walker & C. Hennessy Hagan (Eds.), *Growing older quality of life in old age* (pp. 209–224). Berkshire, England: Open University Press.

Webster's Ninth New Collegiate Dictionary. (1983). Springfield, MA: Merriam-Webster.

World Health Organization. (2012). *Interesting facts about ageing*. Retrieved from http://www.who.int/ageing/about/facts/en

Zhan, H. L. (1992). Quality of life: Conceptual and measurement issues. *Journal of Advanced Nursing, 17*(7), 795–800.

2 PERSON-CENTERED CARE

Ann Coyle

Subjective

"It's the Lord's way."

Objective

Mrs. Betty Baker is 94 years old and describes herself as a mother, grandmother, and homemaker. She came to live in the long-term care facility 14 months ago, having come directly from an acute hospital following repeated bouts of pneumonia. Mrs. Baker was married, has raised four sons, and is now widowed. She has a lifelong interest in politics, likes talking to people, enjoys music, and loves being outdoors. She also describes herself as being deeply religious. She is pragmatic about her incapacity to live alone and states that she is resigned to her situation and grateful for the care she receives. She recounts a daily routine where staff help her to wash and get dressed, after which she sits beside her bed or goes to the day room, where she occasionally reads the newspaper or watches TV. From her perspective, these are long uneventful days where each one is the same as the next, and she says she has little purpose in her life.

Mrs. Baker's son Seamus expresses concerns about her lack of social interaction and stimulation, but considers this to be an inevitable outcome of living in a long-term care setting. He reports that, despite his hopes, she has not made friends with any of the other residents. Although she shares a room, communication is limited due to her roommate's hearing impairment and her own voice being very weak. Seamus lives an hour's drive away and visits once a week. Her other sons live further away and visit when they can.

Mrs. Baker describes her relationship with staff as cordial—based on seeking and receiving support for activities of daily living and health care interventions. She knows little about their personal lives, and does not believe she has any right to. However, she talks animatedly about her relationship with one staff member, Marion, who is the daughter of a neighbor and whom she has known since Marion was a child. Seamus recalls how comforting it was for her to know that she had a connection with one person when she was admitted. While Marion is not scheduled to work in the unit that Mrs. Baker lives in, she visits her occasionally in her own time and buys toiletries for her when she needs them.

Mrs. Baker expresses anxiety at not being able to attend religious events as often as she would like to but states that she does not want to ask for assistance to attend as the *"staff are busy."* Nor does she ask for additional assistance from her family as she feels *"they have their own lives to lead."* While clearly able to express choice in relation to food or when to get up or retire, she describes little involvement in the "running of the day," stating that this is the role and domain of staff. She expresses no resistance to this or to the scheduled bathing and meal times, accepting these as inevitable elements of communal living. When asked about her hopes for the future, Betty talks about her desire for *"a happy death."*

According to her care plan, Mrs. Baker weighs 47 kg (104 lbs.) with a body mass index (BMI) of 20 and has been assessed as having a high risk of malnutrition. Her blood pressure (BP) is 110/70, temperature 36.5, pulse 80, respiration 20, and oxygen saturation is 98. She has a history of diverticular disease and urinary tract infections, and has fallen several times. She has a high risk of skin breakdown with a Waterlow score of 19 and is incontinent at night. She uses a wheelchair and requires the assistance of one person in dressing and for transfers, but can eat independently.

Her care plan also contains biographical information about her life, providing information about her childhood, adolescence, adulthood, and retirement, as well as her likes and dislikes. When asked about her routines and requirements for support, she states that she is *"more used to looking after everyone else."* In relation to meaningful activities, she has been assessed using the POOL Activity Level (PAL) checklist and has an individualized program of meaningful activities: religious worship, cookery, knitting, newspaper, chatting with family and staff, arts and crafts, and going out with family. Over time, Mrs. Baker's capacity to participate in cookery, knitting, art and crafts, and going out with family has declined owing to physical frailty. She still retains a strong religious faith, and enjoys music and talking to people.

Literature Review

The term *person-centered care* is used widely in health and social care discourse and is commonly employed in the articulation of policy, at both governmental and professional levels (Brownie & Nancarrow, 2013; Dow, Haralambous, Bremner, & Fearn, 2006). In the context of older people in long-term care settings, it challenges task-oriented processes and an overemphasis on biomedicine, and promotes a shift in emphasis to holistic, collaborative, relationship-based care environments that focus on quality of life (Bellchambers & Penning, 2007; McGilton et al., 2012).

The roots of person-centered care can be traced back to the philosophy of personhood that can be found within theological, ethical, and social-psychological discourse. This philosophy identifies the uniqueness of each human being, obliging us to treat each person with respect and as an end in himself or herself rather than as a means to some other end (Kitwood, 1997; McCormack, 2004). The humanistic psychological approach to psychotherapy is seen as a precursor to person-centered practice, emerging from the work of Carl Rogers (1951). Rogers acknowledges the subjective experience of all individuals and the need to adopt a facilitative approach to supporting individuals, who are considered experts in their own lives, toward growth and fulfilment (Brooker, 2003; Brownie & Horstmanshof, 2012; McCormack, 2004). Kitwood (1997) is considered by many to be the initiator of theory and discourse in respect of person-centered care in gerontology and, more specifically, the field of dementia. Person-centered care has several interrelated and overlapping attributes and dimensions and is described as a "multidimensional concept based on the subjective feelings of individuals" (Edvardsson, Fetherstonhaugh, & Nay, 2010, p. 2612). McCormack et al. (2010) developed the following definition:

> Person-centeredness is an approach to practice established through the formation and fostering of therapeutic relationships between all care providers, older people and others significant to them in their lives. It is underpinned by values of respect for persons, individual right to self-determination, mutual respect and understanding. It is enabled by cultures of empowerment that foster continuous approaches to practice development. (p. 13)

While various definitions and descriptions of person-centered care exist, in general, the concept focuses on maintaining identity, promoting autonomy, having a partnership- or relationship-based approach, and delivering flexible services based on individual needs and preferences within positive social environments (Brooker, 2003; Edvardsson et al., 2010; Edvardsson, Winblad, & Sandman, 2008; Hill, Kolanowski, Milone-Nuzzo, & Yevchak, 2011; Slater, 2006).

Maintaining the identity of individuals who are vulnerable to a loss of personhood due to cognitive difficulties and/or institutionalization is considered a key element of person-centered care, and it is suggested that by adopting a proactive approach to this, the life and values of the older person become central, therefore driving a change in how care is organized and delivered (Buron, 2010; McKeown, Clarke, Ingleton, Ryan, & Repper, 2010). Autonomy is centrally located within the professional discourse of person-centered care, where it is proposed that individuals should be actively included and involved in a partnership process with carers "doing with" as opposed to "doing to" older people (Bellchambers & Penning, 2007; Dewing, 2004; Kitwood, 1997). From an organizational perspective, promoting autonomy is interrelated with concepts of having choices, shared decision making, and interdependency (Agich, 2003; McCormack & McCance, 2010; Welford, 2012).

Relationships are considered central to the aspiration of person-centered care as an antidote to routine and depersonalized care (Brown Wilson, 2009; Buckley & McCarthy, 2009; Cooney, Dowling, Gannon, Dempsey, & Murphy, 2013). Lack of relationships or connectedness to others can result in feelings of loneliness and associated feelings of isolation and depression in older people living in long-term care settings. Several authors have highlighted the importance of interpersonal relationships between residents and staff in the delivery of person-centered care (Brooker, 2003; Cook, 2006; Heliker & Hoang Thanh, 2010; Kitwood, 1997; McCormack & McCance, 2010). Reciprocal relationships, whereby residents can equally show feelings of care and reciprocity for staff, have been connected to better physical and emotional adjustments and closer caregiving attachments (Brown Wilson, 2009; Heliker & Hoang Thanh, 2010).

Creating positive social environments where individuals are valued and nurtured is considered fundamental to the provision of person-centered care (Kitwood, 1997; McCormack & McCance, 2010; Røsvik, Brooker, Mjorud, & Kirkevold, 2013). This can refer to both the physical infrastructure of residential care, including whether the environment reflects normal or homelike characteristics (Hill et al., 2011; Molony, Evans, Jeon, Rabig, & Straka, 2011; te Boekhorst, Depla, de lange, Pot, & Eefsting, 2009), and to the way care is organized, how decisions get made, and the ethos of care (Brannon, Kemper, Heier-Leitzell, & Stott, 2010; McCormack & McCance, 2010). "Creating community" has been identified as a way of shifting from environments where residents are seen as passive recipients of care to ones where people are engaged in mutually supporting each other (Brown Wilson, 2009). Greater involvement of residents and families in decision making and having opportunities to engage in everyday activity are seen to contribute to positive social environments and the promotion of a sense of purpose (Brooker, 2003; Edvardsson et al., 2010; Edvardsson, Petersson, Sjogren, Lindkvist, & Sandman, 2014; Morgan-Brown, Newton, & Ormerod, 2013).

Role and Cultural Considerations

Person-centered care is now commonly cited in policy documents, mission statements, and promotional materials of service providers across the world (Love & Pinkowitz, 2013; National Institute for Clinical Excellence, 2013; World Health Organization, 2007). There is an increasing body of literature reporting positive outcomes. However, the multidimensional nature of the concept and a lack of clarity in relation to its definition have led to difficulty in providing clear implementation guidelines. While the number of studies continues to grow, there remains a dearth of literature from the perspective of older people and family members (Dow et al., 2006; Edvardsson & Innes, 2010).

Solutions and Strategies for Changing Practice

In order to address the key goal of person-centered care, that of maintaining identity, it is important to identify the previous roles and strengths that each individual resident has as well as to establish what is important to them currently. From this, the potential for maintaining previous routines or the development of new routines of choice can be explored and planned for. Maintaining Mrs. Baker's identity as a homemaker and carer of others could be incorporated into her care plan alongside other biomedical and meaningful activity goals. While physically frail, Mrs. Baker retains the capacity to converse and pray, and as such could perhaps provide company and spiritual support to residents who are ill or unable to communicate verbally. Such a role would enhance her own status, shifting from that of a passive recipient of care to a contributing community member and increase her sense of purpose. Her stated experience, knowledge, and skill as a homemaker could be drawn upon in the exchange of knowledge between younger staff members supporting the concept of intergenerational social exchange and reciprocity (Thomas, 2004).

Supporting residents to participate more fully in the everyday life of a facility can be challenging in the light of low expectations and perceived lack of interest (Mattiasson & Andersson, 1997; O'Hanlon & Coleman, 2004; Owen & Meyer,

2012). While Mrs. Baker acknowledges that she has choices in relation to food and when to get up and retire, she had no expectation of continuing with previous routines, including her religious worship. McCormack and McCance (2010) contend that in a context of low expectations and ill health, supporting older people to make choices may require more than eliciting knowledge about likes and dislikes or providing superficial choices about care routines, but rather requires skilled negotiation and actively seeking to understand the values of the individual. Mrs. Baker has no expectation of being involved in developing the routines of the facility as she considered this to be the domain of staff. Regulators demand evidence of involvement by residents and relatives in the life of long-term care facilities, and consumer forums are a common mechanisms employed to address this (Pillinger, 2012). However, a number of authors suggest that the impact of these is limited because of institutional constraints, the competing agenda of staff and residents, and bureaucratic management systems (Braithwaite, 2008; Meyer, 1991; O'Dwyer & Timonen, 2010). If the goal of shared decision making is to be realized, more immediate forms of daily decision making are required. Decisions that involve residents in the everyday life of facilities, such as engagement with household tasks or other personally meaningful domestic activities, can provide opportunities for engagement and reciprocity (Edvardsson et al., 2014; Morgan-Brown et al., 2013).

Practices of scheduling could be reconstructed to include a greater focus on relationships. Consistent assignments have been found to have a positive impact on person-centered relationships from the perspective of both residents and staff (Castle, 2013; Yeatts & Cready, 2007). Defined as the same staff caring for the same residents every time they are on duty, this has been connected to the promotion of person-centered care both in the context of improving relationships between residents and staff (Brown Wilson, 2009), improved staff satisfaction (Yeatts & Cready, 2007), and to reduced turnover of staff and absenteeism (Castle, 2013). McGilton and Boscart (2007) suggest that managers should take into account which residents and staff "click" and incorporate this into the development of staff schedules. Existing systems could be augmented with knowledge about previous community connections, as, for example, the connection Mrs. Baker had to Marion, who came from her locality and with whom she had a shared history and common cultural values.

Conclusion

The concept of person-centered care, which is promoted as both a philosophy and a set of practices, has developed rapidly as a theory of practice for health professionals and has become a watchword for good quality of care and quality of life. Adopting this stance requires organizational structures that offer opportunities for reciprocity and a continued sense of purpose, as well as promote shared decision making and the fostering of nurturing relationships. Recent studies have shown that this approach has resulted in a more positive experience for both residents and staff.

Clinical Reasoning Questions

1. How can existing and previous routines of individuals be incorporated into the daily routines of the facility?
2. What skills do staff require to elicit information about values and goals of residents where expectations are low?
3. How can shared decision-making systems be developed?
4. How can staff scheduling systems reflect the principles of developing mutuality and reciprocal relationships?

References

Agich, G. (2003). *Dependence and autonomy in old age: An ethical framework for long term care.* Cambridge, UK: Cambridge University Press.

Bellchambers, H., & Penning, C. (2007). Person-centered approach to care (PCA): A philosophy of care and management for carers. *Contemporary Nurse: A Journal for the Australian Nursing Profession, 26,* 196–197.

Braithwaite, J. (2008). *Regulatory capitalism: How it works, ideas for making it work better.* Cheltenham, UK: Edward Elgar.

Brannon, S. D., Kemper, P., Heier-Leitzell, B., & Stott, A. (2010). Reinventing management practices in long-term care: How cultural evolution can affect workforce recruitment and retention. *Generations, 34,* 68–74.

Brooker, D. (2003). What is person-centered care in dementia? *Reviews in Clinical Gerontology, 13,* 215–222.

Brownie, S., & Horstmanshof, L. (2012). Creating the conditions for self-fulfilment for aged care residents. *Nursing Ethics, 19,* 777–786.

Brownie, S., & Nancarrow, S. (2013). Effects of person-centered care on residents and staff in aged-care facilities: A systematic review. *Clinical Interventions in Aging, 8,* 1–10.

Brown Wilson, C. (2009). Developing community in care homes through a relationship-centered approach. *Health and Social Care in the Community, 17,* 177–186.

Buckley, C., & McCarthy, G. (2009). An exploration of social connectedness as perceived by older adults in a long-term care setting in Ireland. *Geriatric Nursing, 30,* 390–396.

Buron, B. (2010). Life history collages: Effects on nursing home staff caring for residents with dementia. *Journal of Gerontological Nursing, 36,* 38–48.

Castle, N. G. (2013). Consistent assignment of nurse aides: Association with turnover and absenteeism. *Journal of Aging & Social Policy, 25,* 48–64.

Cook, G. (2006). The risk to enduring relationships following the move to a care home. *International Journal of Older People Nursing, 1,* 182–185.

Cooney, A., Dowling, M., Gannon, M. E., Dempsey, L., & Murphy, K. (2013). Exploration of the meaning of connectedness for older people in long-term care in context of their quality of life: A review and commentary. *International Journal of Older People Nursing, 9*(3), 192–199.

Dewing, J. (2004). Concerns relating to the application of frameworks to promote person-centeredness in nursing with older people. *Journal of Clinical Nursing, 13,* 39–44.

Dow, B., Haralambous, B., Bremner, F., & Fearn, M. (2006). *What is person centered healthcare? A literature review.* Victoria, Austraila: Government Department of Human Services.

Edvardsson, D., Fetherstonhaugh, D., & Nay, R. (2010). Promoting a continuation of self and normality: Person-centered care as described by people with dementia, their family members and aged care staff. *Journal of Clinical Nursing, 19,* 2611–2618.

Edvardsson, D., & Innes, A. (2010). Measuring person-centered care: A critical comparative review of published tools. *The Gerontologist, 50*, 834–846.

Edvardsson, D., Petersson, L., Sjogren, K., Lindkvist, M., & Sandman, P. O. (2014). Everyday activities for people with dementia in residential aged care: Associations with person-centeredness and quality of life. *International Journal of Older People Nursing, 9*(4), 269–276.

Edvardsson, D., Winblad, B., & Sandman, P. (2008). Person-centered care of people with severe Alzheimer's disease: Current status and ways forward. *The Lancet Neurology, 7*, 362–367.

Heliker, D., & Hoang Thanh, N. (2010). Story sharing: Enhancing nurse aide-resident relationships in long-term care. *Research in Gerontological Nursing, 3*, 240–252.

Hill, N. L., Kolanowski, A. M., Milone-Nuzzo, P., & Yevchak, A. (2011). Culture change models and resident health outcomes in long-term care. *Journal of Nursing Scholarship, 43*, 30–40.

Kitwood, T. (1997). *Dementia reconsidered. The person comes first*. Berkshire, England: Open University Press.

Love, K., & Pinkowitz, J. (2013). *Dementia care: The quality chasm*. Retrieved from http://www.ccal.org/wp-content/uploads/DementiaCareTheQualityChasm_020413.pdf

Mattiasson, A. C., & Andersson, L. (1997). Quality of nursing home care assessed by competent nursing home patients. *Journal of Advanced Nursing, 26*, 1117–1124.

McCormack, B. (2004). Person-centeredness in gerontological nursing: An overview of the literature. *International Journal of Older People Nursing in Association With Journal of Clinical Nursing, 13*, 31–38.

McCormack, B., Dewing, J., Breslin, L., Tobin, C., Manning, M., Coyne-Nevin, A., . . . Peelo-Kilroe, L. (2010). *Implementation of a model of person centered practice in older persons settings—Final report*. Dublin, Ireland: National Council for the Continuing Professional Development of Nursing and Midwifery and Health Service Executive.

McCormack, B., & McCance, T. (2010). *Person centered nursing theory and practice*. Oxford, England: Wiley-Blackwell.

McGilton, K. S., & Boscart, V. M. (2007). Close care provider–resident relationships in long-term care environments. *Journal of Clinical Nursing, 16*, 2149–2157.

McGilton, K. S., Heath, H., Chu, C. H., Boström, A.-M., Mueller, C., Boscart, V. M., . . . Bowers, B. (2012). Moving the agenda forward:

A person-centered framework in long-term care. *International Journal of Older People Nursing, 7*, 303–309.

McKeown, J., Clarke, A., Ingleton, C., Ryan, T., & Repper, J. (2010). The use of life story work with people with dementia to enhance person-centered care. *International Journal of Older People Nursing, 5*, 148–158.

Meyer, M. H. (1991). Assuring quality of care: Nursing home resident councils. *Journal of Applied Gerontology, 10*, 103–116.

Molony, S. L., Evans, L. K., Jeon, S., Rabig, J., & Straka, L. A. (2011). Trajectories of at-homeness and health in usual care and small house nursing homes. *Gerontologist, 51*, 504–515.

Morgan-Brown, M., Newton, R., & Ormerod, M. (2013). Engaging life in two Irish nursing home units for people with dementia: Quantitative comparisons before and after implementing household environments. *Aging & Mental Health, 17*, 57–65.

National Institute for Clinical Excellence. (2013). Quality standard for supporting people to live well with dementia. Retrieved from https://www.nice.org.uk/guidance/qs30

O'Dwyer, C., & Timonen, V. (2010). Rethinking the value of residents' councils: Observations and lessons from an exploratory study. *Journal of Applied Gerontology, 29*, 762–771.

O'Hanlon, A., & Coleman, P. (2004). Attitudes towards aging: Adaptation, development and growth into later years. In J. F. Nussbaum & J. Coupland (Eds.), *Handbook of communication and aging research* (2nd ed., pp. 31–63). Mahwah, NJ: Lawrence Erlbaum Associates.

Owen, T., & Meyer, J. (2012). *My home life: Promoting quality of life in care homes*. York, England: Joseph Rountree Foundation.

Pillinger, J. (2012). *Designated centers for older people: An analysis of inspection findings during the first 15 months of inspection*. Dublin, Ireland: Health Information and Quality Authority.

Rogers, C. (1951). *Client centered therapy*. London, England: Constable.

Røsvik, J., Brooker, D., Mjorud, M., & Kirkevold, O. (2013). What is person-centered care in dementia? Clinical reviews into practice: The development of the VIPS practice model. *Reviews in Clinical Gerontology, 23*, 155–163.

Slater, L. (2006). Person-centeredness: A concept analysis. *Contemporary Nurse, 23*, 135–144.

te Boekhorst, S., Depla, M. F. I. A., de Lange, J., Pot, A. M., & Eefsting, J. A. (2009). The effects of group living homes on older people with dementia: A comparison with traditional nursing home care. *International Journal of Geriatric Psychiatry, 24,* 970–978.

Thomas, W. H. (2004). *What are old people for? How elders will save the world.* St. Louis, MO: VanderWyk & Burnham.

Welford, C. (2012). *Exploring and enhancing autonomy for older people in residential care.* Galway, Ireland: National University of Ireland.

World Health Organization. (2007). *People centered health care: A policy framework.* Retrieved from http://www.wpro.who.int/health_services/people_at_the_centre_of_care/en

Yeatts, D. E., & Cready, C. M. (2007). Consequences of empowered CNA teams in nursing home settings: A longitudinal assessment. *Gerontologist, 47,* 323–339.

3 AUTONOMY

Claire Welford and Catherine Sweeney

Subjective

"How did I get here?"

Objective

Mr. Charlie Cox was admitted to a rural nursing home, close to the home he had lived in for the past 25 years with his wife and three daughters. He does not recall all the details of his admission to the nursing home, but states that he feels trapped and tricked into this admission by his wife and daughters, as he could "live perfectly well at home." He believes his family are not listening to him, that he could manage at home, and that quality of life (QOL) in the nursing home is poor, as he cannot do the things that are important to him. He explained that he was a good cyclist in his younger days and still cycled indoors using his turbo cycle up to the time of his admission. Mr. Cox was the owner and director of a factory that employed 25 staff members, and he was always in control of his work and his life, but now all decisions are made for him. He misses cycling, but his requests to do this are constantly refused by staff who cite "health and safety issues." He believes that staff think he is stupid and incapable just because he is older and a bit confused at times. He finds life in the nursing home difficult and feels as if "everything important has been taken away and I have no longer any control of my life." He would like to be called Mr. Cox, but finds that some staff still call him Charlie. Mr Cox feels that "if he is not free to make decisions about his own life," then he may as well not be alive.

Mr. Cox was admitted to an acute hospital following a fall at home, and from there was admitted to a nursing home after an occupational health assessment found he could not be discharged home because of his confusion, risk of falling again, and weight loss. He is 82 years old with a history of a right-sided cerebrovascular accident (CVA) and increasing memory problems. On admission, his baseline assessments revealed that he was "medium dependency," and his Barthel score was 11. He requires help with transfer from bed to chair and with sitting to standing. While he can walk unaided with a Zimmer frame, his gait is unsteady and his STRATIFY score is 2, putting him at high risk of falling. Mr. Cox has lost weight over the last year—all his adult life he was around 168 lb. (76 kg), but he is currently 142 lbs. (142 kg)—and his height is 5 feet 11 in. (180 cm). His appetite has been poor, and his nutritional status using the Malnutrition Universal Screening Tool (MUST) is at a score of 1, indicating medium risk of malnourishment. On admission, his blood pressure (BP) was 127/81, his pulse was 69, and he was afebrile. Over the first week of his admission, Mr. Cox presented a number of behavioral challenges. He experienced nightmares, from which he woke up confused and upset and was then very aggressive with the staff. Recently, Mr. Cox has become increasingly withdrawn, tearful, and noncommunicative. His score on the Geriatric Depression Scale (Cornell) is 10. He was referred to the Psychiatry of Later Life Team, who diagnosed him with depression, paranoia, and frontal lobe dementia. Mr. Cox was commenced on memantine 20 mg OD, sertraline 100 mg OD, and donepezil 10 mg OD. As the months progressed, Mr. Cox presented with increasing episodes of frustration, depression, agitation, and confusion, for which a PRN dose of Quetiapine 12.5 mg (po) was added to the medication regime. His family wanted Mr. Cox to continue using his turbo cycle while in the home as they found it "settled him" and improved his mood. They were aware of the risk of falling, but felt the benefits to mood were worth the risks.

Literature Review

Researchers who have specifically focused on QOL in residential care have found that autonomy, choice, and control are central to QOL (Ball et al., 2000; Edwards, Courtney, & O'Reilly, 2003;

Kane & Kane, 2000; Murphy, O'Shea, & Cooney, 2007; Tester, Hubbard, Downs, MacDonald, & Murphy, 2004). Further evidence suggests that older people themselves feel that autonomy is important for good QOL (Barkay & Tabak, 2002; Edwards & Staniszewska, 2000; Edwards, Staniszewska, & Crichton, 2004). The United Nations (UN) Madrid International Plan of Action on Ageing (MIPAA, 2002 and 2008) recognized that there is global acknowledgment of the need to include older adults in autonomous decision-making processes.

Autonomy is complex. The first known use of the word *autonomy* was documented in 1623. It was derived from the Greek word *autonomia*, or the freedom to live by one's own laws—"autos" meaning "self" and "nomos" meaning "rule," translating literally into the term *self-rule*. Welford, Murphy, Casey, and Wallace (2010) presented a concept analysis of resident autonomy and delineated six key attributes; these include encouraging and maintaining residents' capacity by involving them in decision making; recognizing that residents should delegate their care needs on the basis of their right to self-determination; and ensuring negotiated care planning, which is encouraged through open and respectful communication and which includes families or significant others when the resident is cognitively impaired. The residential unit should operate a culture and atmosphere of flexibility within an ethos of maintaining resident dignity, and meaningful relationships should be enabled by the presence of regular and motivated staff. Several authors have tried to explain autonomy by defining its opposite concept—paternalism—and by illustrating and describing different "types" of autonomy, which include "basic and ideal, subjective and objective." Boyle (2008) explained that while some older people may not have the "capacity" to exercise autonomy, it does not mean that they no longer have the "need" to exercise autonomy. It should not be assumed that the absence of physical health, functional capacity, or cognitive capacity in older people is a barrier to their being, at least, somewhat autonomous. Boyle (2008) further states that while mental health may be a prerequisite of autonomy, impaired autonomy can in turn lead to mental ill health for the older person. In other words, mental health or capacity enables the person to exercise freedom, independence, and self-government (autonomy), but being prevented from doing this may contribute to depression or apathy in the older person. Similarly, Harnett and Greaney (2008) state that current explanations of autonomy do not encompass the complexities involved in respecting autonomy when caring for patients with diminished capacity (e.g., Alzheimer's or dementia in old age).

Rodgers and Neville (2007) argue that a major problem in enabling personal autonomy in residential care facilities is that of communal interests, whereby organizational needs are privileged over the rights of individuals. They add that while institutional routines maximize efficient use of staff time and provide care efficiently and economically, they are highly likely to interfere with the autonomy of those cared for. Cook (2010) adds that these routines affect residents' identity and autonomy. Some years ago, Agich (1990) called for a refurbished concrete concept of autonomy that would systematically attend to the history and development of persons. "We need to learn how to acknowledge their habits and identifications" (Agich, 1990, p. 12). Yet more recently, a review by Pearson and Peels (2009) revealed that most articles published are expert opinion articles rather than articles reporting change initiatives, interventions, or examples of how to acknowledge residents' habits and identifications, and research studies continue to report residents feel that staff do not know them or communicate with them as "persons" rather than "patients."

There is much discussion in the literature about the importance of recognizing the subjective element of autonomy that recognizes older people's needs, values, goals, and personal preferences. When the subjective element of autonomy is recognized, the health care professional and the resident together can negotiate care. Open and respectful communication must also be maintained in this process (Beauchamp & Childress, 1994; Collopy, 1988), and imbalanced power relationships can affect this. Residents must be involved in decision making (Agich, 1990; Collopy, 1988; Faulkner & Davies, 2006; Hofland, 1994), and dignity should be maintained as it is suggested to be integral to autonomy (Agich, 2004). Table 3.1 delineates key essential strategies from the literature that are needed in order to facilitate autonomy for older people in nursing homes. Further details will now be explored.

TABLE 3.1: Strategies to Promote and Prohibit Autonomy for Older People in Nursing Homes

Promoting Factors	Prohibitive Factors
The Person	
Education/specialism	Lack of education/specialism
Resident independence	Resident dependence
Enable decision-specific capacity	Prevent decision-specific capacity
Sharing power	Not sharing power
The Personality	
Desire to work with older people	Does not choose to work with older people
Positive attitude toward older people	Negative attitude toward older people
Being open, motivated, and flexible	Being closed, demotivated, and inflexible
Person to Person	
Good interpersonal skills	Poor interpersonal skills
Good relationships between residents, between staff and residents, between staff, and between staff and family members	Poor relationships between residents, between staff and residents, between staff, and between staff and family members
Listening	Not listening
Knowing the person: past, present, and future	Not knowing the person: past, present, or future
Biographical care planning	Medicalized care planning
Being Personal	
Negotiation	Lack of negotiation
Agreed routines	Imposed routines
Care planning	Lack of care planning
Flexibility	Inflexibility
Time	Little or no time
Friendly ward atmosphere	Unfriendly ward atmosphere
Good skill mix	Poor skill mix
Motivated	Demotivated
Teamwork	No teamwork
Being Personalized	
Meaningful recreational activity	Meaningless recreational activity
Appropriate language (e.g., care plans are nonpaternalistic and write about "doing with")	Inappropriate language (e.g., care plans are paternalistic and write about "doing to")
Including the resident and their family member in care planning	Not including the resident and their family member in care planning

Role and Cultural Considerations

Different terminology is used in different countries to describe the various housing and health care service options for older people. Recently, Howe, Jones, and Tilse (2012) reported that *nursing home* is the most common and least ambiguous term used that has common meaning across five countries (the United Kingdom, the United States of America, Canada, Australia, and New Zealand). The review by Howe et al. (2012) revealed that "nursing home" always related to facilities in which skilled nursing care is available on a 24/7 basis and whereby nursing care is received by a high proportion of residents.

Assessment and Strategies

Mr. Cox felt that he lacked autonomy over his life. One strategy that was used, therefore, was to rewrite his care plan and to involve him in the main decisions and priorities. It was decided to review the risk assessment in relation to using the turbo cycle, as this was Mr. Cox's main priority. A further risk assessment was undertaken in which Mr. Cox was fully involved, and a new care plan was developed with Mr. Cox that reflected his perception of needs and priorities. Following negotiation with his family, the risk assessment concluded that Mr. Cox could use his turbo cycle provided he was supervised.

Care planning in residential care should adopt a gerontological rather than acute care approach; these differences are outlined in Table 3.2. It is the staff's motivation that enables flexible and innovative approaches to care, and their commitment that drives them to want to understand the person they are caring for (McCormack & McCance, 2006; Reed, Inglis, Cook, Clarke, & Cook, 2007). Nolan, Davies, Brown, Keady, and Nolan (2004) support the view that care planning with older people is underpinned by successful relationships between the older person and the health care professional. The success of the relationship is determined by the level of negotiation and mutual recognition of each other's beliefs. Mr. Cox believed that nobody was listening to him, and staff had failed initially to negotiate with him about his activities. Butterworth (2012), Cook (2010), and Kellett, Moyle, McAllsiter, King, and

TABLE 3.2: Differences in Terminology Between Acute Care and Gerontological Care

Acute Care	Gerontological Care
Nursing process: assessment, planning, implementation, evaluation, documentation	Nursing process: assessment, planning, implementation, recheck, evaluation, documentation
Patient problem	Resident need
Nurse intervention	Agreed actual and potential needs
Nurse dominant	Resident dominant
Clinical style	Biographical/Narrative style
Often preprepared	Individually prepared

Gallagher (2010) suggested that care planning for older people should adopt a biographical approach that aims to understand the older person, look beyond their diagnosis, and better explain their presenting behaviors, while improving communication and relationships with care staff and families.

One month after the implementation of the new care plan, Mr. Cox's Geriatric Depression Scale score dropped from 10 to 5. The care plan template used was devised by staff and specifically focused on ways to enable resident autonomy. The core principles on which the plan was based are outlined in Table 3.3. A key element of this strategy was the use of a core daily life care plan. Each activity of daily living (ADL) is addressed within this core care plan. Staff note something positive about each ADL—for example, something that the resident can do for him- or herself or determine or delegate for him- or

TABLE 3.3: Core Principles for Care Planning in Residential Care

Care Plan Core Principles
Commence with a positive statement of what the resident can do for himself or herself
Determine level of ability for each activity of living rather than designing care plan from summative assessment of dependency
Clarify the nursing diagnosis in simple terms from the medical diagnosis and how it impacts upon daily life
Describe the agreed actual and potential needs

herself—and the resident's level of ability. The Barthel scores and the Mini Mental State Examination (MMSE) scores are still used to determine dependency from an organizational and reporting perspective, but specifying the level of ability for each AL (e.g., level 1 is able, level 2 is able but has some difficulty, level 3 needs assistance, level 4 not able but can delegate, and level 5 is not able) and determining what residents can do for themselves has resulted in increased autonomy for residents.

Another strategy used was to discuss with the resident and/or family and agree the potential and actual needs for the AL and then what would be done to meet those needs. Rather than "doing for or doing to," it is important to "do with." For Mr. Cox, participation in decision making was essential to improving his QOL.

There is no doubt that challenges in facilitating autonomy for older people in long-term care will continue. The population is aging, and right now many of this population find themselves in large homes where multiple needs are balanced on a daily basis. We can start to make the experiences of residential care better by adopting real, not tokenistic, care planning strategies, as well as by admitting at the outset that we cannot enable everything and thus establish a mutual understanding with the resident and his or her family that respects the "person" sharing our home.

Key Considerations

- An organization's approach to care is central to positive resident experiences of care. There are powerful connections between structure, process, and outcomes in an organization's approach to care, and these ultimately affect a resident's autonomy. Routine and task-based care impact negatively on residents' autonomy. An approach to care that recognizes the importance of decision making is essential to developing partnerships, sharing power, and ultimately enhancing residents' autonomy and QOL.
- Staff, residents, and residents' families often have contradictory perceptions of care, and it is therefore important to find common ground. Family members possess important information about the biography or life story of the resident, and

this should be utilized to enhance resident autonomy. Autonomy is recognized as an integral ingredient in providing person-centered care, and person-centered care is viewed as essential to the achievement of QOL. Knowing the person is essential to person-centered care, and this involves knowing the older person's needs, wants, values, and history, thus leading to the development of a negotiated life plan.

- Gerontological nurse expertise is important to enhancing residents' autonomy and QOL.
- Nurse leaders need to promote professional knowledge and practice regarding relationship building and client-centeredness if nurses and clients are to be empowered.
- Positive staff attitudes are associated with the type of care experienced. Staff attitudes may be positively influenced by education.

Clinical Reasoning Questions

1. Based on the information in this case study, what strategies would you suggest to promote the maximum autonomy for Mr. Cox?
2. What institutional changes can be made to promote autonomy for clients across environments of care?
3. What if Mr. Cox had bipolar disorder? How would this complicate his goal to become more autonomous?
4. What impact do caregivers have in promoting autonomy among clients?

Acknowledgment

The author wishes to acknowledge the support of Mowlam Healthcare.

References

Agich, G. J. (1990, November/December). Reassessing autonomy in long-term care. *Hastings Center Report, 20*(6), 12.

Agich, J. (2004) *Dependence and autonomy in old age: An ethical framework for long-term care*. Cambridge, UK: Cambridge University Press.

Atkins, K. (2006) Autonomy and autonomy competencies: A practical and relational approach. *Nursing Philosophy*. 7, 205–215.

Ball, M. M., Whittington, F. J., Perkins, M. M., Patterson, V. L., Hollingsworth, C., King, S. V., & Combs, B. L. (2000). Quality of life in assisted living facilities: Viewpoints of residents. *Journal of Applied Gerontology, 19*, 304–325.

Barkay, A., & Tabak, N. (2002, August). Elderly residents' participation and autonomy within a geriatric ward in a public institution. *International Journal of Nursing Practice, 8*(4), 198.

Beauchamp, T. L. & Childress, J. F. (1994) *Principles of biomedical ethics.* Oxford, UK: Oxford University Press.

Boyle, G. (2008, June). Autonomy in long-term care: A need, a right, or a luxury? *Disability & Society, 23*(4), 299–310.

Butterworth, C. (2012, October). How to achieve a person-centered writing style in care plans. *Nursing Older People, 24*(8), 21–26.

Collopy, B. J. (1988) Autonomy in long term care: Some crucial distinctions. *The Gerontologist* 28(Supplement), 10–17.

Cook, G. (2010). Ensuring older residents retain their unique identity. *Nursing & Residential Care, 12*(6), 290–293.

Edwards, C., & Staniszewska, S. (2000). Accessing the user perspective. *Health and Social Care in the Community, 8*(6), 417–424.

Edwards, C., Staniszewska, S., & Crichton, N. (2004). Investigation of the ways in which patients' reports of their satisfaction with healthcare are constructed. *Sociology of Health and Illness, 26*(2), 159–183.

Edwards, H. E., Courtney, M., & O'Reilly, M. (2003). Involving older people in research to examine quality of life in residential aged care. *Quality in Ageing: Policy Practice and Research, 4*, 38–43.

Faulkner, M. & Davies, S. (2006) The CARE (combined assessment of residential environments) profiles: a new approach in improving quality in care homes. *Quality in Ageing – Policy, Practice and Research,* 7(3), 15–25.

Harnett, P. J., & Greaney, A. M. (2008). Operationalizing autonomy: Solutions for mental health nursing practice. *Journal of Psychiatric and Mental Health Nursing, 15*, 2–9.

Hofland, B. F. (1994, Winter). When capacity fades and autonomy is constricted: A client-centered approach to residential care. *Generations, 18*(4), 31–36.

Howe, A. L., Jones, A.E., & Tilse, C. (2012). What's in a name? Similarities and differences in international terms and meanings for older people's housing with services. *Ageing and Society 33*(4), 547–578.

Kane, R. L., & Kane, R. A. (Eds.). (2000). *Assessing older people: Measures, meaning, and practical applications*. New York, NY: Oxford University Press.

Kellett, U., Moyle, W., McAllsiter, M., King, C., & Gallagher, F. (2010). Life stories and biography: A means of connecting family and staff to people with dementia. *Journal of Clinical Nursing, 19*, 1707–1713.

McCormack, B., & McCance, T. V. (2006). Development of a framework for person-centered nursing. *Journal of Advanced Nursing, 56*(5), 472–479.

Murphy, K., O'Shea, E., & Cooney, A. (2007). Quality of life for older people living in long-stay settings in Ireland. *Journal of Clinical Nursing, 16*, 2167–2177.

Nolan, M., Davies, S., Brown, J., Keady, J., & Nolan, J. (2004). Beyond "person-centered" care: A new vision for gerontological nursing. *International Journal of Older People Nursing, 13*(3a), 45–53.

Pearson, A., & Peels, S. (2009). Effective documentation in residential aged care facilities. *Referencia, 2*(10), 113–132.

Reed, J., Inglis, P., Cook, G., Clarke, C., & Cook, M. (2007). Specialist nurses for older people: Implications from UK development sites. *Journal of Advanced Nursing, 58*(4), 368–376.

Rodgers, V., & Neville, S. (2007). Personal autonomy for older people living in residential care: An overview. *Nurse Praxis in New Zealand, 23*(1), 29–36.

Tester, S., Hubbard, G., Downs, M., MacDonald, C., & Murphy, J. (2004). Frailty and institutional life. In A. Walker & C. Hennessy Hagan (Eds.), *Growing older quality of life in old age* (pp. 209–224). Berkshire, England: Open University Press.

United Nations, Madrid International Plan of Action on Ageing. (2002 and 2008). *Guiding framework and toolkit for practitioners and policy makers.* Department of Economic and Social Affairs [Division for Social Policy and Development]. Retrieved from http://www.un.org/esa/socdev/ageing/documents/building_natl_capacity/guiding.pdf

Welford, C., Murphy, K., Casey, D., & Wallace, M. (2010). A concept analysis of autonomy for older people in residential care. *Journal of Clinical Nursing, 19*, 1226–1235.

4 REAL CHOICE

KATHY MURPHY

Subjective

"I am so breathless and exhausted."

Objective

Mrs. Dyer is a 78-year-old woman admitted to long-term care 6 months ago following her discharge from an acute hospital, where she had been admitted with severe pneumonia. Although this was resolved, her FEV1/FVC had reduced to 28, and an occupational therapy assessment prior to discharge from the hospital determined that she was not capable of independent living.

On examination, Mrs. Dyer has severe dyspnea; her oxygen saturation levels are 65% at rest, dropping to 55% following mild exertion; and her extremities appear cyanosed. She can walk slowly with the help of her walker, but sometimes experiences a panic attack as a result of her breathlessness. She is 148 cm (58 in.) in height and weighs 190 lbs. (86 kg). Her BP is 170/90, her pulse is 120, respirations 30 per minute. She is afebrile with a temperature of 97.8°F. She has hyperinflation of the chest and an audible wheeze. She is often breathless at rest. Cardiac exam reveals a regular heart rate; S1, S2; and no adventitious sounds. Her abdomen is soft and nontender, and her bowel sounds are present in all four quadrants and her bowel movement regular. Her skin is dry, thin, and intact; she has marked bruising on her arms and legs, and there is some dehydration evident. She has pedal edema. Examination of her eyes reveals a cataract in her left eye, but pupils equal, round, reactive to light and accommodation (PERRLA). Her ears reveal normal tympanic membranes bilaterally; her hearing is normal in her right ear but reduced slightly in her left ear. Her mouth is dry, and her oral mucosa is spotted with thrush present. This is being treated at present with nystatin suspension. Neurological exam reveals 2+ deep tendon reflexes bilaterally and equal strength. Her standing balance is poor as a result of a stroke 3 years ago, from which she has recovered, but there is residual muscle weakness of her left leg. Her current medications include Lisinopril, Spiriva 500 mcg OD, Seretide 200 mcg BD, Ventolin 200 mcg PRN, and Exforge 100 mg OD.

Mrs. Dyer states that her main problem is breathlessness; she finds it difficult to get in or out of bed, dress, or wash without help. She has oxygen by her bedside that she uses frequently at a rate of 4 L/minute. She has not been prescribed portable oxygen. She had been taught pursed lipped breathing and other breathing techniques, and although these are helpful, she still finds any exertion difficult and distressing.

Mrs. Dyer has always been a very independent person, and it is very important to her that, despite her breathlessness, she does the things for herself that she can. She does not like to be rushed, as her breathlessness gets worse. She would prefer to be left alone first thing in the morning, to take her morning medications, get her lungs cleared, and to eat her breakfast. She finds her coughing is worst in the mornings and finds it embarrassing; therefore, she likes to be on her own during this time. When asked about her life in a long-term care environment and the choices she can make each day, she is very clear about what matters and what does not. When Mrs. Dyer was admitted, she was asked about the time she rose in the morning, and she said that she had always been an early riser and liked to be up at 7 a.m., but that now she is awake most mornings from 6 a.m., awakened by the residents in the other rooms rising and ringing their bells for help. She finds such early waking leaves her tired by midmorning. However, she is philosophical about this as "that is the way it is when you live with 30 other people." Mrs. Dyer usually goes to the dining room for breakfast around 8:30 a.m. because that is the time that staff like you to have breakfast, but her choice would be to have breakfast in her room.

Mrs. Dyer needs help with personal hygiene, and she finds that the worst part of the morning is waiting for the nurse to come to help her—the time is variable, sometimes too early and sometimes too late. She is clear about how she would like her morning organized. If she had a choice she would get up around 7 a.m., have her breakfast by her bed, take her medications, get her lungs cleared, and shower around 11 a.m. She feels this would be better as her breathing usually settles after her medications and her use of coughing techniques to clear mucus. The nurses often turn up to help her before she is ready, and she feels it is difficult to ask them to come back later as they are so busy and have so many other people to care for. Mrs. Dyer feels all of this has resulted in her being able to do less for herself, and she is unhappy about that.

Mrs. Dyer has lunch each day at 12:30 p.m., but if she had her choice she would have a snack at this time and dinner later in the day. She finds that a large meal at this time makes her sleepy and sluggish. She is very happy with the choice of food, which she describes as very good indeed, but would like her dinner later in the day. Mrs. Dyer was a great reader in the past and loved to listen to the debates on the radio. She finds it difficult, however, to concentrate on reading these days, particularly as she can often hear the TV blaring from next door. She was aware that the unit had an activities program and that there were cards, music, and arts classes in the afternoon, but she found the struggle of getting to these classes too much for her. When asked about her choice of bedtime, Mrs. Dyer stated that her choice would be to stay up until the news is over at 9 p.m. but that was possible only on some days because there is less staff to help in the evenings. If she opted to stay up each evening, then it was sometimes very late when staff were free to get her back to bed and that was a problem for her, so she tended to go back to bed around 6 p.m. Mrs. Dyer felt that she did have choices about her day but that they were limited by the reality of living in a unit with so many people and busy staff; she felt that all her choices had consequences, and she therefore tried to balance the choice with what happened if she made that choice.

Literature Review

The literature suggests that choice over what you do each day is an important element of quality care for older people living in long-term care environments (Bartlett & Stephanie, 1998; Davies, Laker, & Ellis, 1997; Kitson, 1991; Murphy, 2007). Researchers have found that choice and control are central to perceptions of a good quality of life (Ball et al., 2000; Edwards, Courtney, & O'Reilly, 2003; Kane & Kane, 2001; Murphy, O'Shea, & Cooney, 2007; Tester, Hubbard, Downs, MacDonald, & Murphy, 2004). Dyer and Sinclair (1997) found that individualized systems of care that promote patient participation in determining care routines lead to older people experiencing more autonomy, and that care areas therefore need to facilitate resident choice. Randers and Mattiasson (2004) suggested a person's right to choose, decide, and take responsibility for her or his own life is fundamental to good care for older people. As far back as 1991, Kitson identified the right to choose as a concept at the core of good care for older people. McCormack (2003) stressed that the rights of the individual to self-determination, including full participation in decision making, is central to person-centeredness, a philosophy of care promoted by many researchers and policy makers. McCormack (2001) emphasized the need to create a culture in long-term care that requires nurses to include the choices of the older person in determining care routines.

Researchers, however, continue to find over many decades (Norton, 1967; Murphy et al., 2007; Wade, 1999; Waters, 1994; Welford, Murphy, Rodgers, & Frauenlob, 2012; Wells, 1980) that care for older people is routinized, participation in decision making is curtailed, and choice is limited. Many researchers have found that older people have little control over their day-to-day lives while in residential care (Bellis, 2010; Lothian & Philip, 2001; McCormack, 2001; Randers & Mattiasson, 2004) and that despite policy imperatives in many countries focused on the need to provide person-centered care, routines are enduring. McCormack, Mitchell, Cook, Reed, and Childs (2008) found that many older people felt disempowered by a system of care planning and delivery that did not include them in the decision making about their care or treatment. Murphy (2007) found that care in many practice areas in Ireland was not patient centered and that choice and involvement in decision making was limited. Some areas therefore engendered dependency rather than independence, resulting in reduced autonomy and control. Murphy (2007) argued that many care areas need to examine the ways in which choice can be facilitated and the need to focus on the quality of life of the residents rather than on organizational task-based routines. Davies et al. (1997) found that over time many older people come to adopt a position of "resigned passivity," resulting in a lack of expectation or desire to be involved in decisions about care. Burack, Reinhardt, and Weiner (2012) undertook a study in the United States aimed at transforming care within care homes. They utilized a culture change model to try to transform traditional care to a model that was more person centered. They measured choice using the Duncan choice index, and found that while choice scores increased at time point one in the research, over time they decreased, bringing into question the long-term sustainability of this change initiative. Welford et al. (2011), in a study focused on resident autonomy, found that knowledge about residents' choices, evidence of participation in decision making, and overall knowledge of the person's preferences and abilities were very limited.

Role and Cultural Considerations

Around the world, choice within care homes has been an issue. Sometimes, nurses do not perceive that they have the time to enable choice, and at other times, the ethos is simply dictated by the preferences of staff rather than residents. The ward leader creates the ethos of care, and nurses therefore have a vital role in changing practice.

Strategies for Changing Practice

In our experience, there are two main issues that impact resident choice—the first is related to knowing the person, and the second focuses on the ethos of the care environment. Knowing the person is central to facilitating choice as it enables one to understand what is important to the person and to use this knowledge to determine care patterns. It was important, therefore, to have undertaken a detailed life history and assessment with Mrs. Dyer when she was admitted to long-term care. The life history should have detailed Mrs. Dyer's normal routines, preferences, and interests, and described them in sufficient detail so that another person reading Mrs. Dyer's history would get a real understanding of her, her preferences, and her interests. In our experience, the nursing assessment often lacks the specificity required to understand the issues of real importance to the person. An important strategy, therefore, is to agree with the older person a plan for the day—the plan would detail preferences, issues of importance, and the choices of the day's routine, and it would be clearly documented, agreed upon, and signed. If Mrs. Dyer had been asked to describe how she liked to plan her morning, she could have described the importance of clearing her lungs, the need for privacy during this time, and the time she would like to attend to her hygiene needs. Of course, over time a person's preferences may change and regular review of the initial assessment needs to be undertaken. Also, nurses sometimes make assumptions about what is most important to a person to do but this can easily be addressed by asking and checking. We find that asking individuals to identify one thing about their day that was most important to them enables more resident-focused priorities to shape the day.

The second issue is related to the ethos of the care environment. This matters because, ultimately, it shapes staff perspectives about the importance of choice and the status of residents. Changing the routine has been no easy matter across many long-term care environments worldwide. Cheater (2009), however, suggests that while implementation strategies focused on change in long-term care have led only to small improvements in care, there is some evidence that these gains can be increased if there is a systematic identification of the barriers to be overcome and specific strategies to do this identified. A focus on the ethos of the care environment is therefore essential. A systematic identification of the barriers to facilitating choice should be undertaken. For example, staffing rosters can restrict resident choice because they are scheduled around high activity levels in the morning with fewer staff allocated to afternoon or evening shifts, necessitating residents to fit in with staffing rather than staffing facilitating resident choice.

Rosters of kitchen staff, cleaning staff, and activity coordinators can also impact on the daily organization. Staff attitudes to flexibility within care also need to be explored as many studies have found some staff resistant to change (Murphy, 2007). The ethos of a care unit can also determine the extent to which residents are involved in deciding what day activities are offered in a facility. A systematic analysis of the issues within a unit, therefore, may reveal the barriers to change and provide a menu for change. This systematic analysis may include a review of care plans, an analysis of staff rosters, a resident survey, and a documentary review. Observation of care focused on what it is like for Mrs. Dyer could also help staff see the day from the perspective of the resident. Schnelle et al. (2013) found that specific staff training around facilitating resident choice does contribute to a significant increase in resident choices, so a focus on staff training is also important.

Clinical Reasoning Questions

1. What would be your plan for enabling Mrs. Dyer to have more choice in her day?
2. What other tools could be used to measure choice?
3. What if Mrs. Dyer also had heart failure?
4. What staff training would be required within your care unit if resident choices were to be facilitated?

References

Ball, M. M., Whittington, F. J., Perkins, M. M., Patterson, V. L., Hollingsworth, C., King, S. V., & Combs B. L. (2000). Quality of life in assisted living facilities: Viewpoints of residents. *Journal of Applied Gerontology, 19*, 304–325.

Bartlett, H., & Burnip, S. (1998). Quality of care in nursing homes for older people: Providers' perspectives and priorities. *Nursing Times Research, 3*(4), 257–268.

Bellis, A. D. (2010, April–May). Contemporary nurse: Australian residential aged care and the quality of nursing care provision. *A Journal for the Australian Nursing Profession, 35*(1), 100–113.

Burack, O. R., Reinhardt, J. P., & Weiner, A. S. (2012, October–December). Person centered care and elder choice: A look at implementation and sustainability. *Clinical Gerontologist, 35*(5), 390–403.

Cheater, F. M. (2009). Overcoming the barriers to optimum continence care: The need for an expanded approach to implementation. *International Journal of Older People*, *4*, 70–75.

Davies, S., Laker, S., & Ellis, L. (1997). Promoting autonomy and independence for older people within nursing practice. *Journal of Advanced Nursing, 26*(4), 408–417.

Dyer, C. A. E., & Sinclair, A. J. (1997). A hospital-based case-control study of quality of life in older asthmatics. *European Respiratory Journal, 10*(2), 337–341.

Edwards, H. E., Courtney, M. D., & O'Reilly, M. T. (2003). Involving older people in research to examine quality of life in residential aged care. *Quality in Ageing—Policy Practice and Research, 4*, 38–43.

Kane, R. L., & Kane, R. A. (2001). What older people want from long-term care and how they can get it. *Health Affairs, 20*(6), 114–127.

Kitson, A. L. (1991). *Therapeutic nursing and the hospitalised elderly*. Middlesex, England: Scutari Press.

Lothian, K., & Philip, I. (2001). Maintaining the dignity and autonomy of older people in the healthcare setting. *British Medical Journal, 322*, 668–670.

McCormack, B. (2001). *Negotiating partnerships with older people: A person centred approach*. Gateshead, England: Ashgate Publishing.

McCormack, B. (2003). A conceptual framework for person-centred practice with older people. *International Journal of Nursing Practice, 9*(3), 202–209.

McCormack, B., Mitchell, E. A., Cook, G., Reed, J., & Childs, S. (2008). Older persons' experiences of whole systems: The impact of health and social care organizational structures. *Journal of Nursing Management, 16*(2), 105–114.

Murphy, K. (2007). Nurses' perceptions of quality and the factors that affect quality care for older people living in long term care setting in Ireland. *Journal of Clinical Nursing, 16*(5) 873–884.

Murphy, K., O'Shea, E., & Cooney, A. (2007). The quality of life for older people living in long-stay settings in Ireland. *Journal of Clinical Nursing, 16*(11), 2167–2177.

Randers, I., & Mattiasson, A. C. (2004). Autonomy and integrity: Upholding older patients' dignity. *Journal of Advanced Nursing, 45*, 63–71.

Reid, E. (1988). An overview of quality assurance: The concept and the reality. *Recent Advances in Nursing, 19*, 64–97.

Rudd, T. N. (1964). *The nursing of the elderly sick*. London, England: Faber and Faber.

Schnelle, J. F., Rahman, A., Durkin, D. W., Beuscher, L., Choi, L., & Simmons, S. F. (2013, May). A controlled trial of an intervention to increase resident choice in long term. *Journal of the American Medical Directors Association, 14*(5), 345–351.

Tester, S., Hubbard, G., Downs, M., MacDonald, C., & Murphy, J. (2004). Frailty and institutional life. In A. Walker & C. Hagan Hennessy (Eds.), *Growing older quality of life in old age*. Berkshire, England: Open University Press.

Wade, S. (1999). Promoting quality care for older people: Developing a positive attitude to working with older people. *Journal of Nursing Management, 7*(6), 339–348.

Waters, K. R. (1994). Getting dressed in the early morning: Styles of staff/patient interaction on rehabilitation wards for elderly people. *Journal of Advanced Nursing, 19*, 239–248.

Welford, C., Murphy, K., Rodgers, V., & Frauenlob, T. (2012). Autonomy for older people in residential care: A selective literature review. *International Journal of Older People Nursing, 7*(1), 65–69.

Wells, T. J. (1980). *Problems in geriatric nursing care*. London, England: Churchill Livingstone.

5 INDEPENDENCE

Kathy Murphy

Subjective

"I feel so rocky. I have lost my independence. Can you help me get over to that chair?"

Objective

Mrs. Ellen Evans is a 75-year-old woman who has lived in a long-term care facility for just over a year. She was admitted following her discharge from an acute-care hospital where she had been admitted following a left hemisphere middle cerebral artery cerebrovascular accident (CVA). An occupational therapy assessment prior to discharge from the hospital determined that she could not return home. Before her admission, Mrs. Evans was a very independent woman who had worked in the family business. She describes herself as a happy person generally, but feeling low in mood since her admission to long-term care, her loss of independence, and husband's death 6 months ago.

On assessment, Mrs. Evans is 5 foot 2 in. (157 cm) in height, and weighs 160 lbs. (72 kg). Her BP is 180/95, her pulse 90 and regular, respirations 20 per minute. She is afebrile with a temperature of 97.8°F. Her color is good, her breathing sounds are normal, and her pupils are equal and reacting to light. There is marked weakness of the facial muscles with asymmetry of the left and right sides present. When asked to smile, Mrs. Evans is unable to move the right side of her face, and there is also some deviation of the right eye gaze. Mrs. Evans has a hemiparesis of her right side, resulting in problems getting in or out of bed, transferring to a chair, dressing, washing, and eating. Cardiac exam reveals a regular heart rate, S1, S2, and no adventitious sounds. Her abdomen is soft and nontender, and her bowel sounds are present in all four quadrants; her bowel movements are irregular, and she suffers from constipation. She has occasional problems with urinary continence. Mrs. Evans's grip strength, though normal on the left side, is very poor on the right with significant muscle wasting evident. Her sensory awareness of light touch is markedly reduced down her right side with poor detection of pain stimuli in the right arm. Neurological exam reveals 3+ brisk reflexes in the right leg. There is also a positive dorsiflexion Babinski response present. Her skin is intact and dry with visible bruising on the right leg caused by bumping into objects that she finds difficult to see or feel. Further examination of the visual fields revealed a homonymous hemianopia, resulting in spatial and depth perception problems. Her ears reveal normal tympanic membranes bilaterally; her hearing is reduced slightly in her right ear, corrected with the use of a hearing aid. The oral mucosa and swallowing reflex are normal. Mrs. Evans speech is hesitant and sometimes slurred; she cannot name some common objects when asked to do so, and struggles at times to find the right word. However, if given sufficient time, Mrs. Evans can communicate well. Her current medications include Lisinopril 20 mg po daily, aspirin 50 mg.

When Mrs. Evans was first admitted to long-term care, she needed help with all activities of living, but she is gradually regaining some of her physical capacity and skills following a course of physiotherapy and occupational therapy. She would like to be asked about what she needs help with, what clothes she would like to wear, and what activities she would like to participate in. Mrs. Evans, while not able to complete tasks unaided, feels she could do much more if allowed. She feels that if her clothes were loose enough and if she did not have fiddly buttons, she would be able to mostly dress herself. Mrs. Evans also thinks she could feed herself if a plate guard was used and her food cut up. She feels she could also walk to the toilet if given help to stand, had fewer things to maneuver around, and was moved closer to the toilet. Although Mrs. Evans describes herself as quite dependent, she is keen now to do more for herself. However, she finds it frustrating that one nurse encourages her to do things for herself, which she likes, but the next nurse does everything for her.

Literature Review

There are no commonly accepted definitions of dependence or independence within the literature (Murphy, O'Shea, Cooney, & Casey, 2007). Some authors assume that these concepts are fully understood and therefore do not define them (Secker, Hill, Villennaux, & Parkman, 2003), leading to a lack of conceptual clarity and difficulty in comparing research findings. Researchers who do define these concepts take one of two main approaches: a functional approach or a capacity approach.

Researchers who take a functional approach define the concept of dependence or independence by identifying what individuals can or cannot do for themselves. This approach is evident in the work of Goodwin and Coleman (2003) and Covinsky et al. (2003), who define dependence in terms of the extent to which a person is reliant on others for care, and independence as the ability to self-care or a lack of reliance on others. Falter, Gignac, and Cott (2003) claim that the functional approach to defining dependence and independence has been shaped by a medical model of care that is mainly concerned with physical function and disease and fails to account for the complexity of these concepts. Many researchers therefore criticize the functional approach because it fails to appreciate the broader, more holistic and subjective nature of independence (Falter et al., 2003).

In contrast, researchers who take a capacity approach stress the complexity and subjective nature of independence and dependence (Falter et al., 2003). They argue that these terms cannot be seen in absolute terms (Bowers, 2001) and should focus on a range of dimensions, including physical, social, and emotional functioning, as well as economic circumstances. According to this approach, physical capacity is then only one dimension of what independence is about (Falter et al., 2003; Secker et al., 2003). Some researchers make a crucial distinction between executional and decisional independence (Bowers, 2001; Falter et al., 2003; Secker et al., 2003). While the former does focus on the actual physical capacity to undertake activities of living, the latter relates to the extent to which a person can exercise control and autonomy and make decisions over what he or she does. Mrs. Evans feels she has lost her independence and believes she could do more for herself; it may be that the focus has been on executional independence rather than decisional independence and that this may have compounded her view of herself as very dependent. Falter et al. (2003) researched older people's perceptions of independence and dependence and found that perceptions of independence cannot be explained by the extent of disability alone. These researchers found that some older people who were highly dependent categorized themselves as highly independent. They suggested, therefore, that dependency was about more than the ability to do; it was also about the capacity for autonomous decision making. Åberg, Sidenvall, Hepworth, Oreilly, and Lithell (2005) examined the relationship between independence and life satisfaction and found that independence was important to life satisfaction; however, for people with high levels of dependency, being allowed to decide and having influence over what you do was of key importance. Hillcoat-Nallétamby (2014) undertook a large qualitative study exploring older people's understanding of independence and found that older people's feeling of independence was connected to the resources they had access to. She recommended that the concept of independence needed to be expanded to encompass concepts of relative independence and spatial and social independence.

The relationship between dependence and independence is also far from clear. While many researchers present the relationship as inversely correlated, in that any increase in dependence results in a consequent decrease in independence, Secker et al. (2003) found that this was not necessarily the case. Their research revealed that people may be highly dependent on others for care but could perceive themselves to be highly independent. These findings suggest that the relationships between these concepts are not necessarily inversely related and that although they may be connected, the relationship is complex and individually determined.

A number of factors have been identified that influence the extent to which independence can be maintained. Some researchers suggest that social and environmental factors are key determinants of independence/dependence. Good social networks and connectedness and good environmental design can enhance independence, whereas poor design will compound dependence. For Mrs. Evans, the height of the bed, space around furniture, and distance to the toilet or day rooms can impact on the ability to do more or less.

Some researchers have examined the impact of specific interventions on levels of independence. Senior et al. (2014) undertook a randomized controlled trial to examine the effectiveness of a promoting independence intervention on functional ability outcomes measured by the interRAI–HC, and compared these with usual care. The intervention included comprehensive geriatric assessment and multidisciplinary care planning. They did not find a significant difference in outcomes between intervention and control; however, the study did not achieve statistical power; 240 participants were required for this but only 105 were recruited, and this was decreased further by attrition throughout the trial. In contrast, Beswick, Gooberman-Hill, Smith, Wylde, and Ebrahim (2010) undertook a systematic review of interventions designed to maintain the independence of older people across care settings. They identified six outcomes related to independence, including living at home, death, hospital admission, falls, physical function, and reduction in mortality. They found that there was good high-quality evidence demonstrating the effectiveness of many complex interventions for maintaining the independence of older people and concluded that all older people should be given the chance to receive appropriate preventative strategies.

Strategies for Changing Practice

In our experience, there are two main issues that impact on resident independence. The first is related to the detailed assessment of a person's abilities, and the second focuses on the ethos of promoting independence within the care environment.

Nursing assessment sometimes lacks the specificity required for caregivers to identify exactly what a person can and cannot do for him- or herself. Assessment should be detailed enough so that a caregiver, independent of the person who undertook the assessment, would be able to pinpoint what she or he needs to do and what a person can do for him- or herself.

Nursing documentation should enable this level of detail to be documented, evaluated on an ongoing basis, and updated. For example, it may be that Mrs. Evans can clean her teeth if someone helps to put the toothpaste on the brush, so it is important to put exactly such a note on the care plan. Giving this level of specificity is important so that care is consistent and help is focused on what is required so that Mrs. Evans's skills are maintained. Mrs. Evans was very frustrated because of inconsistent care—one nurse would encourage her to do the things she could do, and then the next nurse would do everything for her. Nurses need to promote independence by helping individuals do what they can for themselves and by ensuring that all caregivers are clear about the goals of care and then implement them.

Careful consideration of assistive technologies that may help to facilitate independence is also important—for example, special cutlery, plate guards, and careful selection of clothes can make a difference. Good assessment by the multidisciplinary team matters, with the occupational therapist providing expert advice on what could be done to enable Mrs. Evans to do more for herself. Enabling decisional independence is also important and is about encouraging Mrs. Evans to make decisions for herself—what she wishes to wear, what she would like to do, what she wants to eat. Strategies such as asking how Mrs. Evans likes things done before starting care routines, always giving her a choice, helps her feel more independent. In addition, questions to Mrs. Evans need to be phrased succinctly and time given for her to answer because of her communication problems. Other care interventions that could be considered include some of the evidence-based interventions included in the Beswick et al. (2010) systematic review—for example, those designed to maintain physical functioning or prevent falls.

The second issue related to promoting independence is the ethos of the care environment. The ethos of the care environment matters to promoting independence because, ultimately, it shapes staff perspectives about the importance of enabling residents to do things for themselves. For example, if staff are expected to complete physical care within specified time periods in the morning, they may find that allowing residents to dress themselves slows them down. Helping a resident to dress him- or herself may take more time, at least initially, than it would if staff did it for the resident, so the ethos does matter. Staff need to agree that promoting independence matters and work together as a team to promote this. A focus on the ethos of the care environment is therefore essential to promoting independence, and a systematic identification of the barriers to promoting independence may help identify factors that need to be addressed.

Clinical Reasoning Questions

1. What needs to be changed about the assessment documentation you use to enable detailed assessment of what a resident can and cannot do for himself or herself?
2. What is the difference between executional and decisional independence?
3. What can you do to enable decisional independence?
4. What needs to be changed in the environment to enable a resident to do more for herself or himself?

References

Åberg, A. C., Sidenvall, B., Hepworth, M., O'Reilly, K., & Lithell, A. H. (2005). On loss of activity and independence, adaptation improves life satisfaction in old age—A qualitative study of patients' perceptions. *Quality of Life Research, 14*, 1111–1125.

Beswick, A. D., Gooberman-Hill, R., Smith, A., Wylde, V., & Ebrahim, S. (2010). Maintaining independence in older people. *Reviews in Clinical Gerontology, 20*, 128–153. doi:10.1017/S0959259810000079

Bowers, H. (2001). Promoting interdependence: A new challenge in developing services for older people? *Journal of Integrated Care, 9*(6), 34–39.

Covinsky, K. E., Palmer, R. M., Fortinsky, R. H., Counsell, S. R., Stewart, A. L., Kresevic, D., . . . Landefeld, C. S. (2003). Loss of independence in activities of daily living in older adults hospitalized with medical illnesses: Increased vulnerability with age. *Journal of the American Geriatrics Society, 51*, 451–458.

Falter, L.-B., Gignac, M. A. M., & Cott, C. (2003). Adaptation to disability in chronic obstructive pulmonary disease: Neglected relationships to older adults' perceptions of independence. *Disability & Rehabilitation, 25*, 795–806.

Goodwin, J. A., & Coleman, E. A. (2003, December). Exploring measures of functional dependence in the older adult with cancer. *Medsurg Nursing, 12*(6), 359–366.

Hillcoat-Nallétamby, S. (2014). The meaning of "independence" for older people in different residential settings. *Journals of Gerontology, Series B: Psychological Sciences and Social Sciences, 69*(3), 419–430. doi:10.1093/geronb/gbu008 [Advance Access publication February 27, 2014].

Murphy, K., O'Shea, E., Cooney, A., & Casey, D. (2007). *Quality of life of older people with a disability in Ireland*. Dublin, Ireland: National Council on Ageing and Older People.

Secker, J., Hill, R. T., Villennaux, L., & Parkman, S. (2003). Promoting independence: But promoting what and how? *Ageing and Society, 23*, 375–391. doi:10.1017/S0144686X03001193

Senior, H. E. J., Parsons, M., Kerse, N., Chen, M.-H., Jacobs, S., Hoorn, S., . . . Craig S. (2014, May). Promoting independence in frail older people: A randomised controlled trial of a restorative care service in New Zealand. *Age & Ageing, 43*(3), 418–424.

6 DIGNITY

CYNTHIA S. JACELON

Subjective

"Okay, well. I'll tell ya. I must have been in a bad way. My Don came and got me over [to the doctor's office] within about 20 minutes. He [the doctor] examined me—he could hear the pneumonia. The doctor said 'I'm gonna take you to the hospital.' Well, I gave some arguments, but he didn't pay much attention to me. I went straight from the doctor's office; I was in the hospital by quarter to 10. I was in the emergency room for about 8 hours. I was kind of disgusted. The doctor gave me a slip of paper that indicated I should go to emergency and go straight up to the floor. Somebody did not read the paper right, so I had to sit and watch all that in the emergency department.

"Then they kicked me out of there [the acute care unit]—told me that I had about a half hour to get my stuff together to go down [to the skilled unit]. It wasn't even 10 minutes. It happened much faster than I thought it was going to. They could have had Don take my clothes home. Instead the staff came in with these two paper bags. It was terrible. I have a new coat that I like. They took my coat and my boots and just rolled 'em up and shoved them in the bags—just like you were nothing. I mean I don't understand that. They were so disrespectful of my things. I just think that wasn't very nice.

"And tellin' me how wonderful it was gonna be on the skilled unit. So that was a lie. I don't think that it is necessary to lie. Tell the truth. Right? See, I had two bad roommates [in the acute unit], and they pretended that's why they were moving me. That wasn't it. They wanted the bed.

They said, 'You won't have bad roommates down there.' So, I came down to this. This roommate is bad, too. When they were wheeling me in, I couldn't get in. She [the roommate] had my way blocked. I was pushed way over in the corner with no room most of the time. I think they could've been more honest with me."

Objective

Mrs. Frieda Feiffer is an independent 84-year-old woman. She had moved from the Sun Belt to western New England 4 years ago to be closer to her only son, Don. She lived in an apartment in a small town that was within walking distance to stores and church and that would permit Mrs. Feiffer to have a dog. She engaged in an active family life with her son and grandson and their families, but her closest companion is her dog, Dottie. Dottie was a very small dog who had been Mrs. Feiffer's constant companion for the past 2 years.

Mrs. Feiffer has had significant asthma for many years. In 2005, she had a stroke resulting in mild weakness on her left side. She used a cane when she took the dog outside for a walk. In addition to breathing problems, during the past year she has had two or three falls, one in which she broke her ankle and another where she needed stitches on the bridge of her nose. She was admitted to the hospital this time for pneumonia. Mrs. Feiffer was in the hospital for a total of 26 days. The first 6 days were on a medical–surgical acute care unit. Mrs. Feiffer was then transferred to a skilled nursing facility located within the hospital. While Mrs. Feiffer was in the hospital, Dottie stayed alone in their apartment. Don went to the apartment twice a day to walk Dottie and play with her. Dottie visited Mrs. Feiffer in the hospital every other day.

When the nurse practitioner made her first visit, Mrs. Feiffer was sitting upright in her hospital bed with two pillows behind her. She was wearing a hospital gown; she had an IV flowing into her right forearm, and an oxygen cannula in her nose. Between spasms of a very wet sounding cough, Mrs. Feiffer was trying to eat some dinner. The tray had been brought from the kitchen 2 hours earlier, and the food was now cold. Mrs. Feiffer's black leather pocketbook and a packet of admitting information lay haphazardly on the windowsill.

When Mrs. Feiffer was admitted to the hospital, she had been quite dehydrated. At admission, the physician ordered 500 mL of normal saline bolus to be followed by continuous IV set at the rate of 100 mL/hour. During the first 24 hours of being in the hospital, Mrs. Feiffer received almost 3,000 mL of fluid. By the third day, Mrs. Feiffer was having significant stress incontinence. She explained it this way: "I'm so full of fluid that every time I cough I wet the bed. I'm not used to having all of this fluid."

Seventy-two hours after admission, the IV fluids were discontinued, and the stress incontinence gradually resolved. By that time, Mrs. Feiffer had taken to sitting on the commode all of the time she was out of bed so as not to urinate on herself and her clothing. In bed she was using waterproof pads and changing them independently when the pads became wet. Her perception was that the nurses were not interested in her incontinence; she was having a hard time getting the staff to respond to her needs for dryness. She said, "I just threw one of those things (incontinence pads) under the bed, the staff don't care."

Mrs. Feiffer had very definite ideas about how hospital personnel should treat patients. She believed that the staff should be respectful of patients and their things, be honest, and treat them with respect. Mrs. Feiffer preferred to be called Mrs. Feiffer rather than her first name. Most of the staff called her that, although they tended to call most patients by first names. The staff members of whom Mrs. Feiffer thought the most highly were those staff members who conveyed genuine caring. These staff members showed interest in Mrs. Feiffer. One such staff member was the medical resident who admitted Mrs. Feiffer. He took his time with Mrs. Feiffer and went out of his way to arrange for Dottie to come and visit. Another was a respiratory therapist who conveyed an aura of calm and competence. Mrs. Feiffer liked several of the nurses. They were usually the older ones; she thought they had more compassion.

There was one nurse's aide on the skilled unit that Mrs. Feiffer particularly did not care for. She described his behavior this way: "He comes in and shouts at me. I'm not deaf. And he comes in and tries to give my glasses. I have almost 20/20 vision. I don't need to have my glasses on for breakfast. He's always pushing everyone to get done. See, he just wants to get finished so that he can hang out with the girls down at the desk." It was the impression that he gave that he had other things to do, rather than attend to the immediate client, that contributed to Mrs. Feiffer's dislike of him. This aide called Mrs. Feiffer by her first name even though she had asked him not to.

Mrs. Feiffer tried to maintain her dignity throughout her hospital stay by reminding herself that she had been in tough situations before and had survived, by being pleasant to the hospital staff and trying not to be too demanding, and by asserting her will when she felt that not to do so would place her in peril.

Literature Review

Dignity is a concept that is widely discussed in relation to older adults. Achieving and maintaining dignity is thought to be a developmental task of old age (Erikson, Erikson, & Kivnick, 1986), and important for wellness (Jacelon, 2003). Over the last several years, there has been increasing interest in exploring the concept of dignity for older adults in various contexts and across cultures. Attention has been focused on dignity in cognitively intact older adults (Jacelon & Choi, 2014), cognitively impaired older adults (Sørensen, Waldorff, & Waldemar, 2008), and at the end of life (Chochinov et al., 2006). Another area of interest with regard to dignity has been the effect of health care on the dignity of older individuals (Baillie, 2009; Baillie, Ford, Gallagher, & Wainwright, 2009).

Dignity in community dwelling, cognitively intact older adults has been defined as an attributed, dynamic sense of self-value, behavior of self in relation to others, perceived value from others, and behavior that demonstrates respect toward self and others (Jacelon, 2012). Attributed dignity is a manifestation of human dignity that is sensitive to human interaction, including interventions by health care providers. Older adults manage their attributed dignity by using introspective, interactive, and active strategies to maintain or recover dignity when it is threatened (Jacelon, 2014).

In a qualitative study exploring dignity in seriously ill older adults, researchers (vanGennip, Pasman, Oosterveld-Vlug, Willems, & Onwuteaka-Philipsen, 2013) found that personal dignity, a concept similar to attributed dignity (Jacelon & Choi, 2014) described previously, was affected by the illness. Three types of self—the individual self, the relational self, and the societal self—were important. Becoming a patient and developing the symptoms of illness affected individual dignity. Individual dignity was related to sense of control, and was only possible in cognitively intact individuals. Relational dignity was associated with changes in social roles. Being of value to significant others was critical to maintaining relational dignity. Interactions with people outside a patient's immediate social circle could have a negative effect on dignity. These people often responded to the symptoms of the illness and not the individual.

When working with older adults who have dementia, their self-perceived, attributed dignity may not be the standard by which to measure an individual's dignity. For these individuals, the concept of human dignity is more appropriate. Using a conceptual model such as Nordenfelt's (2004) in which dignity is conceptualized as *Menschenwürde,* the intrinsic value of being human, and dignity of identity, moral stature, and merit, provide a framework by which to think about the dignity of these individuals.

There is a large body of research exploring issues of Alzheimer's disease through the perceptions of formal and informal caregivers. The body of research focused on the individuals experiencing the disease is more modest. This is, in part, related to the challenges of conducting research with cognitively impaired individuals, and may inadvertently affect the *Menschenwürde* of these individuals.

Conducting interviews with older adults in the early stages of dementia living at home with their spouses, Sørensen, Waldorff, and Waldemar (2008) found these individuals perceived decline in their personal dignity and value. The perceptions of decline were increased when the individuals experienced well-known places that were familiar and strange at the same time; words were recognized, but the meanings were not understood; actions that had been easy to perform in the past now became difficult or impossible; and spouses responded to the individuals in new ways (p. 294). In order to protect themselves from this decline, individuals in this study described using strategies such as talking less to avoid making errors, minimizing the importance and impact of the disease, and recounting their life story to enhance their personal dignity. They also limited their social interactions and relied on the relationship with their spouse for social support.

Heggestad, Nortvedt, and Slettebø (2013) used qualitative research methods to describe the experience of individuals with dementia living in a nursing home. Using a combination of observation and interviews, they found that these individuals wanted to be seen and heard as individuals, felt they were captives of the nursing home, and were homesick living among strangers in an institution. Often, individuals are not seen as whole individuals, but only in relation to their diminished cognitive capacity. This can lead to older people feeling marginalized and not respected. Focusing on the individual's abilities rather than limitations may help confirm the individual's wholeness and uniqueness as a human being.

Recently, there has been a lot of attention focused on dignity at the end of life. Researchers have identified factors threatening the dying individual's dignity, including frailty, dependence, and the need for physical care, adequate communication, and to leave a legacy.

Chochinov and colleagues have led the way in extensively exploring the issues of dignity at the end of life. They found that the most significant threat to dignity at the end of life was "feeling life no longer had meaning or purpose" (p. 670). Dying individuals indicated that "not being treated with respect or understanding" and "feeling a burden to others" (p. 669) also diminished dignity at the end of life (Chochinov et al., 2006). Based on these findings, Chochinov et al. (2006) developed dignity therapy, a short-term research-based psychotherapy for individuals at the end of life. Dignity therapy can be conducted by any professional care provider who has been trained in the therapy, and is guided by a list of questions developed in previous research. The session is recorded and transcribed. The transcription is given to the dying individual to share with individuals of his or her choice. These individuals reported that dignity therapy was more beneficial than standard palliative care or client-centered care in supporting dignity at the end of life (Chochinov et al., 2011). Another group of scientists evaluated the value of the transcribed documents to families of dying individuals in care homes. Even though memory problems of the residents affected their ability to engage in dignity therapy, family members found the document helpful in promoting dignity at the end of life (Goddard, Speck, Martin, & Hall, 2013).

Like Mrs. Feiffer in the case study, older individuals interacting with the health care system want to be treated with respect. Matiti and Trorey (2008) interviewed over 100 patients to find out how these individuals thought their dignity was compromised in the health care setting. Although most individuals reported that their dignity had been adequately maintained, protection of privacy of person and confidentiality of information, appropriate communication and information sharing, the inclusion of the patient in care choices, being addressed as one chose, and being treated with respect were critical for protecting dignity.

Role and Cultural Considerations

Research findings regarding the need for dignity with older adults are remarkably consistent across countries and cultures. This research on dignity in older adults has been conducted in many different countries including Australia (Henderson et al., 2009), Canada (Chochinov et al., 2011; Jacobsen, 2009; Montross, Winters, & Irwin, 2011), Germany (Pleschberger, 2007), the United Kingdom (Arino-Biasco, Tadd, & Boiz-Ferrer, 2005; Baillie & Gallagher, 2011; Brown, Johnston, & Ostlind, 2011), Scandinavia (Jakobsen & Sørlie, 2010), Taiwan (Lin, Tsai, & Chen, 2011), and the United States (Periyakoil, Noda, & Kraemer, 2010).

The need to be treated with dignity may actually increase as the individual ages. Recently, Jacelon (2013) discovered that individuals who were 75 years old and older reported higher attributed dignity scores than their younger seniors. It seems that the oldest individuals in our society may be more sensitive to slights to their dignity than younger individuals. Mrs. Feiffer is a good example of this. She was sensitive to many actions of the staff that she perceived as disrespectful.

In another recent study, Jacelon (2013) found that the strategies that older adults used to restore their dignity varied according to race. Although all individuals interviewed used introspective strategies to restore their dignity, only African American women reported that they "took it to God."

Strategies for Changing Practice

Person-centered care—care that meets the specific needs, values, and beliefs of patients (McMillan et al., 2013)—holds promise for supporting the dignity of older adults in care settings. According to Morgan and Yoder (2012), patient-centered care is holistic, individualized, respectful, and empowering. Person-centered care inherently enhances the dignity of the individual by incorporating the interventions identified previously.

Patient-centered care is more challenging when the patient cannot fully participate in the process. In order to determine the best interventions to promote dignity in individuals with dementia, a group of scientists conducted a metasynthesis of qualitative studies (Tranvag, Petersen, & Naden, 2013). Two major intervention strategies were identified:

- Interventions advocating for the person's autonomy and integrity. These activities include:
  - Having compassion for the person
  - Confirming the person's worthiness and sense of self
  - Creating a humane and purposeful environment (p. 867)
- Interventions that balance "individual choices in persons no longer able to make sound decisions, against the duty of making choices on behalf of the person" (p. 868). The bulleted activities below require a balance between autonomy and safety and can be incorporated into the overarching philosophy of "Sheltering Human Worth" (p. 877). Care providers in these situations are responding to the individual's *Menschenwürde.*
  - Employing persuasion
  - Exerting a certain degree of mild restraint (p. 868)

Implementing patient-centered care in acute care settings may be challenging. Hunter and Carlson (2014) identify nine strategies for creating a patient-centered environment. These nine actions are focused on improving care and respecting the individual and creating a partnership with the patient. They include activities to promote quality care:

- Creating a calm and quiet healing environment
- Care coordination conferences
- Hourly rounding
- Bedside report
- Activities focused on enhancing the participation of patients and their families
- Personalized care
- Engaging patients as care partners
- Open medical record policy
- Encouraging family presence at all times including during procedures and resuscitation (p. 42)

Employing these actions in the acute care environment will fundamentally change the way care is delivered, and will promote the dignity of all individuals, patients, family members, and care providers.

In interactions with the health care system, older adults expect to be treated like competent individuals whose wants and needs are taken into account in the care situation. Care providers can enhance the health and dignity of these patients by treating them as individuals, respecting their wishes and choices, and demonstrating respect for their person, property, and information by maintaining their privacy. Remembering to be polite using "please" and "thank you" liberally goes a long way toward improving patient satisfaction and maintaining an individual's dignity. Mrs. Feiffer's dignity was enhanced by those care providers who made it possible for Dottie, the dog, to visit regularly, as well as those who addressed her as she wanted to be addressed, were truthful with her, and helped her maintain privacy. Dignity is nurtured and supported in the interpersonal space that exists between people in relationship (Street & Kissane, 2001). The care providers that nurtured Mrs. Feiffer's dignity did not require additional time to do so; they incorporated dignity-preserving care into all of their interactions.

Clinical Reasoning Questions

1. What is dignity? How is it affected by interaction with the health care system?
2. How would you advise the nurses' aide on the skilled unit to change his behavior? Why?
3. What are the critical components of interaction that you should include in every encounter with an older individual?
4. How might dignity needs vary by cognitive status or severity of illness?

References

Arino-Biasco, S., Tadd, W., & Boiz-Ferrer, J. A. (2005). Dignity and older people: The voice of professionals. *Quality in Ageing, 6*(1), 30–36.

Baillie, L. (2009). Patient dignity in an acute hospital setting: A case study. *International Journal of Nursing Studies, 46*, 23–37.

Baillie, L., Ford, P., Gallagher, A., & Wainwright, P. (2009). Nurse's views on dignity in care. *Nursing Older People, 21*(8), 22–29.

Baillie, L., & Gallagher, A. (2011). Respecting dignity in care in diverse care settings: Strategies of UK nurses. *International Journal of Nursing Practice, 17*, 336–341.

Brown, H., Johnston, B., & Ostlind, U. (2011). Identifying care actions to conserve dignity in end-of-life care. *British Journal of Community Nursing, 16*(5), 238–245.

Chochinov, H. M., Kristjanson, L. J., Breitbart, W., McClement, S., Hack, T. F., Hassard, T., & Harlos, M. (2011). Effect of dignity therapy on distress and end-of-life experience in terminally ill patients: A randomised controlled trial. *Lancet Oncology, 12*, 753–762.

Chochinov, H. M., Kristjanson, L. J., Hack, T. F., Hassard, T., McClement, S., & Harlos, M. (2006). Dignity in the terminally ill: Revisited. *Journal of Palliative Medicine, 9*(3), 666–672.

Erikson, E. H., Erikson, J. M., & Kivnick, H. Q. (1986). *Vital involvement in old age*. New York, NY: W. W. Norton.

Goddard, C., Speck, P., Martin, P., & Hall, S. (2013). Dignity therapy for older people in care homes: A qualitative study of the views of residents and recipients of "generativity" documents. *Journal of Advanced Nursing, 69*(1), 122–132.

Heggestad, A. K., Nortvedt, P., & Slettebø, Å. (2013). "Like a prison without bars": Dementia and experiences of dignity. *Nursing Ethics, 20*(8), 881–892.

Henderson, A., Van Eps, M., Pearson, K., James, C., Henderson, P., & Osborne, Y. (2009). Maintainance of patients' dignity during hospitalization: Comparison of staff–patient observations and patient feedback through interviews. *International Journal of Nursing Practice, 15*, 227–330.

Hunter, R., & Carlson, E. (2014). Finding the fit: Patient-centered care. *Nursing Management, 45*(1), 38–43.

Jacelon, C. (2003). The dignity of elders in an acute care hospital. *Qualitative Health Research, 13*(4), 543–556.

Jacelon, C. S. (2012). *The evolution of the concept of attributed dignity*. Council for the Advancement of Nursing Science 2012 State of the Science Congress on Nursing Research, September 13–15, 2012, Washington Hilton Hotel, Washington, DC.

Jacelon, C. S. (2013). *Attributed dignity, optimal aging, and health*. Gerontological Society of America 66th Annual Scientific Meeting, New Orleans, LA.

Jacelon, C. S. (2014). Strategies used by older adults to maintain or restore attributed dignity. *Research in Gerontological Nursing, 7*(6), 273–283.

Jacelon, C. S., & Choi, J. (2014). Evaluating the psychometric properties of the Jacelon Attributed Dignity Scale. *Journal of Advanced Nursing, 70*(9), 2149–2161.

Jacobsen, N. (2009). Dignity violation in health care. *Qualitative Health Research, 19*(11), 1536–1547.

Jakobsen, R., & Sørlie, V. (2010). Dignity of older people in a nursing home: Narratives of care providers. *Nursing Ethics, 17*(3), 289–300.

Lin, Y.-P., Tsai, Y.-F., & Chen, H.-F. (2011). Dignity in care in the hospital setting from patients' perspectives in Taiwan: A descriptive qualitative study. *Journal of Clinical Nursing, 20*, 794–801.

Matiti, R. M., & Trorey, G. M. (2008). Patients' expectations of the maintenance of their dignity. *Journal of Clinical Nursing, 17*, 2709–2717.

McMillan, S. S., Kendall, E., Sav, A., King, M. A., Whitty, J. A., Kelly, F., & Wheeler, A. J. (2013). Patient-centered approaches to health care: A systematic review of randomized controlled trials. *Medical Care Research and Review, 70*(6), 567–596.

Montross, L., Winters, K. D., & Irwin, S. A. (2011). Dignity therapy implementation in a community-based hospice setting. *Journal of Palliative Medicine, 14*(6), 729–734.

Morgan, S., & Yoder, L. H. (2012). A concept analysis of person-centered care. *Journal of Holistic Nursing, 30*, 6–15.

Nordenfelt, L. (2004). The varieties of dignity. *Health Care Analysis, 12*(2), 69–81.

Periyakoil, V., Noda, A., & Kraemer, H. (2010). Assessment of factors influencing preservation of dignity at life's end: Creation and the cross-cultural validation of the preservation of dignity card-sort tool. *Journal of Palliative Medicine, 13*(5), 495–500.

Pleschberger, S. (2007). Dignity and the challenge of dying in nursing homes: The residents' view. *Age and Ageing, 36*, 197–202.

Sørensen, L., Waldorff, F., & Waldemar, G. (2008). Coping with mild Alzheimer's disease. *Dementia, 7*(3), 287–299.

Street, A. F., & Kissane, D. W. (2001). Constructions of dignity in end-of-life care. *Journal of Palliative Care, 17*(2), 93–101.

Tranvag, O., Petersen, K., & Naden, D. (2013). Dignity-preserving dementia care: A metasynthesis. *Nursing Ethics, 20*(8), 861–880.

vanGennip, I., Pasman, H., Oosterveld-Vlug, M., Willems, D., & Onwuteaka-Philipsen, B. (2013). The development of a model of dignity in illness based on qualitative interviews with seriously ill patients. *International Journal of Nursing Studies, 50*, 1080–1089.

7 RISK ENGAGEMENT

KATHY L. RUSH AND MARY KJORVEN

Subjective

"Without a certain amount of risk there is no progress, but sometimes I overestimate my capabilities. Then, when something happens, it's fait accompli."

Objective

Mr. George Green is an 83-year-old man who lives independently in a supportive housing facility. He receives medication support four times a day, is independent with showering and dressing, has grabs in the shower, uses a four-wheeled walker and cane, and uses a scooter to get to appointments. He has a history of falls, myocardial infarction, metastatic prostate cancer, chronic obstructive pulmonary disease, diabetes, arthritis, depression, and hypertension. He has some short-term memory loss, adequate vision, and denies alcohol use. His medications include: ASA chewable 80 mg po OD; Amlodipine 5 mg po OD; Bisoprolol 2.5 mg po OD; Domperidone 10 mg TID; Fluoxetine 10 mg po OD; Valsartan 80 mg Q 12h.

George was admitted to the hospital by ambulance after a fall at his facility. Although George was reluctant to go to the hospital, stating that "it's not serious and I'm fine," facility staff noticed that he was in significant pain when he attempted to mobilize. They convinced him to go by ambulance to the hospital emergency department (ED). An x-ray of his right hip was "suspicious for a subcapital femoral neck fracture," and clinical correlation was recommended.

The nurses' notes indicated that his temperature was 36.6°C; blood pressure was 186/108; pulse was 92 and irregular; respirations were 16, and SpO_2 was 94% on room air. His Glasgow Coma Scale score was 15/15; his blood sugar via glucometer was 11.4; and his right hip pain rated 2/10. George's pedal pulses were positive bilaterally with slight bilateral ankle and pedal edema and no shortening or external rotation of his right leg. His sensory status and movement were satisfactory.

George was anxious to go home, continuing to underreport his pain (2/10) and expressing confidence in being able to manage with what appeared to be a "soft tissue injury." Within 12 hours of returning home, staff at his facility convinced him to return to the ED, where a radiologist confirmed that his hip was broken.

Prior to surgery, George and his daughter (Mary) had a discussion with the surgeon about using spinal anesthesia owing to George's risk of respiratory infection and avoiding the use of a urinary catheter due to his risk of urinary tract infections. George went into an uncomplicated surgery and returned to the orthopedic patient care ward. During a conversation with one of the nurses who worked the previous day, Mary discovered that the nurses were concerned about George going home the previous day, collectively knowing he was at high risk for becoming a "bounce back." Yet they could not prevent the discharge.

While in the hospital, George followed all of the rules and did all of the exercises; his goal was to get home, and with great relief he finally did. Once home, George relaxed on the exercise regime despite encouragements from his family. Two weeks later, he boarded an airplane with two of his children to attend the funeral of a family member. He managed well with his walker as he moved from place to place in unfamiliar environments and unpredictable winter weather. Feeling confident in his progress after he returned home, he visited the gym in his facility and attempted to use the treadmill. He was the only one in the gym at the time and he forgot to turn on the lights. Afterward, he stated, "It started up at a nice, easy pace but speeded up quickly and got away from me." He fell and broke both of his arms.

Literature Review

Risk is a high-priority concept in Western culture and around the globe, permeating all levels of society, including health care. Although risk is typically associated with the probability of an event occurring that may produce harmful outcomes or loss, constructive outcomes of taking risks have been documented (Rush, Murphy, & Kozak, 2012; Waring, 2000). Risk is often referenced in terms of behavior, but more recently it has been conceptualized as a process. The Model of Risk in Aging describes risk as a process of mediating quality of life (QOL) for older adults who negotiate choices, decisions, and agency along a continuum of risk taking and avoiding (Clarke & Members of the International Collaborative Research Network on Risk and Ageing Populations, 2006). The older adult engages with risk as an outcome of interaction with multiple and increasingly broader spheres of enabling or disabling influences, extending from family, to service providers, to the health system organization, and to society. These complex spheres of influence that are culturally specific and interdependent (Clarke & Members of the International Collaborative Research Network on Risk and Ageing Populations, 2006) were evident in George's situation as he navigated the risk continuum.

Older adults, like George, have been targeted as an "at risk" group because of several risk factors, such as age, multiple chronic diseases, polypharmacy, and history of falls, which all predispose to deficit accumulation and hospitalization for an acute event (Rockwood & Mitnitski, 2011). Age has been identified as a major predictor of risk, with 75% of older adults in the top three risk categories (moderate, high, very high) and high-risk older adults demonstrating a proportionately higher incidence of physical and mental health conditions (Bestsennyy, Kibasi, & Richardson, 2013). Risk stratification has been used widely in health care circles for early risk detection and interventions. Mehta and colleagues (2011) found that their clinical index predicted new onset disability in hospitalized older adults, like George, who had been independent 2 weeks prior to hospitalization. Seven risk factors were predictive of disability: age; premorbid instrumental ADLs and admission ADLs; mobility;

acute stroke/metastatic cancer; severe cognitive impairment; albumin. George scored 5 out of 15 on the index; 45% of study participants with this score developed new onset disability. This index may be useful for both generalist and advanced practice nurses (APNs) for early intervention to prevent functional decline that accompanies hospitalization (Volpato et al., 2007).

Although risk stratification is a valuable tool, its pervasiveness has served to organize, define, and structure the personal spaces in which to grow old. The "being at risk" designation creates the older adult's identity as vulnerable, passive, dependent, and powerless (Furedi, 2011). As such, it may impinge on the everyday lives of older adults, diminishing their agency and placing them in the role of victim in need of protection such as institutionalization (Furedi, 2011; Slade, Fear, & Tennant, 2006; Lupton, 2013). Powell, Wahidan, and Zinn (2007) describe the challenge among older adults to reduce risk amid a deeply held value of autonomy. Risk surveillance often threatens older adults' independence that they value more than personal risk (Kilian, Salmoni, Ward-Griffin, & Kloseck, 2008). Faulkner (2012) found that the risk of losing independence, coupled with the increased risk of institutionalization, was of greater concern to older adults than other risks such as health and safety. George resisted the scrutiny of others, as evidenced by his reluctance to go to the hospital and his lack of engagement in exercises he was being encouraged to do; these threatened his choice and decision making. The tension between safety and autonomy has been well documented in the health care literature (Hunt & Ells, 2011). The risk of institutionalization was very real for George, given comments by his family and physician that he might need a higher level of care than the supportive housing he was now receiving.

Risk discourse is prominent in the language and practice of health care. Despite the prevalence of the term "risk" in health care, it does not appear in older adults' vernacular in the same way (Furedi, 2011). George had difficulty in applying language about risk to his situation. Furedi (2011) noted the absence of any reference to "risk," "risk taking," "choice," or any of the terms that policy makers use in relation to the care and support of older adults. Older adults use other language to describe risk such as "common sense" (Kilian et al., 2008) and "rights" (Furedi, 2011) that may be interpreted as indirect reflections of risk. This has implications for risk communication or the "exchange of information concerning the existence, nature, form, severity or acceptability of health or environmental risks" (Government of Canada, 2006, pp. 2–5). Evidence shows that the way communication is framed influences patients' risk perceptions and decisions (Edwards, Elwyn, Covey, Matthews, & Pill, 2001). Therefore, risk communication with older adults must take account of the language they use and can relate to.

Society expects older adults to identify and manage their personal risks through risk avoidance at the expense of risk taking, creating tensions and contradictions for the older adult. When older adults fail to acknowledge their risks and take action to contain and diminish them, they often become targets of criticism. Research shows some tendency for older adults to deny risk, regard it impersonally, and view it as applicable to others (Kilian et al., 2008). By downplaying the risks related to his falls and pain and saying all was fine, George was protecting his capabilities and diverting attention away from the appearance of being disabled. This practice of passing, or making things seem normal, has been described as a way of "not disturbing the peace [and] containing the matter which is potentially out of place" (Campbell, 2009, p. 25). However, there is also risk in passing, or failing to disclose perceived or actual danger (Leary, 1999), for in seeking to self-protect and safeguard, the individual may be hiding valuable information that has the potential to decrease risk. Understanding this tendency for older adults to equate risk with competence and ability can help nurses frame and support care according to older adults' abilities and strengths rather than emphasizing losses.

Even though risk is not in their everyday language, research has suggested that older adults have a balanced approach to risk. Older adults acknowledge a range of objects, activities, and situations associated with risk and are specific in judging certain behaviors and situations as risky (Rush et al., 2012). Rush and colleagues (2012) found that community-living older adults preferred risk taking but balanced it by avoiding risks in specific situations. They were not reckless but often adapted, modified, or set boundaries in taking risks or embraced opportunities for growth and social engagement.

Taking risks is critical to the older adult's sense of self and self-worth (Faulkner, 2012). This was true for George, who equated risk with progress. Despite the potential risk of another fall, shortly after returning home, George decided to attend a family funeral in another province made possible with several accommodations. Nurses can explore ways to help older adults take risks by helping them adapt activities in order to do them safely (Rush et al., 2012).

There is considerable variability in older adults' responses to risks, with over- or underestimation commonly observed (Denscombe, 1993). Differences in risk estimation, such as George's tendency to underestimate, are not due to cognitive appraisal alone, but involve emotions and values (Finucane & Holup, 2006; Loewenstein, Weber, Hsee, & Welch, 2001; MacCourt & Tuokko, 2010). Risks are judged using a number of heuristics, or mental strategies, including perceived control, affect (e.g., fear), awareness, vulnerability, and vividness (Rush et al., 2012; Visschers, Meertens, Passchier, & DeVries, 2007). Further, the patient's subjective, situated, sociocultural, and biographical context plays a role in older adults' interpretations and perceptions of risk (Morden, Jinks, & Ong, 2012; Zinn, 2005). These are all important considerations for generalists and APNs when helping older adults, like George, navigate risk. For example, it is important for nurses to work with George to decrease his sense of "fait accompli" and give him as much control as possible to grow his confidence and agency in managing his risks.

Knowing the patient has been identified as an important strategy to address risk with hospital patients (Groves, Finfgeld-Connett, & Wakefield, 2012). Knowing the patient involves gathering information through interaction to understand the patient as a complete person rather than as a group of diagnoses and physical assessment data, and may be supplemented with valuable biographical information from the family that the patient may have missed. The use of an interactive, supported decision tool as a means of guiding and documenting choices and decisions involving risk may enhance nurses' ways of knowing George. The Department of Health (DoH, 2007) in the United Kingdom developed a 21-question support tool to assess the individual's decision-making situation. The tool helps to elicit specific information from patients about who and what is important to them; what is working/not working and could be improved; difficulties and their impact; barriers to doing what they want to do; risks they identify and how they could be reduced; what they/family/organization need to do; and what/who could help and support. The use of such a tool is highly encouraged in situations involving older adults with complex needs, or those who are undertaking activities that appear risky (DoH, 2007), and where there are differences among older adults, their families, and/or providers as to risk-related decisions. Use of such a tool may help patients and health providers, including nurses, to reconcile their views of risk and give patients the power to influence decisions.

Family is often involved in matters of risk related to the older adult, but has often been absent in the study of risk (Kilian et al., 2008). In some instances, family assumes the primary responsibility for speaking to risk in managing the older adult's care. Tensions can arise when perceptions of risk differ between families and patients, such as George's decision to discontinue his exercise program at home. Kilian et al. (2008) found polarized views on fall risk in their study of older adults and their adult children, with older adults not acknowledging risk, in contrast to their adult children's perceptions of risk. Adult children used a variety of strategies to deal with perceived risk, including standing back to allow the parent to make the decisions, sharing the decision making, and secretly acting behind the parent's back. Conversely, other evidence suggests the tendency for families with a cognitively impaired older adult to cover potential risk and to give the appearance of normalcy (Adams, 2001). It is important for nurses to assess the families'/caregivers' perceptions of risk and their resources and preferred strategies as a basis for planning approaches, such as the shared decision making that occurred pre-operatively involving George, Mary, and the physicians.

Nurses must be sensitive to families' needs for information and support and access their expertise of the older adult. Families have important collateral information to add to assessment data in managing risk; Mary may have provided insight and knowledge about George's pain denial. Davis (2013) encourages health care providers to listen to the patient and the family as their most readily available resource; to treat them with respect, caring, and compassion; and to give them voice by including them as equal partners when developing policies and practices. Programs such as Safer Health Care Now! and Patients for Patient Safety Control, led by the Canadian Patient Safety Institute (CPSI), have developed under the umbrella of the World Health Organization to support organizations to improve patient safety and to allow patients and families to share their voices (McIver & Wyndham, 2013). Health care organizations are beginning to recognize the patient voice as an untapped resource for contributing to safety directives to prevent adverse events and promote a culture of learning rather than blame (CPSI, 2012; McIver & Wyndham, 2013).

Health care practice has historically been based on a culture of risk avoidance, reduction, and management. This risk-averse approach is often driven by accepted societal values; organizational policy; and concerns about legal liabilities and moral, ethical, and professional obligations to protect safety, with limited resources allocated to support risk taking (Moats & Doble, 2006). Risk avoidance and removal have been critiqued for ignoring the older adults' needs and values that contribute to QOL (Clarke et al., 2006). Yet, increasingly, the shift to patient- and family-centered care has prompted greater attention to promoting the patient's autonomy and right to live at risk. While the rhetoric is to support the patient's decision, many contextual realities are often at play that may take the decision making away from the patient. For example, decreasing readmission to the hospital is a priority of policy makers, yet moving patients through the system may outweigh decisions that put the older adult at risk. One such contextual reality is pay-for-performance models that have emerged in developed nations to reward physicians, hospitals, medical groups, and other health care providers for meeting certain quality and efficiency performance measures (Boyd, Ritchie, Tipton, Studenski, & Wieland, 2008). Nurses often experience tensions between their obligations to patients/families, the interprofessional team, and their organizations. Nurses caring for George experienced this system pressure; they knew he was not ready for discharge during his first hospitalization but felt powerless to prevent it. Health care providers need to adopt a true philosophy of interprofessional practice where differences are addressed in an equitable rather than hierarchical manner, with no profession having trumping rights over another. A unified and coordinated approach had the potential to achieve better outcomes for George and his family, including reducing his risk of readmission.

Role and Cultural Considerations

Culture is central to the meaning risk has for older adults and families; nurses must take account of this in their assessments (Clarke et al., 2006; Siaki, Loescher, & Trego, 2012). Nurses are well positioned to address risks specific to older adults, but may underestimate risks because of an acute care culture that fails to value the specialized nature of caring for this heterogeneous population. In this culture, the important educative and consultant role of the APN is to build capacity in the acute care nurses' gerontological expertise that allows them to better contextualize risk. A greater understanding of available resources, including the roles of APNs, may support decision making with complex cases such as George's (MacDonald-Rencz & Bard, 2010). The importance of generalist and APNs collaborating across and within care sectors is vital to reduce risk for this vulnerable population.

Strategies for Decreasing Risk

1. Poor judgments about risks (or underestimating risks) related to the patient's desire to remain independent should be avoided; therefore:
   - Assess mental strategies, emotions, values, and past experiences in influencing risk appraisal.
   - Use interactive assessment and support tools to gather risk data.
   - Adapt activities to allow for safe risk engagement, thus supporting patients' beliefs and values related to progress.
   - Give control in risk decision making.
   - Use available resources to balance risks with abilities.

2. Withholding information about the patient's risks relates to a desire to appear normal; therefore:
   - Assess for a pattern of downplaying risks such as saying that all is fine or diverting attention away from risks.
   - Understand the purpose of passing about risks for the older adult.
   - Support use of abilities and strengths to address the fear of losing them.
   - Gain collateral information from the family to address gaps in information the patient may have missed.
   - Communicate with him or her about risk in language he will understand.

Clinical Reasoning Questions

1. What are some of George's risk factors associated with this hospitalization?
2. What would you include in George's patient-specific care plan?
3. What is your plan for follow-up with George as he transitions from hospital to home?

References

Adams, T. (2001). The social construction of risk by community psychiatric nurses and family carers for people with dementia. *Health, Risk & Society, 3*(3), 307–319.

Bestsennyy, O., Kibasi, T., & Richardson, B. (2013). *Understanding patients' needs and risk: A key to a better NHS.* Retrieved from http://www.mckinsey.com/~/media/mckinsey%20offices/united%20kingdom/pdfs/understanding%20patients%20needs%20and%20risk%20%20a%20key%20to%20a%20better%20nhsfinal.ashx

Boyd, C. M., Ritchie, C. S., Tipton, E. F., Studenski, S. A., & Wieland, D. (2008). From bedside to bench: Summary from the American Geriatrics Society/National Institute on Aging Research Conference and Multiple Morbidity in Older Adults. *Aging Clinical & Experimental Research, 20*(3), 181–188.

Campbell, F. K. (2009). *Contours of ableism: The production of disability and abledness.* New York, NY: Palgrave Macmillan.

Canadian Patient Safety Institute. (2012). *Safer health care now*. Retrieved from http://www.saferhealthcarenow.ca/EN/Pages/default.aspx

Clarke, C. L., & Members of the International Collaborative Research Network on Risk and Ageing Populations. (2006). Risk and ageing populations: Practice development research through an international research network. *International Journal of Older People Nursing, 1*, 169–176.

Davis, D. (2013). Vance's gift. In S. McIver & R. Wyndham (Eds.), *After the error: Speaking out about patient safety to save lives* (pp. 155–162). Toronto, ON, Canada: ECW Press.

Denscombe, M. (1993). Personal health and the social psychology of risk taking. *Health Education Research, 8*(4), 505–517.

Department of Health. (2007). *Independence, choice and risk: A guide to best practice in supported decision making*. Retrieved from www.dh.gov.uk/publications

Edwards, A., Elwyn, G., Covey, J., Matthews, E., & Pill, R. (2001). Presenting risk information: A review of the effects of framing and other manipulations on patient outcomes. *Journal of Health Communication: International Perspectives, 6*(1), 61–82.

Faulkner, A. (2012). *The right to take risks: Service user's view of risk in adult social care*. Retrieved from www.jrf.org.uk

Finucane, M. L., & Holup, J. L. (2006). Risk as value: Combining affect and analysis in risk judgments. *Journal of Risk Research, 9*(2), 141–164.

Furedi, F. (2011). *Changing societal attitudes, and regulatory responses, to risk-taking in adult care*. Retrieved from www.jrf.org.uk

Government of Canada. (2006). *Strategic risk communications framework*. Retrieved from http://www.riskcommunications.gc.ca

Groves, P. S., Finfgeld-Connett, D., & Wakefield, B. J. (2012). It's always something: Hospital nurses managing risk. *Clinical Nursing Research*. Advance online publication. doi:10.1177/1054773812468755

Hunt, M. R., & Ells, C. (2011). Partners towards autonomy: Risky choices and relational autonomy in rehabilitation care. *Disability and Rehabilitation, 33*(11), 961–967.

Kilian, C., Salmoni, A., Ward-Griffin, C., & Kloseck, M. (2008). Perceiving falls within a family context: A focused ethnographic approach. *Canadian Journal on Aging, 27*(4), 331–345.

Leary, K. (1999). Passing, posing, and "keeping it real." *Constellations, 6*, 85–96.

Loewenstein, G. F., Weber, E. U., Hsee, C. K., & Welch, N. (2001). Risk as feelings. *Psychological Bulletin, 127*(2), 267–286.

Lupton, D. (2013). *Risk* (2nd ed.). London, England: Routledge.

MacCourt, P., & Tuokko, H. (2010). Marginal competence, risk assessment and care decisions: A comparison of values of health care professionals and older adults. *Canadian Journal of Aging, 29*(2), 173–183.

MacDonald-Rencz, S., & Bard, R. (2010). The role for advanced practice nursing in Canada [Special issue]. *Nursing Leadership, 23*, 8–11.

McIver, S., & Wyndham, R. (2013). *After the error: Speaking out about patient safety to save lives*. Toronto, ON, Canada: ECW Press.

Mehta, K. M., Pierluissi, E., Boscardin, W. J., Kirby, K. A., Walter, L. C., Chren, M. M., . . . Landefeld, C. S. (2011). A clinical index to stratify hospitalized older adults according to risk for new-onset disability. *Journal of the American Geriatric Society, 59*(7), 1206–1216.

Moats, G., & Doble, S. (2006). Discharge planning with older adults: Toward a negotiated model of decision-making. *Canadian Journal of Occupational Therapy, 73*(5), 303–311.

Morden, A., Jinks, C., & Ong, B. N. (2012). Rethinking "risk" and self-management for chronic illness. *Social Theory & Health, 10*(1), 78–99.

Powell, J., Wahidan, A., & Zinn, J. (2007). Understanding risk and old age in Western society. *International Journal of Sociology and Social Policy, 27*(1/2), 65–76.

Rockwood, K., & Mitnitski, A. (2011). Frailty defined by deficit accumulation and geriatric medicine defined by frailty. *Clinics in Geriatric Medicine, 27*, 17–26.

Rush, K. L., Murphy, M. A., & Kozak, J. (2012). A photovoice study of older adults' conceptualizations of risk. *Journal of Aging Studies, 26*, 448–458.

Siaki, L. A., Loescher, L. J., & Trego, L. L. (2012). Synthesis strategy: Building a culturally sensitive mid-range theory of risk perception using literary, quantitative, and qualitative methods. *Journal of Advanced Nursing, 69*(3), 726–737.

Slade, A., Fear, J., & Tennant, A. (2006). Identifying patients at risk of nursing home admission: The Leeds Elderly Assessment Dependency Screening tool (LEADS). *BMC Health Services Research, 6*(31), 1–9.

Visschers, V. H. M., Meertens, R. M., Passchier, W. F., & DeVries, N. K. (2007). How does the general public evaluate risk information? The impact of associations with other risks. *Risk Analysis, 27*(3), 715–727.

Volpato, S., Onder, G., Cavalieri, M., Guerra, G., Sioulis, F., Maraldi, C., . . . Italian Group of Pharmacoepidemiology in the Elderly Study. (2007). Characteristics of nondisabled older patients developing new disability associated with medical illnesses and hospitalization. *Journal of General Internal Medicine, 22*, 668–674.

Waring, A. (2000). Constructive risk in the care of the older adult: A concept analysis. *British Journal of Nursing, 9*(14), 916–924.

Zinn, J. O. (2005). The biographical approach: A better way to understand behaviour in health and illness. *Health, Risk & Society, 7*(1), 1–9.

8 SEXUALITY

MEREDITH WALLACE KAZER

Subjective

"It seems that every time my husband and I make love, I come down with one of these infections. Can't you make it stop?"

Objective

Mrs. Hedda Hyde is an 85-year-old woman who lives at home with her husband, Matthew. She was admitted to the home care service after a brief hospital stay, where she had been admitted for a severe urinary tract infection (UTI). As she reported at the beginning of this chapter, this was not her first UTI. But the others were managed at home with antibiotics once symptoms began. This time, she was in the hospital for 3 days on intravenous (IV) antibiotics. She was discharged the day before her first follow-up home care visit by a nurse practitioner.

Upon physical examination, Mrs. Hyde appears alert and oriented and ambulates independently. She is 60 in. (152 cm) in height, and weighs 110 lbs. (50 kg). Her blood pressure is 122/74; her pulse is 80, respirations 16/minute. She is afebrile with a temperature of 98. Her oxygen saturation is 95%. Her lungs are clear bilaterally with no adventitious sounds and good expansion. Her cardiac exam reveals a regular heart rate, S1, S2, and no adventitious sounds. Her abdomen is soft, nontender, and her bowel sounds are present in all four quadrants. Her skin is warm, dry, thin, and intact, and her eye examination reveals clear sclera bilaterally and pupils equal, round, reactive to light and accommodation (PERRLA). Her ear examination reveals normal tympanic membranes with slightly reduced hearing bilaterally. Her oral examination reveals normal, moist, pink mucosa with adequate dentition. Neurological exam reveals 2+ deep tendon reflexes bilaterally and equal strength bilaterally. Her current medications include Metoprolol 25 mg po qd, Lipitor 20 mg by mouth every day, and she is on her second day of a 10-day prescription of Bactrim.

In following up with the patient's chief complaint, the nurse practitioner questioned Mrs. Hyde further on how her sexual life with her husband has changed over the years. Mrs. Hyde replied that the problems began when she went through menopause about 30 years ago and are just getting worse. She reported that the hot flashes bothered her a little bit, and she found herself tired and cranky all the time. However, her mother had warned her about this and she was not too surprised by these symptoms that marked her passage to older womanhood. She and Matt had always had what she regarded as a "good sex life." However, she would be fooling herself if she did not acknowledge the ups and downs they had. When their children were younger, Mrs. Hyde shared that sex was the last thing on her mind and that this was a source of constant argument between the two of them. Also, when her husband had an accident at work in his 60s, it was too painful for him to have sex for about a month.

Despite their continued desire for each other, Mrs. Hyde reported that she did not respond to her husband's touch with much lubrication anymore. When he tried to penetrate her during intercourse, she was very dry and in obvious discomfort. Mrs. Hyde reported that she could hardly stand the pain and could not wait until it was over, and then she almost always ended up with one of these infections. At this point, she thought it would be best to avoid intimacy with her husband.

Literature Review

While it is commonly believed that older adults decrease or limit sexual activity as they age, the literature published since the Masters and Johnson study (1966) indicates that the opposite is true. In a well-powered cohort study of 3,005 older adults, regular sexual activity was assessed in 73% of individuals aged 57 to 64, 53% of those aged 65 to 74, and 26% of research participants aged 75 to 84 (Lindau et al., 2007). More recently, Trompeter, Bettencourt, and Barrett-O'Connor (2012) discovered in their study of 806 older women that 50% of participants with a mean age of 67 described sexual activity within the last month. These research studies support that sexuality is a continuing human need throughout the life span.

Sexuality is defined as "a central aspect of being human throughout life and encompasses sex, gender identities and roles, sexual orientation, eroticism, pleasure, intimacy and reproduction" (World Health Organization, 2006). However, in a population with increasing health problems (Fiest, Currie, Williams, & Wang, 2011), older adults may experience a variety of challenges in fulfilling their sexual needs and desires (Derogatis & Burnett, 2008). Sexual health may be promoted through nursing interventions provided by generalist and advanced practice nurses that will promote quality of life (QOL) among older adults (Gianotten, Whipple, & Owens, 2006).

As a result of menopause, women experience a significant reduction in estrogen that may impact sexual health and function (Berman, 2005). Estrogen in women results in significant sexual changes. Most important, estrogen is responsible for maintaining the integrity and lubrication of the walls of the vagina. As estrogen decreases, the vaginal walls become thinner, and women experience decreased or delayed vaginal lubrication, or dryness, in response to sexual stimulation. Research reveals that many women experience vaginal dryness during and after "going through the change" (McNicoll, 2008). During sexual intercourse, the vaginal walls that are thinner and not protected by rich lubricants may tear, which may lead to pain during intercourse. Some bleeding may also be seen as a result of small tears in the vagina. The tears in the vagina, along with an increase in the pH level associated with decreased estrogen, put older women at high risk for vaginal infections and UTIs as a result of intercourse (Berman, 2005).

Other sexual changes that occur as women age result in changes to the female anatomy. In older women, the vagina shortens, and the cervix may descend into the vagina. During sexual intercourse, the penis may be more likely to come in contact with the walls of the shortened vagina and the lower cervix. Thus, penetration, with or without the presence of vaginal lubrication, may cause further pain and discomfort. Research has also shown that vaginal contractions are fewer and weaker during orgasm in older women after menopause. After sexual intercourse is completed, older women are more likely to return to the prearoused stage faster than they would at an earlier age.

As a result of the normal age-related changes that older women experience as part of the aging process, aging women may experience some changes in sexual health and function. Health care providers rarely ask about these changes during routine or illness-related health assessments. What often happens is that women (and their partners) suffer in silence (Wallace, 2000, 2003). The pain resulting from anatomical changes and vaginal dryness often causes women to avoid sexual intercourse in order to prevent painful intercourse. The decline in vaginal lubrication may cause partners to assume that the women are no longer sexually interested.

Despite the documented barriers to sexual health among older adults, there are ways in which to counteract some of the normal aging changes that occur. First and most importantly, women should take the time to understand these changes and how this will make them look and feel. Health care providers must also understand these changes. If women are comfortable doing so, an appointment may be scheduled to discuss sexual health issues and strategies for improvement.

There are a number of treatments available for the most common symptoms of vaginal dryness (Berman, 2005). Topical estrogen is available by prescription only. The product works by replacing some of the estrogen that is reduced as a result of menopause. It works to relieve the vaginal dryness symptoms through application directly into the vagina. Consequently, these treatments do not put as much estrogen into the system as oral estrogen hormone therapy.

There are three ways in which the topical estrogen can be applied, and women who are interested may choose the method that works best for them: (1) The vaginal estrogen ring is a soft, flexible ring that is inserted directly into the vagina by a health care provider. Once inserted, the ring releases a steady emission of estrogen directly to the vaginal wall. Health care providers replace the ring every 3 months to facilitate a constant stream of estrogen into the vagina. (2) Women may also administer vaginal estrogen tablets directly in the vagina themselves using a disposable applicator (similar to the way tampons are inserted). Once treatment is started, the tablet is inserted daily for 2 weeks, then twice a week. (3) Finally, women may also choose to use a vaginal estrogen cream instead of a tablet. The cream is administered via an applicator (similar to the tablet and/or a tampon), and is usually inserted once a day for the first week or two and then according to package instructions thereafter.

It is important to note that any type of estrogen product may result in adverse effects, such as vaginal bleeding and breast pain. Moreover, while topical estrogen may be a great solution to relieve vaginal dryness in some women, it is not recommended for women with a history of breast cancer, endometrial cancer, or dysfunctional vaginal bleeding of unknown origin (Simon, 2011). Unfortunately, there is not a great deal of research on the long-term effects of topical estrogen. However, at this point, most health care providers believe they are a safe and effective treatment for vaginal dryness.

In addition to topical estrogen available by prescription only, there are a number of over-the-counter products that may be helpful in lubricating the vagina. Water-based lubricants (such as K-Y) are available in tubes and via gel caps that can be inserted by hand or applicator into the vagina. Lubricants can also be applied directly to the male penis for added lubrication. This process may increase arousal of both partners. Older women are advised to avoid using douches and taking frequent bubble baths, as they may increase vaginal dryness. Many scented soaps and lotions also contain alcohol, which will worsen dryness, and so should not be used on sensitive vaginal tissues.

Many older adults lack knowledge regarding normal changes of aging that impact sexuality. A study by Baumgartner et al. (2008) revealed the need for increased sexual information and education among a sample of 81 community-dwelling older adults. If women feel pain or experience vaginal or urinary bleeding, itching, odor, or discharge after sexual intercourse, they should always contact their health care provider, as these are symptoms of infection. If antibiotics are prescribed, they should be taken as ordered and the entire dose completed to prevent reinfection.

In order to prevent UTIs from recurring chronically, a few simple steps may be helpful. First, women should always urinate immediately after intercourse, which will help flush away any bacteria that surround the urinary meatus. Women should be taught to wipe from front to back to prevent the spread of any organisms from the anal or vaginal area toward the urinary meatus. Patients should be instructed to make sure to empty the bladder completely. Substituting cotton underwear for synthetic fibers, drinking plenty of water, and adding cranberry supplements may also be helpful in the case of patients like Mrs. Hyde with chronic UTIs.

While it is Mrs. Hyde's inclination to stop sexual intercourse because of the pain, one of the most important preventive measures older adults can take to reduce the impact of normal aging changes on sexual health is to continue to engage in sexual activity. The old adage, "use it or lose it," is true when it comes to sex. Despite the normal aging changes to impact couples, continuing sexual relations will actually help to reduce the impact of these changes on overall sexual health and functioning.

The key to true intimacy in any relationship is communication. Women should talk to their partners about changes they have experienced and how they feel about them. This is often a difficult task, but sharing personal information is important to building strength. Despite the best efforts of menopause to deter vaginal lubrication, the more aroused a woman is, the greater the chance she will produce vaginal lubrication. The lubrication may need some assistance from topical estrogens or over-the-counter products. However, there is no harm in creating a mood in which sexual arousal results.

Planning for more time during sexual activities, being sensitive to changes in one another's bodies, and using aids to increase stimulation and lubrication, as well as the exploration of foreplay, masturbation, sensual touch, and different sexual positions, along with education about these common changes associated with sex and aging, may help immensely. By doing so, changes in sexual response patterns are less likely to occur. Eating healthy foods, getting adequate amounts of sleep, exercising, stress-management techniques, and not smoking are also very important to sexual health.

While there are no treatments for the anatomical changes that occur to women during the sexual process, some sexual positions may be more comfortable than others. Sexual partners are encouraged to engage in some experimentation to determine which positions are most comfortable.

Role and Cultural Considerations

Most nurses are not provided with an adequate amount of education on the changing health needs of older adults, how to assess these needs, and strategies for improving the sexual health and QOL of older adults. More education is needed, and nurses at both generalist and advanced practice levels must understand the importance of sexual health among older adults and conduct effective sexual health assessments. Standardized tools, such as the Geriatric Sexuality Inventory (Kazer, Grossman, Kerins, Kris, & Tocchi, 2013), may be effective in promoting sexuality assessments and provide a framework for integrating strategies to promote sexual health.

Despite the persistent sexual health needs of older adults, not all older adults will be comfortable discussing sexuality. Cultural norms and values must also be considered when addressing sensitive sexual health issues. In the case of Mrs. Hyde, she and her husband practiced the Roman Catholic religion, which supports that sexuality is part of a marital relationship for procreation only. While time spent among other religious cultures may have resulted in a certain level of acculturation that may influence their beliefs, they may not be comfortable discussing continuing sexual practice that is not consistent with their belief system. It is important to approach discussions of sexuality, especially the risk of sexually transmitted diseases and need for protection, sensitively.

Solutions and Strategies

In order to treat Ms. Hyde, the nurse practitioner will implement the following plan:

- Vaginal dryness related to postmenopausal changes
  - Prescribe and teach use of topical estrogen application
  - Suggest water-based lubricants (such as K-Y)

1. Chronic UTI
   - Provide teaching regarding early signs/symptoms of infection
   - Provide teaching regarding postcoital hygiene
   - Encourage good diet to maintain nutritional and hydration status
   - Consider cranberry supplements as necessary
   - Prescribe antibiotics as necessary to prevent/treat UTI
2. Sexual dysfunction secondary to pain during intercourse and risk of UTIs
   - Encourage continued sexual health and activity, assuring patients of the safety and health benefits of a good sex life.
   - Encourage good communication with partner
   - Consider referral to couples' therapist as needed
   - Provide teaching on increasing time for sexual activity and alternatives to sexual intercourse
   - Provide teaching on and lifestyle choices

Clinical Reasoning Questions

1. What is your plan for follow-up care of Mrs. Hyde?
2. Are any referrals needed in this case? If so, to whom?
3. What if Mrs. Hyde was also diabetic, hypertensive, or depressed?
4. Are there any standardized guidelines that you could use to assess or treat Mrs. Hyde?

References

Baumgartner, M. K., Hermanns, T., Cohen, A., Schmid, D. M., Seifert, B., Sulser, T., & Strebel, R. T. (2008). Patients' knowledge about risk factors for erectile dysfunction is poor. *Journal of Sexual Medicine, 5*(10), 2399–2404.

Berman, J. R. (2005). Physiology of female sexual function and dysfunction. *International Journal for Impotence Research, 17*, S44–S51.

Derogatis, L. R., & Burnett, A. L. (2008). The epidemiology of sexual dysfunctions. *Journal of Sexual Medicine, 5*(2), 289–300.

Fiest, K. M., Currie, S. R., Williams, J. V., & Wang, J. (2011). Chronic conditions and major depression in community-dwelling older adults. *Journal of Affective Disorders, 131*(1–3), 172–178.

Gianotten, W., Whipple, B., & Owens, A. (2006). Sexual activity is a cornerstone of quality of life: An update of "the health benefits of sexual expression." In M. Tepper & A. F. Owens (Eds.), *Sexual health: Vol 1 psychological foundations* (pp. 128–142). Westport, CT: Prager.

Kazer, M. W., Grossman, S. G., Kerins, G., Kris, A., & Tocchi, C. (2013). Validity and reliability of the geriatric sexuality inventory. *Journal of Gerontological Nursing, 39*(11), 38–45.

Lindau, S. T., Schumm, L. P., Laumann, E. O., Levinson, W., O'Muircheartaigh, C. A., & Waite, L. J. (2007). A study of sexuality and health among older adults in the United States. *The New England Journal of Medicine, 357*, 762–764.

Masters, W. H., & Johnson, V. E. (1966). *Human sexual response.* Boston, MA: Little & Brown.

McNicoll, L. (2008). Issues of sexuality in the elderly. *Geriatrics for the Practice Physician, 91*(10), 321–322.

Simon, J. A. (2011). Identifying and treating sexual dysfunction in postmenopausal women: The role of estrogen: Identifying and treating sexual dysfunction. *Journal of Women's Health, 20*, 1453–1466.

Trompeter, S. E., Bettencourt, R., & Barrett-O'Connor, E. (2012). Sexual activity and satisfaction in healthy community-dwelling older women. *The American Journal of Medicine, 125*(1), 137–143.

Wallace, M. (2000). Sexuality and intimacy. In *Textbook of gerontological nursing* (2nd ed., pp. 217–231). St. Louis, MO: Mosby Year Book.

Wallace, M. (2003). Sexuality in long term care. *Annals of Long Term Care, 11*(2), 53–59.

World Health Organization. (2006). *Defining sexual health: Report of a technical consultation on sexual health, 28–31 January 2002.* Geneva, Switzerland: Author.

II

CARE DELIVERY THAT ENHANCES QUALITY OF LIFE

MEREDITH WALLACE KAZER

As individuals age, a number of normal and pathological processes may impact the ability to live independently. Illness, decline in functional status, the loss of a spouse or significant other, and changes in economic status caused by death of the family provider or retirement are all reasons why an older adult may need to make changes to his or her current environment. Older adults reside in a variety of environments of care. The majority of older adults remain at home throughout life, with or without assistance from family or external caregivers. The Administration on Aging (2013) reports that approximately half of older women aged 75 and over live alone. In addition, the report states that roughly 28% (12.1 million) of noninstitutionalized older adults also live alone (8.4 million women, 3.7 million men).

While older adults prefer to stay in their homes, many older adults also transition to more supportive living environments including senior housing, nursing homes, assisted living communities, or continuing care retirement communities. Regardless of the reason an older adult changes environments or where they reside, relocation is a significant life event that has a strong influence on overall quality of life (QOL). Thus, attention to various issues that occur across care settings is essential in order to promote the highest possible QOL for all older adults.

This middle section of the book is devoted to an exploration of issues that occur across care settings. The cases illustrated reveal the experiences of older adults at home and in assisted living and nursing home environments. The chapters provide background on the problems that may occur and, in many cases, strategies to prevent the problems from occurring.

Through an exploration of the cases and the supporting literature, nurses will increase their understanding of issues that extend across environments of care and can be proactive in assessment and management. The cases in this section cover a broad breadth and depth of issues impacting older adults. Using the case study framework, nurses will develop enhanced clinical knowledge regarding the impact of these care issues on the QOL of older adults.

This section of the book is organized around 15 chapters that focus attention on a number of environmental issues that impact the QOL of older adults. Chapter 9 explores the case of an older man who had worked hard all his life as a farmer. Now, plagued with numerous medical conditions, he struggles with how to find activities that are meaningful in his life. Through the review of literature, Dr. Coyle explores the concept of occupational balance among older adults and provides strategies to keep patients engaged in meaningful activity throughout the life span. In Chapter 10, Dr. Quell explores the impact of animals on the QOL of older adults. She illustrates the evolving body of literature that supports the roles of pets and animals in maintaining QOL and suggests essential interventions to involve animals in planning care for older adults across care environments.

In Chapter 11 the purpose of life for an older adult man is considered. Amid a life of work, caring for family, and meaningful activity, entering a nursing home provides a number of challenges to one's purpose in life. Relevant exploration of the literature into the purpose of older adulthood is provided in this chapter. The solution to finding purposeful activity may be found in the philosophy of "questing," in which aspirations may be modified and activities provided to explore new, purposeful ambitions. The ability to express oneself in nursing home environments is explored in the next chapter of this book. In Chapter 12, Drs. Ramió and Rodríguez challenge caregivers to find ways to facilitate individualism amid institutional climates. Chapter 13 continues to explore the pursuit of individualism in institutional environments as Cooney and O'Shea write about "Keeping Me."

The next chapters of this book explore the complex issues of social isolation, social stigma, staffing patterns, nurse–physician communication, and elder abuse among older adults. Chapter 14 addresses issues of social isolation among older adults. In this chapter, Lovanio and O'Neil-Meyers present an emotional case of isolation and provide strategies and solutions for addressing this issue to improve QOL. Social stigma has been a longstanding issue that impacts the care of older adults across care settings, especially among cognitively impaired older adults. In Chapter 15, Ford and co-authors present current literature and solutions to combat stigma for this population. In Chapter 16, Dr. Kris explores the impact of staffing patterns on the QOL of older adults and provides compelling suggestions for ideal staffing to promote QOL. Similarly, Chapter 17 addresses the impact of poor nurse–physician communication. Authors Yamauchi and Mostone show how improved communication can improve quality of care and consequently quality of life. In Chapter 18, O'Tuathail presents the care of an older adult who was abused. This devastating, yet far too common issue is addressed through the current literature, and strategies for prevention and early detection are provided.

As the section continues, readers are drawn to the home environment, where the majority of older adults continue to reside. In Chapter 19, Bartlett and Carroll present the case of a socially isolated older adult living at home. The authors use the literature and their clinical experiences to provide solutions to connecting community-dwelling older adults with others. In Chapter 20, Hunter takes us back to residential care and the specific challenges caregivers experience in building relationships with cognitively impaired older adults. Gannon continues to explore these challenges in Chapter 21, in which suggestions and strategies are provided to enhance resident–resident relationships in institutional care environments. Ryan expands this work in Chapter 22, where she writes about promoting family connections among nursing home residents and their significant others. In the final chapter of the section, Doyle, Hunter, and White present their original and compelling research, completed with 70 family caregivers, on family caregiving.

The many case studies and evidence-based literature reviews contained within this section expand the discussion of care environment issues substantially. The authors of these chapters use clinical experience and sources to enhance understanding of issues that impact the QOL of older adults. The solutions and strategies contained herein are, in many cases, easily implementable and can significantly impact care for older adults and their families. Each chapter presents a unique care environment issue and uses the case study approach to broaden understanding of nurses and, consequently, promote QOL for older adults.

Reference

Administration on Aging. (2013). *Profile of older Americans.* Washington, DC: Author. Retrieved from http://www.aoa.gov/Aging_Statistics/Profile/2013/docs/2013_Profile.pdf

9 THERAPEUTIC ACTIVITY

Ann Coyle

Subjective

"I can't hold the newspaper together with one hand; parts of it fall on the floor, and the nurse needs to pick it up, but they don't have the time."

Objective

Mr. Isaac Inisfree is a farmer, a keen conversationalist, and a devout Catholic. He came to live in a long-term care facility following a stroke that resulted in a right-sided hemiplegia. Prior to this, he had lived on his own, following the death of his wife. Although he would have preferred to live with his brother following his stroke, he understood that, because he was a large heavy man, his brother would be unable to lift him.

Mr. Inisfree can decide when he wants to get up in the morning, although he says it takes him a bit of time to "come to life" and that the staff are "always in a hurry." He gets up most days, and after his personal care routine, he is taken to the day room, where he sits in front of the television and watches "whatever comes on." He likes to read the newspaper, but finds it difficult to hold or turn the pages due to his hemiplegia. For this reason, he does not read as often as he would like. He makes no objection to this and states that he just "goes with the flow" as a means of coping with communal living.

As a farmer, he was used to working hard and is frustrated by his current lack of activity. After he retired from farming, he continued to grow vegetables, and he retains an interest in agriculture. He enjoys talking to people and having the opportunity to discuss how much life has changed since he was young. Although he considers himself lucky to be well looked after physically, he would like it if the staff had more time to engage in conversation with him. Mr. Inisfree spends long periods of time sitting alone or sleeping in the dayroom. He occasionally joins in the scheduled activities, although he states that music, bingo, and art are not for him. He usually goes back to bed in the afternoon or early evening as he finds sitting for long periods of time uncomfortable. Here he spends a lot of time in prayer. He shares a room with another resident and complains about the constant noise from the television when he is trying to pray. His favorite time of the day is evening when "everything calms down."

Mr. Inisfree is an 80-year-old man who has lived in a long-term care setting for 2 years. He was admitted directly from an acute care setting following a right-sided cerebral vascular accident. He also has been diagnosed as having hypertension, right-sided carotid stenosis, and chronic obstructive pulmonary disease. Mr. Inisfree weighs 306 lbs. (106 kg), his BP is 140/70, his pulse is 72, respirations 20/minute. His oxygen saturation levels are 96%.

Mr. Inisfree requires assistance with all activities of daily living. He is unable to walk or move independently, has poor sitting balance, and requires frequent repositioning while in bed. He is incontinent of bladder and bowel and requires the assistance of two people and a full hoist for transfers to his wheelchair, bed, toilet, and shower. He has a mild oropharyngeal dysphagia with a delayed swallow and has been assessed as requiring thickened fluids and a soft diet. He has had repeated chest infections and ongoing problems with skin integrity and constipation. He complains of a poor sleep pattern, for which he is given seroxat at night.

Mr. Inisfree has been assessed for meaningful activity using the Pool Activity Level (PAL) profile, and has been identified as being able to engage in activity at an exploratory level. This means he can engage in familiar tasks in familiar settings and carry out more complex tasks if they are broken down into two to three steps. Using this assessment, a profile of activities was drawn up and included in this care plan. These include reading the paper, exercise/games, eating/drinking, parties, talking about farming, visits by his brother, and religious worship.

Literature Review

Being engaged in some kind of meaningful activity has been identified as important to older people, as is continuing to make a contribution to society and feeling valued as a result (Gabriel & Bowling, 2004). Having opportunities to engage in activity and having a sense of purpose are seen to contribute to the well-being of older people in long-term care settings (Brooker, 2003; Edvardsson, Petersson, Sjogren, Lindkvist, & Sandman, 2014; Nolan, Davies, & Brown, 2006).

Meaningful activity represents interaction between a person and his or her context. The concept of social interaction connects the ideas of meaningful activity and participation together, as it is through the involvement in meaningful activity and occupation that people come together and get involved with other people (Townsend & Wilcock, 2004). Different tasks and activities mean different things to different people, and occupational patterns vary across cultures and communities and the life course (Katz, Holland, Peace, & Taylor, 2011).

The literature has repeatedly shown that levels of social interaction and social activity in residential care settings are low despite evidence of the impact of such inactivity on the self-esteem of residents (Ice, 2002; Mattiasson & Andersson 1997; Nolan, Grant, & Nolan, 1995; Ward, Vass, Aggarwal, Garfield, & Cybyk, 2008). Thomas (2004) suggests that boredom, alongside helplessness and loneliness, rather than ill-health or disability, represent the real scourges of long-term care.

Occupational balance is a concept that describes how an individual balances the need to be engaged in meaningful and productive activity against needs for rest and recreation. This balance is subjectively defined and determined on the basis of an individual's values and obligations. As a concept, it is usually identified with the "all work and no play" idea, where the balance between productivity and leisure is out of kilter. There is a vast literature on the psychological aspects of occupational imbalance and associated patterns of ill-health such as burnout or other stress-related illnesses. The corollary is where the need to be productive or to engage in self-care activity is curtailed or lost through disability or frailty. Occupational loss occurs where people can no longer participate in normal routines and activities as determined through their normal lifetime routines. Losing occupations of choice can lead to emotional distress, depression, and loss of self-identity and self-efficacy (Lou, Chi, Kwan, & Leung, 2013; Polatajko, Townsend, & Craik, 2007; Van Beek, Frijters, Wagner, Groenewegen, & Ribbe, 2011).

The idea of incorporating meaningful activity into everyday life rather than relying on separate scheduled "activities" to counteract boredom and occupational loss has been proposed (Bowers et al., 2011; Edvardsson et al., 2014). The concept of normalization, a term in the disability literature (Race, 2003), connects residents in long-term care settings to meaningful activity through continuing with their previous routines and lifelong habits. This has resulted in the development of domestic-style environments and strategies to move from "care environments"—where residents are passive recipients of services—to ones that promote the development of "home" and "community," based on mutually supportive relationships and more involvement in the decisions about everyday life (Brown Wilson 2009; Edvardsson, Fetherstonhaugh, & Nay, 2010; Edvardsson et al., 2014; Shields & Norton, 2006; Shura, Siders, & Dannefer, 2011).

There is a growing body of evidence supporting the development of domestic-style environments as a means of counteracting the dominance of biomedicine in residential care and as a means of improving social engagement (Kane, Lum, Cutler, Degenholtz, & Tzy-Chyi, 2007; Molony, Evans, Jeon, Rabig, & Straka, 2011; Morgan-Brown, Newton, & Ormerod, 2013; te Boekhorst, Depla, de Lange, Pot, & Eefsting, 2009). However, it has been acknowledged that environmental reconstruction on its own is insufficient to change decision-making systems and routines that prioritize organizational goals of efficiency and clinical governance (Fox, 2007; Jenkens, Sult, Lessell, Hammer, & Ortigara, 2011; Rosemond, Hanson, Ennett, Schenck, & Weiner, 2012). In a recent Irish study, Morgan-Brown et al. (2013) compared the social engagement and interactive occupation of residents with dementia in two Irish nursing homes before and after an intervention to create a household (domestic-style) model of care. The intervention involved staff development, leadership support, and the creation of a "homemaker role," whereby one staff member incorporated housekeeping duties in the communal area, which now had an open plan kitchen, encouraging residents to become involved in domestic roles and activities. The study reported that residents were more socially engaged to a statistically significant level following the intervention.

In a study involving 1,266 residents of long-term care settings who had dementia, Edvardsson et al. (2014) found that only 18% of residents participated in everyday activities such as making coffee, setting or clearing tables, cleaning, or watering plants. They also found that those who participated in these activities lived in more person-centered units. The authors point to the many opportunities that exist within everyday life to engage with residents and support the maintenance of their identity through the engagement in personally meaningful activities.

Strategies for Changing Practice

Lack of time and competing organizational demands have been identified as reasons why staff do not prioritize meaningful activity (McCormack et al., 2010). Many facilities employ activity coordinators who develop schedules of social and recreational programs. While such activities can be enjoyable and stimulating, they often represent only a small portion of the day, and these usually group-based activities cannot meet the needs or wishes of all residents, given their heterogeneity and diverse interests and functional capacity.

An important strategy is to understand the occupational desires of each individual resident, the level of engagement that he or she wishes to have, and to plan accordingly. Given the environmental cues of biomedicine and patienthood that exist in many long-term care settings, this requires the use of facilitation skills to see beyond passivity resignation and loss of self-esteem in order to elicit what is truly important to each individual resident (McCormack & McCance, 2010).

Mr. Inisfree has stated that his most pleasurable activity is engaging in conversations; however, this does not happen as often as he would like as staff are busy moving from resident to resident providing personal and biomedical care. Instead, he sits in the day room, where he states he has little interaction with his fellow residents.

The reconstruction of living environments whereby staff are present and undertaking domestic duties while engaging with residents at the same time as identified in the Morgan-Brown et al. (2013) study suggests the development of more flexible routines whereby programs of activities become less defined, and normal activity and daily rhythms of domestic life take over. This requires a greater flexibility of roles within appropriate professional scope of practice. In an evaluation of frontline practices in Green Houses (small domestic-scale communities of older people) in the United States, Sharkey, Hudak, James, Horn, and Howes (2010) found that staff spent more time engaging directly with residents than in traditional long-term care facilities. Through reshaping roles to incorporate household duties such as meal preparation and laundry alongside personal care and activities, the certified nursing assistants provided consistent and more participative support for residents. Within such models, the need for separate activity coordinators declines as staff and residents begin to live together.

Edvardsson, Fetherstonhaugh, and Nay (2010) propose that promoting a continuation of self and normality and providing meaningful activity are important to people with dementia. They highlight the need to actively translate knowledge about likes and dislikes into real activity, prompting participation and increased self-esteem. Blood and Bamford (2010) and Katz, Holland, Peace, and Taylor (2011) suggest that individuals value the opportunity to make small contributions to communal life, such as setting the table or tending a section of garden.

Seeking out activities that engender a sense of purpose and contribution could enhance Mr. Inisfree's well-being. His lifelong expert knowledge of food production through farming could be channelled into kitchen garden work alongside other residents and staff who have less knowledge but physical capacity to follow his directions.

Connecting such activity to real sustenance of the community as opposed to simulated "activity" would make this more real; however, this might require cooperation with local food safety personnel to overcome regulatory barriers.

Supporting Mr. Inisfree to pursue his interest in farming and current affairs requires a rethinking of how he can read the newspaper. In its existing format, he is unable to turn the pages, and he is concerned about bothering the staff to pick it up should it fall.

Conclusion

The engagement of residents in meaningful activity as a way of improving social interaction and participation can support a sense of purpose and well-being. While competing organizational demands can work against the social interaction between residents and staff, emerging evidence suggests that involving residents in everyday tasks that align with their previous routines, occupational roles, and values may result in improved quality of life.

Clinical Reasoning Questions

1. How could the existing routines of your long-term facility be adapted to create more opportunities for participation by residents?
2. How can the rhythms of the day reflect the goals of residents rather than purely biomedical and organizational goals?

References

Blood, I., & Bamford, S.-M. (2010). *Equality and diversity and older people with high support needs.* York, England: Joseph Rowntree Foundation.

Bowers, H., Mordey, M., Runnicles, D., Barker, S., Thomas, N., Wilkins, A., . . . Catley, A. (2011). *Not a one-way street: Research into older people's experiences of support based on mutuality and reciprocity*. York, England: Joseph Rowntree Foundation.

Brooker, D. (2003). What is person-centered care in dementia? *Reviews in Clinical Gerontology, 13*, 215–222.

Brown Wilson, C. (2009). Developing community in care homes through a relationship-centered approach. *Health and Social Care in the Community, 17,* 177–186.

Edvardsson, D., Fetherstonhaugh, D., & Nay, R. (2010). Promoting a continuation of self and normality: Person-centered care as described by people with dementia, their family members and aged care staff. *Journal of Clinical Nursing, 19,* 2611–2618.

Edvardsson, D., Petersson, L., Sjogren, K., Lindkvist, M., & Sandman, P. O. (2014). Everyday activities for people with dementia in residential aged care: Associations with person-centeredness and quality of life. *International Journal of Older People Nursing, 9*(4), 269–276.

Fox, N. (2007). *The journey of a lifetime: Leadership pathways to culture change in long term care.* Milwaukee, WI: Action Pact.

Gabriel, Z., & Bowling, A. (2004). Quality of life from the perspectives of older people. *Aging and Society, 24,* 675–691.

Ice, G. H. (2002). Daily life in a nursing home. *Journal of Aging Studies, 16,* 345–359.

Jenkens, R., Sult, T., Lessell, N., Hammer, D., & Ortigara, A. (2011). Financial implications of THE GREEN HOUSE® Model. *Seniors Housing & Care Journal, 19,* 3–22.

Kane, R. A., Lum, T. Y., Cutler, L. J., Degenholtz, H. B., & Tzy-Chyi, Y. (2007). Resident outcomes in small-house nursing homes: A longitudinal evaluation of the initial green house program. *Journal of the American Geriatrics Society, 55,* 832–839.

Katz, J., Holland, C., Peace, S., & Taylor, E. (2011). *A better life: What older people with high support needs value.* York, England: Joseph Roundtree Foundation.

Lou, V. W. Q., Chi, I., Kwan, C. W., & Leung, A. Y. M. (2013). Trajectories of social engagement and depressive symptoms among long-term care facility residents in Hong Kong. *Age and Aging, 42,* 215–222.

Mattiasson, A. C., & Andersson, L. (1997). Quality of nursing home care assessed by competent nursing home patients. *Journal of Advanced Nursing, 26,* 1117–1124.

McCormack, B., Dewing, J., Breslin, L., Tobin, C., Manning, M., Coyne-Nevin, A., . . . Peelo-Kilroe, L. (2010). *Implementation of a model of person centered practice in older persons settings* (Final report). Dublin, Ireland: National Council for the Continuing Professional Development of Nursing and Midwifery and Health Service Executive.

McCormack, B., & McCance, T. (2010). *Person centered nursing theory and practice*. Oxford, England: Wiley-Blackwell.

Molony, S. L., Evans, L. K., Jeon, S., Rabig, J., & Straka, L. A. (2011). Trajectories of at-homeness and health in usual care and small house nursing homes. *Gerontologist, 51*, 504–515.

Morgan-Brown, M., Newton, R., & Ormerod, M. (2013). Engaging life in two Irish nursing home units for people with dementia: Quantitative comparisons before and after implementing household environments. *Aging & Mental Health, 17*, 57–65.

Nolan, M., Davies, S., & Brown, J. (2006). Transitions in care homes: Towards relationship-centered care using the "senses framework." *Quality in Aging and Older Adults, 7*, 5–14.

Nolan, M., Grant, G., & Nolan, J. (1995). Busy doing nothing: Activity and interaction levels amongst differing populations of elderly patients. *Journal of Advanced Nursing, 22*, 528–538.

Polatajko, H. J., Townsend, E. A., & Craik, J. (2007). Canadian model of occupational performance and engagement (CMOP-E). In E. A. Townsend & H. J. Polatajko (Eds.), *Enabling occupation II: Advancing an occupational therapy vision of health, well-being & justice through occupation* (pp. 22–36). Ottawa, ON, Canada: CAOT Publications ACE.

Race, D. (2003). *Leadership and change in human services: Selected readings from Wolf Wolfensberger*. New York, NY: Routledge.

Rosemond, C. A., Hanson, L. C., Ennett, S. T., Schenck, A. P., & Weiner, B. J. (2012). Implementing person-centered care in nursing homes. *Health Care Management Review, 37*, 257–266.

Sharkey, S. S., Hudak, S., Horn, S. D., James, B., & Howes, J. (2011). Frontline caregiver daily practices: A comparison study of traditional nursing homes and The Green House Project sites. *Journal of the American Geriatrics Society, 59*, 126–131.

Shields, S., & Norton, L. (2006). *In pursuit of the sunbeam: A practical guide to transformation from Institution to Household*. Manhattan, Kansas: Manhattan Retirement Foundation.

Shura, R., Siders, R. A., & Dannefer, D. (2011). Culture change in long-term care: Participatory action research and the role of the resident. *The Gerontologist, 51*, 212–225.

te Boekhorst, S., Depla, M. F. I. A., de Lange, J., Pot, A. M., & Eefsting, J. A. (2009). The effects of group living homes on older people with dementia: A comparison with traditional nursing home care. *International Journal of Geriatric Psychiatry, 24*, 970–978.

Thomas, W. H. (2004). *What are old people for? How elders will save the world.* Missouri, TX: VanderWyk & Burnham.

Townsend, E., & Wilcock, A. A. (2004). Occupational justice and client-centered practice: A dialogue in progress. *Canadian Journal of Occupational Therapy, 71*, 75–87.

Van Beek, A. P. A., Frijters, D. H. M., Wagner, C., Groenewegen, P. P., & Ribbe, M. W. (2011). Social engagement and depressive symptoms of elderly residents with dementia: A cross-sectional study of 37 long-term care units. *International Psychogeriatrics, 23*, 625–633.

Ward, R., Vass, A., Aggarwal, N., Garfield, C., & Cybyk, B. (2008). A different story: Exploring patterns of communication in residential dementia care. *Aging & Society, 28*, 629–651.

10 ANIMAL-ASSISTED CARE

THERESA TAVELLA QUELL

Subjective

"Cosmo and I are doing just fine—no need to worry about us."

Objective

Mrs. Jane Jenkins, a 75-year-old thin, pale, Caucasian female, presented with complaints of dizziness, balance problems, and systolic blood pressure over 200. She has a history of dementia, and her daughter states that she is having difficulty living independently. The daughter reports that her mother has been living alone, will not leave her house, and it appears that the home has not been cleaned in months. The patient forgets to take her medications, refuses to take a shower, and is sometimes incontinent of urine. Her past medical history includes hypertension, hyperlipidemia, right carotid aortic stenosis, ataxia, hearing impairment with one hearing aid, and transient ischemic attacks.

Although Mrs. Jenkins reports that she has been widowed for 1 year, records indicate that her husband died 6 years ago. She lives alone, is financially self-supporting, but has been having trouble paying bills in a timely manner. She has little food in the refrigerator, often forgets to eat, says she mainly eats cereal and frozen dinners, and refuses meals on wheels. She has a 6-year-old cat, Cosmo, who lives inside the home; the cat is well fed and well groomed, although the litter box area is not well cleaned. Mrs. Jenkins is college educated and taught elementary art until her retirement 11 years ago. She used to volunteer at her church until about 8 months ago when she began having trouble with her balance and tired frequently during the day. The patient states that she does not smoke, drink, or use drugs, although her daughter reports a history of alcohol abuse and frequent falls since the patient's husband died. Visiting nurse services report that the patient does not use her cane, sleeps most of the day, and has significant problems with ADLs. Her daughter, Cynthia, is the only child. Mrs. Jenkins has a 90-year-old sister, who recently moved to a new assisted living facility.

Mrs. Jenkins is alert and awake without agitation, pleasant, friendly, and cooperative throughout her exam. Her hair has not been combed, and her clothing appears to be at least one size too big for her. Although appropriately oriented to month, date, and year, she misstated her age by 4 years. The patient had significant problems copying a simple clock design and was unable to depict the prespecified time setting accurately. Her thought process is disorganized, with poor insight and impaired judgment. Her vital signs are T 98.2°F, P 89, RR 18, BP 180/64, height 5 feet 6 in. (168 cm), weight 128 lbs. (58 kg). She has no known allergies, and her medications include amlodipine, aspirin, calcium with vitamin D, candesartan, carvedilol, omeprazole, and simvastatin (Zocor).

One week after Mrs. Jenkins's evaluation, her daughter arrives at her mother's home and finds Mrs. Jenkins on the floor in the bathroom. She is disoriented, has a bump on her forehead, and says her leg hurts and she cannot stand up. After calling the ambulance and spending the afternoon in the ED, Mrs. Jenkins is diagnosed with a urinary tract infection (UTI) and admitted for further evaluation. The following morning, after feeding Cosmo, Cynthia goes to visit her aunt at the assisted-care facility where Jane's sister now lives. She asks about the possibility of an opening for her mom, and learns that a unit will be available in about 3 weeks.

Cynthia gets to the hospital and finds her mother arguing with Amanda, the PCT, about taking a shower. Amanda promises a nice surprise after she finishes getting washed up. Emerging from the bathroom with a clean nightgown and combed hair, but a frown on her face, Mrs. Jenkins gets back into bed as a woman with a calico kitten enters the room.

"Here is your surprise visitor, Mrs. Jenkins!" Mrs. Jenkins immediately smiles and claps her hands together as the pet therapist steps forward with the cat. Mrs. Jenkins reaches out her hands, and the kitten hops upon the bed and snuggles into her lap.

Literature Review

The human–animal bond has been studied for many decades. Animals are a part of our lives from the time we are children, whether the family cared for a fish, guinea pig, gerbil, or cat. Those without a family pet may have grown up enjoying the company of a friend's dog, or taken pleasure in a visit to the zoo. On the continuum of health to illness, animals can be instrumental in offering comfort, decreasing stress, or providing assistance for activities of daily living. For an older adult like Mrs. Jenkins, an animal such as her cat, Cosmo, could provide company, decrease isolation, and assist in providing cues for a number of activities of daily living (ADL), including toileting, eating, and household cleaning.

Loss of a spouse, a declining pool of friends, or distance from families can leave a deficit in the life of an older adult that can lead to loneliness, depression, and solitude (Krause-Parello, 2008; Vladeck, 2005). Older adults may become withdrawn and distance themselves from family and friends as they lose supportive individuals around them. Providing opportunities to interact with or care for an animal may lead to opportunities to increase socialization and provide comfort.

Especially for those who live alone, having a pet can provide companionship, elevate mood, and increase socialization (Prosser, Townsend, & Staiger, 2008). McColgan and Schofield (2007) conducted a pilot project that explored the relationships between older adults and their dogs. Conversational interviews were conducted with three men and three women, ages 22 to 70, who lived alone with dogs. Results indicated that the participants considered their dogs to be family members that were just as important as other people. The animals served as companions and confidants, and provided emotional support.

Krause-Parello (2008) studied 159 older women living independently with a cat or dog in a housing community. Participants completed three surveys measuring loneliness, general health, and pet attachment. Results supported a positive relationship between pet attachment and loneliness, indicating that pet attachment support could serve as a coping mechanism for loneliness (Krause-Parello, 2008). Pets can also be used to decrease pain and anxiety in some patients. Engleman (2013) conducted a study of 19 patients who met with a psychologist and her therapy dog to assist with pain management. Findings, based on patient self-reports and staff observations, indicated that patients reported a decrease in pain symptoms, distraction from pain symptoms, and relaxation that decreased discomfort after interacting with the therapy dog.

Understanding of the human–animal relationship is found around the world. In a study conducted in seven aged care rest homes in northern Italy, 144 cognitively intact older adults were randomly given a canary, a plant, or nothing. Participants were observed for 3 months to assess whether a pet therapy program had a favorable effect on quality of life (QOL). Results indicated no significant differences in the control groups, while participants caring for a canary had statistically significant improvement in all areas including depressive symptoms, anxiety, and mood (Columbo, Buono, Smania, Raviola, & De Leo, 2006).

In Japan, the 2000 Act on Welfare and Management of Animals recognized that animals—especially cats and dogs—could increase QOL (Kumasaka, Masu, Kataoka, & Numao, 2012). Twenty patients on a palliative care unit of an acute care hospital were given the opportunity to interact with a trained animal for 30 minutes. Using the Loris face scale, the mood of each subject was evaluated before and after the animal interaction. Results indicated that all subjects experienced an increased mood, with almost no difference in gender. Higher "joyfulness" was found in participants who were interested or had pets in the past, as well as those who felt that animals were like family members (Kumasaka et al., 2012). Each of these studies has implications for Mrs. Jenkins, who lives with her cat. While her relationship with her pet needs to be explored, it appears that the animal is a well-cared-for companion. With her current social isolation, Cosmo may be her most significant existing relationship aside from her daughter.

While the benefits of companion animals have clearly been demonstrated in the literature, some challenges must be considered for older adults in the decision to keep or acquire a pet.

In 2010, the Federal Interagency Forum on Aging-Related Statistics reported that 37% of women and 19% of men lived alone (Federal Interagency Forum on Aging-Related Statistics, 2012). The agency projects that by the year 2030, the U.S. population over age 65 will grow to 72 million, or 20% of the American population. Given the number of older adults living alone over age 65, some seniors will experience the loss of one or more pets.

This loss can occur when an older adult moves to another setting where pets are not welcome. In this instance, the individual not only gives up his or her residence, but may also have to leave a pet behind. As the circle of friends and family grows smaller, the loss of a beloved pet can be devastating (Durkin, 2009; Walsh, 2009). Whether the pet dies, or is separated from its owner, practitioners need to have empathy for the adult who has lost yet another member that may considered part of the family. Sometimes, finances become an issue when the cost of feeding and caring for a pet becomes a burden. In the case of Mrs. Jenkins, she has been able to provide and care for her pet as long as her daughter helps with shopping for food and litter. However, one of the reasons she refuses to move in with her daughter is her daughter's allergy to cats. Since Mrs. Jenkins's sister happily resides in a new assisted living community, it will be worth exploring whether the establishment allows pets.

Another concern is the care of pets when seniors are displaced, such as during admission to a hospital or rehabilitation facility. A hospitalized patient worrying about a hungry pet may experience additional stress that can be detrimental to both physical and mental health. Further, an older adult may be reluctant to move into a retirement community or senior housing facility if his or her animal companions are not allowed to live there as well (Krause-Parello, 2008). As the number of older adults continues to climb, retirement and assisted living communities will become increasingly important in optimizing independence, maintaining health, and providing socialization (Brandon & Flury, 2009). This could have important implications for the kind of community support needed to enable older people to keep their companion animals with them either at home or in supported living accommodation.

Caring for a pet, much like caring for another family member, can provide an opportunity for physical activity, offer cues to eat meals, and supply a source of entertainment and companionship. While service animals, protected by the American Disabilities Act, provide assistance with owners who have physical and emotional disabilities, therapy animals work with professionals and clients to improve health and well-being (Horowitz, 2010; Uyemura, 2011).

Substantial research may be found in the literature that supports the health benefits of animal-assisted therapy in a variety of settings (Cangelosi & Sorrell, 2010; Horowitz, 2010). In a study of 30 inpatients with schizophrenia in Taiwan, researchers reported that animal-assisted activities improved self-esteem and emotional symptoms, and increased physical activity when patients began to play with the dogs (Chu, Liu, Sun, & Lin, 2009). A therapist might talk about the animal's needs for exercise, hygiene, and nutrition, using this as a topic starter for patient self-care (Uyemura, 2011). For a patient like Mrs. Jenkins, who does not like to take a shower, discussing her pet's hygiene can be a way to help her recognize the need for regular bathing.

Animals have been used with positive results in psychiatric, critical care, hospice, and outpatient settings with patients of all age groups. Health care providers need to recognize that, for many older adults, pets can support and enhance QOL. Risley-Curtiss (2010) surveyed 5,012 members of the National Association of Social Workers to investigate knowledge of animal–human relations, inclusion of animals in patient assessments, and history of education regarding animals in social work practice. Results indicated that 97.8% of the participants were familiar with the positive impact of animals on adults, yet only 23.2% asked questions about pets as part of their patient assessments (Risley-Curtiss, 2010). It is critical that health care providers recognize the important role that pets play in the lives of older adults, and provide assistance in nurturing these valuable relationships.

Role and Cultural Considerations

- While animals can be sources of great comfort and happiness, some cultures believe that animals do not belong inside the home and/or in a location serving food; these individuals may be resistant to working with therapy animals.
- Although many individuals treat animals as members of their family, not all individuals feel this way, and may not understand the human–animal bond.
- The loss of a companion animal can be a source of grief that is not well understood by those who have not experienced a strong bond with an animal.

Solutions and Strategies

In working with Mrs. Jenkins, the nurse practitioner will implement the following plan to increase opportunities for exercise, optimize independence, and cue ADLs, using Mrs. Jenkins's pet cat Cosmo.

1. Housing
   - Explore options for pet-friendly assisted living facilities, including the facility where Mrs. Jenkins's sister lives.
2. Meals and medications
   - Have meals delivered to the home while exploring assisted living arrangements.
   - Have medications prepoured for Mrs. Jenkins.
   - Provide cues for Mrs. Jenkins to eat and take her medications when she feeds her cat each morning and evening.
3. Exercise and bathing
   - Create a daily calendar indicating days when Mrs. Jenkins will brush her cat to help her stay clean. Use this exercise to cue Mrs. Jenkins to take a shower after she brushes her cat.

- Set up a schedule for Mrs. Jenkins to play with her cat each day after lunch, increasing the likelihood of her getting at least a minimal amount of exercise.
- Provide a home care aid every other morning to assist with cues to maintain ADLs.

4. Incontinence
   - Mrs. Jenkins says she checks the litter box after each meal and before bed to keep the bathroom clean. Since the litter box is in the bathroom, this activity can be used as a cue to remind Mrs. Jenkins to use the toilet and decrease incidents of incontinence.
5. Social isolation
   - Connect Mrs. Jenkins with other individuals who enjoy pets.
   - Encourage Mrs. Jenkins to attend pet therapy sessions each Thursday and Sunday morning at her sister's assisted care facility.

Clinical Reasoning Questions

1. What changes in behavior do you expect to see in Mrs. Jenkins 1 week after implementing these strategies?
2. Reflect on the frustration of Mrs. Jenkins's daughter. Brainstorm ways to include her in the plan of care.
3. Identify opportunities for Mrs. Jenkins to interact with other older adults who enjoy pets.
4. Consider challenges that Mrs. Jenkins will face if she is unable to find a pet-friendly assisted care facility.
5. Discuss ways to maintain a safe home environment for Mrs. Jenkins until she can be relocated to an assisted living facility.

References

Brandon, B., & Flury, E. (2009). Aging with choice: Coping with a changing marketplace: The inexorable pressure to keep seniors home can present opportunities, not just threats. *Long-Term Living: For the Continuing Care Professional, 58*(1), 14–18.

Cangelosi, P. R., & Sorrell, J. M. (2010). Walking for therapy with man's best friend. *Journal of Psychosocial Nursing, 48*(3), 19–22.

Chu, C. I., Liu, C. Y., Sun, C. T., & Lin, J. (2009). The effect of animal-assisted activity on inpatients with schizophrenia. *Journal of Psychosocial Nursing and Mental Health Services, 47*(12), 42–48.

Columbo, G., Buono, M. D., Smania, K., Raviola, R., & De Leo, D. (2006). Pet therapy and institutionalized elderly: A study on 144 cognitively unimpaired subjects. *Archives of Gerontology and Geriatrics, 42*, 207–216.

Durkin, A. (2009). Loss of a companion animal. *Journal of Psychosocial Nursing and Mental Health Services, 47*, 26–31.

Engleman, S. R. (2013). Palliative care and use of animal-assisted therapy. *OMEGA: Journal of Death and Dying, 67*(1–2), 63–67.

Federal Interagency Forum on Aging-Related Statistics. (2012). *Older Americans 2012: Key indicators of well-being*. Washington, DC: U.S. Government Printing Office.

Horowitz, S. (2010). Animal assisted therapy for inpatients. *Alternative and Complementary Therapies, 16*(6), 339–343.

Krause-Parello, C. A. (2008). The mediating effect of pet attachment support between loneliness and general health in older females living in the community. *Journal of Community Health Nursing, 25*(1), 1–14.

Kumasaka, T., Masu, H., Kataoka, M., & Numao, A. (2012). Changes in patient mood through animal-assisted activities in a palliative care unit. *International Medical Journal, 19*(4), 373–377.

McColgan, G., & Schofield, I. (2007). The importance of companion animal relationships in the lives of older people. *Nursing Older People, 19*(1), 21–23.

Prosser, L., Townsend, M., & Staiger, P. (2008). Older people's relationships with companion animals: A pilot study. *Nursing Older People, 20*(3), 29–32.

Quell, T. T. (2012). Opportunities and challenges of growing old. In J. W. Lange (Ed.), *The nurse's role in promoting optimal health of older adults: Thriving in the wisdom years* (pp. 54-74). Philadelphia, PA: F.A. Davis.

Risley-Curtiss, C. (2010). Social work practitioners and the human-companion animal bond: A national study. *Social Work, 55*(1), 38–46.

Uyemura, B. (2011). The truth about animal-assisted therapy. *PsychCentral*. Retrieved from http://psychcentral.com/lib/2011/the-truth-about-animal-assisted-therapy

Vladeck, B. C. (2005). Economic and policy implications of improving longevity. *Journal of the American Geriatric Society, 53*(9), 304–307.

Walsh, F. (2009). Human-animal bonds II: The role of pets in family systems and family therapy. *Family Process, 48*(4), 481–499.

11 PURPOSEFUL ACTIVITY

GLENDA COOK AND JULIANA THOMPSON

Subjective

"It's all just so pointless. This is just an existence, not a life. I want my life to continue to have meaning, and for what I do to be worthwhile."

Objective

Mr. Kevin Kavanagh is an 82-year-old man who was moved to a nursing home 4 weeks ago after spending 2 months in the hospital, where he had been admitted after suffering a right hemispheric cerebrovascular accident. As a result, Mr. Kavanagh has left-sided hemiparesis, which has led to impaired mobility (he requires the aid of a walking stick to mobilize over short distances, and a wheelchair for longer distances), impaired ability to grasp objects with his left hand, decrease in movement precision, and poor coordination. Mr. Kavanagh's condition is further complicated by the onset of poststroke vascular dementia. This has resulted in short-term memory loss, episodes of confusion, occasional difficulties in verbalizing needs (he has some word-finding difficulty that has improved since the stroke), poor concentration, and visual orientation problems. A Geriatric Depression Scale assessment is indicative of depression. In addition, he reports that he is irritable and has occasional episodes of aggression.

Mr. Kavanagh has never been married and has no children. His next of kin is his nephew David, who is able to visit only once a month. However, during the first week of Mr. Kavanagh's relocation to the nursing home, David stayed in the vicinity to support his uncle with the move, his finances, and the closure of his home.

During this period, the staff were able to gather information from Mr. Kavanagh and his nephew about his life and interests. They ascertained that Mr. Kavanagh had been a cook in the army until his retirement. During his army years, he had generated an impressive collection of army memorabilia, of which he was very proud. After retiring, he had moved to a small rural village. He continued to enjoy cooking, and had acquired an allotment so he could grow, then cook, his own food. He enjoyed DIY projects and was very proficient at house maintenance. Friends and neighbors were always consulting him regarding their own property difficulties. Mr. Kavanagh took a keen interest in current affairs, and listened to the news on the radio every day. He enjoyed discussing the day's news events with Mr. Todd next door. Since retiring, Mr. Kavanagh had developed a passion for field sports, and had obtained permission of a local farmer to shoot rabbits on the farm every Saturday.

Since his move, the staff have noticed that Mr. Kavanagh is withdrawn. He is reluctant to engage with the other residents, and after attending one organized music event, he has refused to participate in any further events. The staff have acquired a radio for him, but he appears to have little interest in it. Mr. Kavanagh has told the staff on a number of occasions that he is frustrated and angry with his situation. He says that he is "existing, not living," and he feels that nothing about his life seems worthwhile.

Literature Review

Quality of life (QOL) and life meaning are significant influences on psychological and social well-being and physical health. Life meaning has been defined as "making sense" of and "having a point" to existence and, characteristically, involves engagement in purposeful activity because such activity contributes to this "sense making" (Eakman, 2013). Purposeful activity is composed of an expanse of subjective experiences. Ludwig, Hattjar, Russell, and Winston (2007) have proposed that it includes social experiences, such as participating in social interactions, and supporting and caring for others. In addition, Eakman, Carlson, and Clark (2010) have suggested that purposeful activities are actions that personally motivate us, such as engaging in interests and activities, having control, succeeding at tasks, and progressing toward valued goals. In the case of Mr. Kavanagh, for example, before his stroke he enjoyed a number of hobbies, and delighted in socializing and helping friends and neighbors. These activities gave a sense of purpose and meaning to his life.

However, after suffering a stroke, Mr. Kavanagh was unable to manage in his own home and moved into a nursing home. As a result of his disability, as well as the move, he could no longer participate in these activities. Indeed, many reports and studies highlight how older care home residents, when deprived of purposeful activity, can experience long and empty days that are devoid of meaning (Cook, 2007; Mozley, 2001; Nolan, Grant, & Nolan, 1995). This has driven the promotion of meaningful activity in the context of service provision for older care home residents.

Older people living in nursing homes have a vision for a good life in long-term care that includes being supported in the pursuit of purposeful activities that fulfill life's meaning (Bowers et al., 2009). Indeed, studies that have explored the QOL of residents have concluded that participation in purposeful activity has significant positive implications for well-being. For example, residents with dementia in Phinney, Chaudhury, and O'Connor's (2007) research reported that "doing" activities, and connecting with others, led to feelings of enjoyment and happiness, and a sense of belonging. Residents in Cook and Stanley's (2009) study recounted how participating in "meaningful activity" contributed to their "lived" QOL by supporting their sense of identity, biography, and autonomy. These studies highlighted that residents often struggle to achieve purposeful activity without the support of care home staff.

So what constitutes purposeful activity within the nursing home environment? It may include solo or group activities, and it may be active or sedentary. In other words, purposeful activity could comprise any type of activity. Bergland and Kirkevold's (2006) study found that what makes purposeful activity distinctive is that it is person-specific, rather than one-size-fits-all.

It is based upon individual residents' preferences and choices, and it provides stimulation and pleasure for the participant.

Government policies and care standards acknowledge the importance of purposeful activity to QOL (e.g., Australian Aged Care Quality Agency, 2014; Great Britain Department of Health, 2003; Medizinischer Dienst der Krankenversicherung, 2014; UK Care Quality Commission, 2013; U.S. Department of Health and Human Services, 2013). As such, these policies offer directives and guidelines that promote nursing home residents' choice, self-determination, and opportunities for stimulation through the provision of appropriate activities. For example, the Great Britain Department of Health's (2003) *Care Homes Regulations: National Minimum Standards—Care Home Regulations* requires that, at an absolute minimum, each establishment should facilitate activities "in and outside the home," and cater to individuals' preferences. These regulations also state that individuals' cognitive, sensory, and physical impairments should not be a barrier to the availability and accessibility of preferred activities (standard 12, p. 15).

Although the importance of purposeful activity to QOL is widely recognized, a significant proportion of residents' activities in nursing homes are passive. Observational studies of residents' occupational patterns have revealed that less than a third of activities constitute purposeful activity, while two thirds are comprised of nonactive, nonengaged behaviors (Morgan-Brown et al., 2011; Nolan, Grant, & Nolan, 1995; Wood, Womack, & Hooper, 2009). For example, the study by Morgan-Brown et al. (2011) of two nursing homes providing services for people with dementia found that only 23.75% of residents' time was spent engaged in interactive or social occupations. For the majority of the time (76.25%), residents were nonengaged (sleeping, sitting in front of the television, waiting, doing nothing, receiving care).

Interactive and social occupations that are supported in nursing homes are generally formal and organized by staff. Eyers, Arber, Luff, Young, and Ellmers' (2012) study of the role of organized activity in nursing homes found that activities are usually staff-led rather than resident-led, and depend upon availability of an activities coordinator. As such, residents may be unable to pursue activities during evenings and weekends, when the activities coordinator is absent from the home. The study also reported that organized activities tend to be of short duration, are group based rather than individually tailored, and are restricted to hobby-like pastimes involving music, games, or arts and crafts. Resident participants indicated that they viewed the organized activities on offer as "bland, almost childish and often inappropriate" (p. 67). Participants also felt that activities were arranged to "fit" around the staff's routines, rather than accounting for their individual interests, preferences, and abilities.

Because of these factors, many residents' choices regarding what type of activities they would like to participate in are limited. Harper Ice (2002) and Eyers et al. (2012) have suggested that even the right to choose whether or not to attend organized activities may be denied to residents with physical and cognitive dependencies. This is because staff often "control" the mobility of such residents and, disregarding their wishes, "place" them in activity locations. Harper Ice's (2002) study found that these occurrences result in "attendance," but not necessarily "engagement." In the light of their findings, these two studies concluded that unless residents can derive meaning from formal organized activities, these activities are ineffectual and inadequate. Cooney's (2012) research, which explored residents' perspectives of "finding home" within long-term care settings, suggested that ineffectual and inadequate activities fail to provide stimulation or purposeful engagement for residents, which leads to boredom and a loss of interest in the world outside the self. The study noted that in environments where opportunities for purposeful activity are lacking, many residents demonstrate an "inward gaze" (p. 192) and become reserved and less talkative. Indeed, in the case of Mr. Kavanagh, it appears that the activities on offer in the nursing home are organized events that do not match his preferences and interests. As a result, he has disengaged from the world and feels that life has lost meaning.

Studies that have investigated the impact of workforce issues on the facilitation of purposeful activity in nursing homes have highlighted potential barriers to its implementation. For example, the nurse participants in a study conducted by Bedin, Droz-Mendelzweig, and Chappuis (2013) acknowledged that understanding what is meaningful to residents, and helping residents to formulate meaningful activity projects, is essential to promoting QOL. However, these participants felt that time and resource constraints obstructed their efforts, so that recording residents' preferences at times becomes little more than a paper exercise. They suggested that in order to be successful in their endeavors, staff must be able to influence institutional managers in order to secure the necessary human and material resources. In addition, Shin's (2013) study of staff skill mix in nursing homes found that while an increase in registered nurse hours (with less care assistant hours) led to increased resident functional ability, scores for purposeful activity decreased. Shin (2013) proposed that this indicates that nurses are more concerned with physiological matters and are less concerned with the facilitation of activities as part of their role. Yet the principles of holistic nursing care recognize that individuals are biopsychosocial functioning entities; as such, biological and biographical aspects are both significant. Less attention given to either aspect could have a detrimental impact on QOL; therefore, it could be argued that nurses do have a role in the provision of purposeful activities in the context of nursing homes.

The previous literature review reveals that there are a number of barriers to the facilitation of purposeful activity in care homes. These include:

- Lack of understanding about what defines purposeful activity, and how to resource and facilitate it effectively and efficiently.
- Uncertainty of staff regarding whose role it is to facilitate purposeful activity.
- Staff "controlling" the activities of residents whose physical, sensory, or cognitive abilities are impaired.

Role and Cultural Considerations

Most nursing home nurses have little training regarding what constitutes purposeful activity, its importance to the well-being of residents, or its facilitation. Creative expression and doing something meaningful is important for everyone, but even more important for people living in long-term care settings with chronic illness, disease, and disability for whom other avenues of self-expression can be severely limited. Cutler, Kelly, and Silver (2011), for example, argued that engaging in art forms can offer sensory and tactile pleasures. For instance, a positive focus on color, sound, and light can improve a subjective sense of well-being while enabling individuals to express their inner feelings. However, self-expression and doing something meaningful do not need to be restricted to creative arts. Residents can express themselves in everything that they do, such as making choices regarding their clothes, relationships, and interests. Nurses can play an important role in supporting residents to make and act on their decisions regarding activities, thus affirming their individuality, identity, and autonomy.

What is considered purposeful and meaningful varies from one individual to another. Nurses therefore require skills to identify what individuals consider meaningful, what they want to do, and how they want to do it. These include being able to negotiate with residents, encourage participation, effectively communicate, facilitate creative thinking, deliver purposeful activities, and support reflection on participation and what was accomplished.

Nurses and other staff bring a rich array of personal qualities to their role, from specific interests and talents for art forms to competence in outdoor activities such as gardening and animal husbandry. These personal qualities should be acknowledged and blended with professional competence to support purposeful activity when planning and interacting with residents. This can be effectively achieved through models of work-based and interprofessional learning. Such learning is both active and reflective. For example, nursing staff can continuously develop their knowledge of activities that older residents with various problems can engage with. These might include, for instance, forms of movement and dance that are enjoyable, but which also help to improve balance and gait, thus reducing the risk of falls. Alternatively, emerging technologies such as interactive IT applications enable older people to keep in touch with their social networks, and emotional robots encourage people with advanced dementia to interact with the world around them. Various activities, practices, and innovations can be implemented to determine what is relevant to the current resident population.

Nurses may also learn facilitation techniques by observing and reflecting upon the interaction between residents and visiting health, social care, and arts professionals. For example, the learner may observe how an individual with short-term-memory and word-finding problems is supported with good communication skills, including describing an activity through words/pictures/objects, breaking down the steps required for participation into small parts, and using paraphrasing and summary. The learning acquired through reflection provides insight into the skills required to facilitate a resident's engagement. Reflection also provides insight into the benefits that a creative and skilled approach may achieve, compared with practices that are focused merely on addressing biomedical needs.

As already discussed, purposeful activity must be based upon individuals' interests and preferences if it is to be meaningful. During assessment and care planning processes, it is important to discover preferred activities and continue, wherever possible, to facilitate them. However, some residents may be unable to carry on with their old pursuits because physical, sensory, or cognitive deterioration may impede their abilities, or render participation unsafe. In cases where residents are no longer able to manage old pursuits or undertake them safely, it is important that nursing staff do not "take control" of activity issues. For example, returning to the case study of Mr. Kavanagh, although his failing sensory, cognitive, and physical health does not permit engagement with his former interests, nurses should not assume attendance at a quiz or music event is an adequate or effective substitute. While this may be an alternative activity, for this individual, it may not be a purposeful activity. In these circumstances, nursing staff need to use a different approach.

Strategies for Improvement

Older residents desire to live in communities in which all their needs are met, and where they have opportunities to live a full biographical life that includes opportunities to engage in purposeful activities. How nursing home managers fulfill their leadership role is pivotal to the facilitation of a homelike, personalized culture. Managers influence the nature of daily life through the development and implementation of policy and procedures that encourage personal expression, for example, encouraging residents to maintain and sustain creative activities, helping residents to harness their capabilities to engage in purposeful creative activities, and facilitating purposeful activity by optimizing the physical environment of the home.

Implementation of procedures is possible only if staff and nonstaff resources are available to support purposeful activities. Hence, managers are responsible for ensuring that the home's budget accommodates the real cost of delivering activities by accounting for these costs in annual planning cycles. In terms of staff resources, managers must realize that staff support of purposeful activity is not just about the amount of hours dedicated to the delivery of activities at specified times during the day. Staff must be skilled facilitators ensuring that meaningful activity occurs in every aspect of daily life. This highlights the importance of developing the workforce to be competent both in the delivery of personal care, and in addressing psychosocial needs of residents with the aim of maximizing QOL.

A useful tool is Frank's (1995) "quest" approach. "Questing" is a philosophy that views changes in health and ability as a stimulus for modifying aspirations, and a chance to explore new but purposeful possibilities for future activities. The success of "questing" depends very much upon the attitudes and practices of nurses, and the integration of a "questing" strategy into the care plan. If nurses revise care objectives to include "questing," then they will be able to support residents to devise, and progress toward, achievable goals based upon modified or new interests. For example, a "questing" strategy for Mr. Kavanagh might involve exploring whether he would be interested in participating in an alternative field sport, such as fishing. This activity is still a field sport, and Mr. Kavanagh's current disability would not prohibit participation in this, or the following activities:

- Listening to the news throughout the day: Nurses and health care assistants could encourage Mr. Kavanagh to continue with this activity, and then discuss the day's news with him while assisting him to bed at night.
- Cooking: Nurses could prompt kitchen staff to include Mr. Kavanagh in menu preparation.

- Social contact: Nurses and health care assistants could support Mr. Kavanagh to use Skype to keep in touch with his nephew, neighbors, and friends.
- Working in an allotment: Nurses could ask gardeners to seek Mr. Kavanagh's advice and assistance in the nursing home's garden.
- Army memorabilia: Nurses could encourage domestic staff to arrange Mr. Kavanagh's items for display.

Often, nurses do not view the facilitation of purposeful activity to be part of their role. However, nursing home nurses must recognize that purposeful activity is crucial to the health and well-being of residents, and as such, it is a fundamental aspect of their role. Facilitating purposeful activity can have a direct impact upon an individual resident's mood, emotional health, self-esteem, and confidence. It can also support the maintenance and improvement of mobility, strength, and coordination; stimulate concentration and cognitive skills; and help to preserve and develop social skills, as well as speech and language abilities.

Once nurses acknowledge that the implementation of purposeful activity is part of their remit, it will become an essential and established element of care planning. As such, nursing staff are more likely to incorporate it into resourcing requests to management. In addition, if details of residents' preferences and interests are recorded, this information can be assimilated into the everyday work plans of other staff.

Clinical Reasoning Questions

1. Provide a detailed purposeful activity care plan for Mr. Kavanagh that incorporates a "questing" strategy.
2. How might this care plan/strategy contribute to Mr. Kavanagh's QOL?
3. How would you revise your care plan/strategy if Mr. Kavanagh's physical, sensory, or cognitive health declined further?
4. How might the nurse and activities coordinator work together to improve purposeful activity outcomes for nursing home residents?

References

Australian Aged Care Quality Agency. (2014). *Accreditation standards.* Retrieved from http://www.aacqa.gov.au/for-providers/accreditation-standards

Bedin, M. G., Droz-Mendelzweig, M., & Chappuis, M. (2013). Caring for elders: The role of registered nurses in nursing homes. *Nursing Inquiry, 20*(2), 111–120.

Bergland, Å., & Kirkevold, M. (2006). Thriving in nursing homes in Norway: Contributing aspects described by residents. *International Journal of Nursing Studies, 43*(6), 681–691.

Bowers, H., Clark, A., Crosby, G., Easterbrook, L., Macadam, A., MacDonald, R., . . . Smith, C. (2009). *Older people's vision for long-term care.* York, England: Joseph Rowntree Foundation.

Cook, G. (2007). *Life as a care home resident in later years: "Living with care" or "existing in care"* (Unpublished doctoral dissertation). Northumbria University, New Castle upon Tyne, UK.

Cook, G., & Stanley, D. (2009). Quality of life in care homes: Messages from the voices of older people. *Journal of Care Services Management, 3*(4), 391–407.

Cooney, A. (2012). "Finding home": A grounded theory on how older people "find home" in long-term care settings. *International Journal of Older People Nursing, 7*(3), 188–199.

Cutler, D., Kelly, D., & Silver, S. (2011). *Creative homes: How the arts can contribute to the quality of life in residential care.* Retrieved from http://www.baringfoundation.org.uk/CreativeCareHomes.pdf

Eakman, A. M. (2013). Relationships between meaningful activity, basic psychological needs, and meaning in life: Test of the "meaningful activity and life meaning model." *OTJR: Occupation, Participation and Health, 33*(2), 100–109.

Eakman, A. M., Carlson, M. E., & Clark, F. A. (2010). Factor structure, reliability and convergent validity of the "engagement in meaningful activities survey" for older adults. *OTJR: Occupation, Participation and Health, 30*(3), 111–121.

Eyers, I., Arber, S., Luff, R., Young, E., & Ellmers, T. (2012). Rhetoric and reality of daily life in English care homes: The role of organised activities. *International Journal of Ageing and Later Life, 7*(1), 53–78.

Frank, A. W. (1995). *The wounded storyteller: Body, illness and ethics.* Chicago, IL: University of Chicago Press.

Great Britain Department of Health. (2003). *Care homes for older people: National minimum standards—Care homes regulations.* London, England: The Stationery Office.

Harper Ice, G. (2002). Daily life in a nursing home. *Journal of Aging Studies, 16*(4), 345–359.

Ludwig, F. M., Hattjar, B., Russell, R. L., & Winston, K. (2007). How caregiving for grandchildren affects grandmothers' meaningful occupations. *Journal of Occupational Science, 15*(1), 14–51.

Medizinischer Dienst der Krankenversicherung. (2014). *MDK quality inspections of care facilities.* Retrieved from http://www.mdk.de/1328.htm

Morgan-Brown, M., Ormerod, M., Newton, R., & Manley, D. (2011). An exploration of occupation in nursing home residents with dementia. *British Journal of Occupational Therapy, 74*(5), 217–225.

Mozley, C. G. (2001). Exploring connections between occupation and mental health in care homes for older people. *Journal of Occupational Science, 8*(3), 14–19.

Nolan, M., Grant, G., & Nolan, J. (1995). Busy doing nothing: Activity and interaction levels amongst differing populations of elderly patients. *Journal of Advanced Nursing, 22*(3), 528–538.

Phinney, A., Chaudhury, H., & O'Connor, D. L. (2007). Doing as much as I can do: The meaning of activity for people with dementia. *Aging and Mental Health, 11*(4), 384–393.

Shin, J. H. (2013). Relationship between nursing staffing and quality of life in nursing homes. *Contemporary Nurse, 44*(2), 133–143.

UK Care Quality Commission. (2013). *The national standards.* Retrieved from http://www.cqc.org.uk/public/national-standards

U.S. Department of Health and Human Services. (2013). *National nursing home quality care collaborative change package.* Baltimore, MD: Author.

Wood, W., Womack, J., & Hooper, B. (2009). Dying of boredom: An exploratory case study of time use, apparent affect, and routine activity situations on two Alzheimer's special care units. *American Journal of Occupational Therapy, 63*(3), 337–350.

12 SELF-EXPRESSION

Anna Ramió Jofre and Laura Martínez Rodríguez

Subjective

"I think I would rather live well alone."

Objective

Mr. Lawrence Lorenzo is currently 95 years old. He has spent the last 5 years living in a nursing home. He lived in a rented flat in Barcelona until the age of 90. It contained a dressmaking shop he shared with another man who was 4 years younger. They came from two different towns, each 100 km from the city. They decided to open a business, and thought about the possibility that it should also be their home since they had no family nearby. They spent their lives in the workshop working many hours a day to keep going. They had a circle of friends with whom they would share Sunday dinner, trips, and walks around the city. The two got used to appreciating their independence, the respect they had for one another. When Mr. Lorenzo was 89, his flatmate had an ischemic cerebrovascular accident (CVA); he was hospitalized and died soon after. The situation for Mr. Lorenzo changed completely, and although his family (brother and sister-in-law) gave him emotional support and invited him to live with them, he decided to get on with his life in the same flat. However, he found it was impossible to transfer the rent agreement to his name, and his health and memory were deteriorating; he therefore made the decision to enter a nursing home.

Mr. Lorenzo is a quiet, calm, and cheerful person. He is slim and well-dressed. He likes talking, but he would rather listen and give advice when requested. He presents with a cataract of 5 years' duration, and although he could have had surgery, he had decided not to. He has no known drug allergies or toxic habits. His diagnoses include: (a) long-standing hypertension, in pharmacological treatment, with good control; (b) dyslipidemia in dietary treatment; and (c) mild cognitive impairment for the past 3 years due to vascular dementia. He has been followed for neurology treatment in Barcelona. His regular medications include Hidrosaluretil 50 mg, venlafaxine 150 mg, Adiro 100 mg, lormetazepam 2 mg, and omeprazole 20 mg.

Literature Review

In the 21st century, the nursing discipline faces new challenges to meet new social needs. One of these new challenges is to tackle the demand arising from the world's aging population. According to the United Nations' (UN) population data, from 2003 a quarter of the world's population was over 60 years old, and it is estimated that one in three adults is a person of advanced age (Morphi Samper, 2005).

This entails that the development and improvement of gerontological nursing must be an imperative of the nursing profession. This specialty was defined in 1981 by the American Nurses Association as the profession that encompasses the promotion and maintenance of health, prevention of disease, and self-care promotion in older adults, with the aim of restoring and achieving the maximum degree of autonomy and performance from a holistic approach, including the care of diseases and ensuring the welfare and dignity of the patient until his or her death.

Gerontological nursing is a key element in addressing community needs in terms of age. It promotes conceptual change intended to consider it as a stage of active life, in which one can achieve maximum individual autonomy and the possibility of self-realization (Belenger & Aliaga, 2000; Fillenbaum, 1984, p. 84). It is therefore necessary to consider two aspects: First, nurses must ensure the quality of life (QOL) of older people from a functional perspective, understanding that a healthy older adult is one who is able to face the change process at an appropriate level of functional adaptability and personal satisfaction. Therefore, a view that overcomes the limitations of the biomedical paradigm and a shared comprehensive and personalized plan of activities designed to meet the needs of enhancing functional autonomy of older adults are needed. On the other hand, gerontological nursing must respond to the social challenges of aging. Nurses must not act only on current problems—if the aim is to increase the level of functionality of older people, they should be able to anticipate situations that might jeopardize the preservation of welfare and QOL (Sanhueza Parra, Castro Salas, & Merino Escobar, 2005).

Currently in Spain, the care of older people is carried out either by the family or at nursing homes or residential care homes. Both geriatric nursing and community nursing establish intervention targets such as the development of programs aimed at stimulating functional autonomy, promoting and encouraging self-care as a healthy lifestyle, and promoting social and community involvement from the perspective of the active and valued older person (Sanhueza Parra, Castro Salas, & Merino Escobar, 2005).

The process of nursing care in Spain is based mainly on the conceptual model of Dr. Virginia Henderson, since this is the one that adapts best to the professional competencies of the profession in this country.

Role and Cultural Considerations

Currently, the social needs of older adults require new strategies on several levels: (a) organizational, (b) professional, and (c) caring. Regarding the organization of care and nursing homes, they are considered to provide better quality care if the training of those leading them is focused on health education, as opposed to today's prevailing biomedical model. It is important to recognize that nurses who lead other professionals are the backbone of care (Ramió, 2005). From the professional perspective, we consider that contractual stability, sufficient staff (understanding the ratios qualitatively, that is, as measured by levels of dependency of people served and not by number of users), and nurses' round-the-clock attention are directly related to the quality of care. Regarding assistance, it is advisable to generate protocols that are contextualized and agreed upon by the health teams in what refers to welcome, family visits, and risk of falls, among other examples. Personalized assistance from the very moment that the older person enters the nursing home is essential, as well as his or her follow-up in multidisciplinary clinical sessions. The quality of care has to be assessed both through qualitative and quantitative indicators whether it is perceived or carried out by users (Beltran, 2010). It is important to promote specialization in gerontology nursing to provide an adapted response to the new situation of care required by older people. As Colliere said, in the life cycle, there is a stage that corresponds to the old age, where people need to be cared for again (Colliere, 1996).

Strategies for Improvement

Of the 14 fundamental needs, we will develop only those presenting manifestations of dependency. In the *need to eat and drink,* Mr. Lorenzo follows a 1,500 kcal hypolipidemic soft diet. He tolerates it well, although some days he requests other types of food. He has little appetite, no feeling of thirst, and drinks only when reminded; his weight is 115 lbs. (115 kg); height 5 feet 8 in. (173 cm). He has lower and upper dentures, and he has lately presented problems with his prosthesis fixation, which has generated sores in his mouth. He does not present with any problem of swallowing and digestion. In the *need to eliminate bodily waste,* he presents slight urinary incontinence due to poor muscle tone of the pelvic floor secondary to the aging process, which does not cause concern; he gets up to urinate twice a night, he has a habit of regular defecation, and perspiration is minimal. In the *need to move and maintain desirable postures,* his movement is suitable for his age; some hesitation and weakness in the step is perceived when not carrying the cane. He shows some difficulty getting out of bed or chair, but does not need help. As for the *need to sleep and rest,* he has difficulty sleeping, and needs medication regularly; when he wakes up to urinate, he goes back to sleep immediately.

He sleeps about 6 hours a night, waking around 5 a.m., but is happy to remain in bed quietly until around 8 a.m. During the day, when he is sitting in front of the TV or reading, he often falls asleep. He also usually has a nap for about an hour after lunch. As for the *need to maintain body temperature within normal range,* he presents slight hypothermia secondary to aging that produces a feeling of cold that he alleviates with dress clothes. He presents slight cyanotic coloration in the most distal parts of the hands and feet with pale skin color. His hands and feet are always cold.

As for the *need to keep the body clean and well groomed* and protect the integument, it is concluded that he requires help to groom thoroughly and maintain good hygiene of the skin, nails, and hair. He is very concerned with his personal appearance, and therefore is highly motivated in taking care of his physical appearance and personal hygiene. In the *need to avoid dangers,* he shows that although he is a cautious person, he displays a certain tendency to have accidents, falls, or injuries during ambulation. These accidents are also related to hearing loss and decreased visual field due to his cataract. As for the *need to communicate with others,* he is well adapted to life in the care home; he presents the aforementioned sensory problems, caused by the aging process, as well as a slight but progressive slowdown due to the diagnosed mild dementia. On the *need to work in such a way that there is a sense of accomplishment,* Mr. Lorenzo explains his sadness at not being able to sew owing to loss of vision. There has also been a decrease in participation in daily activities in the care home. In the *need to learn,* insufficient knowledge about the evolution of dementia, drug treatment, and preventive measures for falls is observed.

Nine diagnoses must be addressed as follows: (1) imbalanced nutrition—less than body requirements; (2) risk for deficit fluid volume; (3) functional urinary incontinence; (4) bathing or hygiene self-care deficit; (5) impaired memory; (6) deficient knowledge; (7) risk for falls; (8) impaired dentition; and (9) adult failure to thrive. In the process of the secondary analysis, in which each and every one of the diagnostic labels has been used, four definitive diagnoses have been identified. These include demonstrations of dependence or defining characteristics that Mr. Lorenzo presents, which will help

TABLE 12.1: Care Plan

DIAGNOSIS	
Failure to thrive r/t* unfamiliarity with senses optimization and physical strength.	
Nursing Intervention Classification (NIC)	**Nursing Outcomes Classification (NOC)**
• Feeding • Self-care assistance: bathing/hygiene • Self-care assistance: toileting • Incipient dementia • Family process maintenance	• Appetite • Urinary continence • Memory • Self-care activities of daily living (ADL) • Social involvement
DIAGNOSIS	
Risk of falls r/t* lack of physical strength in muscles and senses; lack of knowledge secondary to mild dementia.	
NIC	**NOC**
• Exercise therapy: ambulation • Exercise therapy: balance	• Fall prevention behavior nursing

*Related to.

the staff of the care home in planning for the general goal of increasing his overall QOL. The four diagnoses are (1) adult failure to thrive, (2) risk of deficit fluid volume, (3) readiness for enhanced sleep, and (4) risk of falls (Table 12.1).

In order to achieve the criteria of the previously established results, we propose the following activities in the nursing diagnoses that Mr. Lorenzo presents. In relation to food, we explore his preferences and offer him choice among several elaborated and attractively presented meals; we also negotiate the possibility of changing his location in the dining room, depending on the guests present, so that he feels more relaxed. While he can attend to his daily hygiene, he requires help to bathe once a week. The nurse will remind him to go to the bathroom and urinate every 3 hours in order to prevent urinary incontinence. Regarding the diagnosis of incipient dementia, we started him on stimulation through music and craft activities, in his case sewing (according to his capabilities), and short walks around the care home grounds supervised by the nurses or the family, which allows us to also work on balance and ambulation exercises while maintaining family involvement.

Clinical Reasoning Questions

1. What are the issues in trying to care for Mr. Lorenzo at home?
2. Are any referrals needed in this case? If so, to whom?
3. What if Mr. Lorenzo was depressed?
4. Are there any standardized guidelines that could be used to assess Mr. Lorenzo's needs?

References

Belenger, M. V., & Aliaga, F. M. (2000). Functional autonomy and management of leisure time by the elderly. *Rol de Enfermería, 23*(3), 231–234.

Beltran, C. (2010). *Quality assistance in nursing management*. Girona, Spain: Documenta universitaria.

Colliere, F. (1996). Caring . . . Ensuring life's maintenance and continuity. *Índex de Enfermería, 18*, 9–14.

Fillenbaum, G. (1984). *The wellbeing of the elderly. Approaches to multidimensional assessment*. Geneva, Switzerland: WHO, Offset Publications.

Morfi Samper, R. (2005). The health of older people in the 21st century. *Revista CubLorenzo Enfermería, 21*(3). Ciudad de la HabLorenzo sep.-dic. Version On-line.

Organización Mundial de la Salud, OPS/OMS. (1985). *Toward the wellbeing of the elderly.* Washington, DC: EE.UU.

Ramió, A. (2005). *Values and professional attitudes: Study of nursing practice in Catalonia.* (Doctoral thesis) Barcelona, Spain: Universitat de Barcelona. Retrieved from http://hdl.handle.net/2445/43007

Sanhueza Parra, M., Castro Salas, M., & Merino Escobar, J. (2005). Older people functioning: A new concept of health. Version On-line, *Ciencia y Enfermería, 11*(2), 17–21.

Staab, A. S., & Hodges, L. C. (1997). *Gerontological nursing.* México: McGraw-Hill Interamericana.

13 KEEPING ME

ADELINE COONEY AND EAMON O'SHEA

Subjective

"I enjoy my breakfast . . . I have porridge, tea and toast, which is what I like for breakfast. I could have a fried breakfast, but I've always liked porridge for breakfast. Did you know you can even have breakfast in bed? I wouldn't like that. I like to be up and doing, I've been like that all my life. It takes me a little time to get going, I'm a bit stiff in the morning, so better to get up and get going. After breakfast I stay behind with a few others to help staff clear the tables. I like to go outside then and do a bit of gardening. I sit down on a little stool when I'm gardening because my knees aren't great. I love flowers, and when I do my garden, everybody tells me it looks lovely. My best hobby of all, though, is playing cards. Four of us play poker and rummy in the little room down the corridor there, and I really enjoy that. We're serious players; Mary (a nurse) called us 'card sharks' the other day [laughing]. *We've become friends and we look out for one another. We're always chatting, you know the usual stuff,* 'In my day . . .'*—we tell stories and have a laugh. You know what I miss? I miss going shopping. I'd love if the four of us could go together, have lunch and look around the shops. Try on a few clothes and dream* [laughs]. *I love clothes . . . I like to look well. My other thing . . . I like to have my hair nice. You can get your hair done here. I like it cut just so; I'm very fussy but they know what I like now, so it's great. I love my room here. I have it all organized the way I like. These pictures are from my home, and I brought this little table with me, and it fits in really well. It's nice to have a place of your own; sometimes you just*

want a little peace and quiet so this is my little haven. On Saturday, I like to clean my room, sweep the floor, dust, and polish. I don't have to do it, but I like to tidy it. I like to do my little bit to help. I'm very happy here; it suits me. It was a good decision to come here."

Objective

Mary Murphy, 86 years old, moved to the long-term care unit 5 years ago. Her reason for moving was inability to self-manage because of progressively worsening osteoarthritis (OA). Her knees are worst affected, and on admission she described the pain as ". . . shocking." Pain combined with stiffness and fatigue (classic symptoms of OA) impacted negatively on all aspects of her day-to-day life, including social participation. Mary explained, "I'd no life . . . I couldn't do anything. I couldn't go out . . . I was a prisoner in my own home. I just couldn't live like that anymore." Mary was diagnosed with idiopathic localized osteoarthritis (OA). Localized OA most commonly affects the hands, feet, knee, hip, and spine (Kalunian, Tugwell, & Ramirez, 2013). OA is a synovial joint disorder characterized by (a) articular cartilage loss, (b) the formation of bony spurs (osteophytes) at the joint margins, (c) synovial membrane inflammation, and (d) thickening of the subchondral bone plate and changes to the underlying trabecular bone (Swift, 2002). Mary complains of joint tenderness, stiffness (worse in the morning), and pain when mobilizing. She has difficulty walking more than 20 minutes because of pain, and her symptoms are exacerbated by kneeling or descending stairs. Functional assessment shows Mary has arthritis-related self-care deficits related to decreased range of movement; for example, she needs assistance with climbing into and out of the bath. Although sitting relieves her pain, she becomes stiff if she stays in one position too long. On observation, she walks slowly but is safe mobilizing independently with the aid of a stick. She has difficulty sitting down or standing up from low chairs and with climbing or descending steps. Mary's plan of care focuses on pain relief and maximizing function and independence. She has been prescribed an anti-inflammatory and analgesia. Appropriate adaptive equipment has been made available with the goal of maximizing her independence, for example, grab rails by the bath, a raised toilet seat, and a seat cushion to heighten the chair. In addition, she attends physiotherapy at least once a week with the goal of (a) increasing range of movement and flexibility, and (b) strengthening the hamstring and quadriceps muscle. Tight hamstrings and weak quadriceps muscles are associated with pain severity and the amount of physical disability in knee OA (Gür et al., 2002), and there is some evidence that strengthening exercises improve functioning and reduce knee pain (Iverson, 2010; Tanaka et al., 2013). To further help maintain Mary's independence, staff have strategically placed chairs and stools around the unit so she (and others) can take a rest break when moving from place to place (energy conservation); for example, a stool has been purposefully left in the garden near a raised flower bed, which makes gardening possible for Mary. On admission, Mary's osteoarthritis was found to limit her social participation. Mary's goal was to be more active and "not to be sitting moping all day." History-taking focused on finding out what activities Mary enjoys. She indicated she enjoyed gardening, playing cards, joining in the singing of songs, watching television, and going shopping. She made clear that making a contribution to the work of the facility was important to her and that she likes to be "busy." Staff have incorporated this into her plan of care; for example, they have arranged some "jobs" for her that she is able to do. To help realize her goal of being active, staff introduced her to a group of women living in the long-term care unit who enjoyed playing cards. Mary is now a member of this group and plays cards every day.

Literature Review

The number of people aged 60 years or over is expected to more than triple by 2100, increasing from 841 million in 2013 to 2 billion in 2050 and almost 3 billion in 2100 (United Nations, 2013). Those aged 80 years and over are the fastest growing population group, with numbers expected to increase almost sevenfold by 2100, increasing from 120 million in 2013 to

392 million in 2050, and to 830 million in 2100 (United Nations, 2013). The demand for long-term care increases exponentially with age, so an increase in the very old (80 years and over) will be matched by an increasing demand for long-term or alternative care options. For example, in Ireland, it is anticipated that each year 2,833 extra people will require residential or formal care at home between 2012 and 2021 (Wren et al., 2012). In contrast, in the United States, the number of people living in nursing homes has declined (Houser, 2007), but this trend should be interpreted with caution. Bernstein et al. (2003) note that in the United States, older people who might previously have moved to a nursing home now have other options such as assisted living and life care communities.

The importance of the physical and social aspects of these environments should not be underestimated. Vogel (2001) comments that it is increasingly accepted by design researchers and practitioners that identity is expressed through interior environments. Rubinstein (1990) also notes the relationship between personal identity and the surrounding environment. The Design in Caring Environments (DICE) study (Parker et al., 2004) examined the impact of the design of nursing homes on residents' quality of life (QOL). This study was carried out in 38 care homes in and around Sheffield and Rotherham in the United Kingdom. The design of the care homes varied—some had been adapted and others were custom built. The care homes were categorized as small (n = 11), medium (n = 14), and large (n = 13). A total of 1,373 long-term residents lived in these homes, and 452 were randomly selected for inclusion in the study. Data were collected on building design and residents' QOL. Data on residents' QOL were assessed using (a) dementia care mapping, (b) structured interviews with cognitively able residents, and (c) questionnaires, which were completed by the care worker who knew the resident best. To contribute to a fuller understanding of residents' QOL, the CAPE Behavior Rating Scale (Pattie & Gilleard, 1979) was used to measure resident dependency; the Pleasant Events Schedule-AD (Logsdon & Teri, 1997) was used to measure frequency and enjoyment of pleasant activities, and the Affect Rating Scale (Lawton, 1994) measured outward signs of emotion. The built environment was evaluated using a tool specially designed for the study, the Sheffield Care Environment

Assessment Matrix (SCEAM). The SCEAM assessed the building under four headings: support for the resident as a person, support for old age, support for cognitive frailty, and support for staff (Torrington, 2007). Residents' QOL was found to be consistently lower for the large homes than for the small and medium homes. For example, the overall well-being scores were highest in the small homes (38%) and lowest in the large homes (13%). The proportion of time residents spent engaged in any activity was highest (46%) in medium-sized homes and lower in small (38%) and large (28%) homes. Large homes had low scores for personalization and high scores for safety/health. Medium homes tended to have high scores for personalization, community, and choice/control. Small homes scored best for comfort, normality, and cognitive support, but less well on staffing levels. These findings suggest that residents' QOL is enhanced when they live with a smaller group of people. Parker et al. (2004) found significant positive relationships between the built environment and residents' QOL in relation to (a) provision within the building design for residents' choice/control—for example, access to indoor and outdoor spaces and facilities was related to resident well-being; (b) the community orientation of the building—for example, connection of the building to the wider community and provision for visitors were related to resident activity and the percentage of time they were active; (c) a supportive environment that compensated for residents' physical frailties and/or sensory impairments was related to residents' ability to control their immediate environment; and (d) the extent to which the building compensated for cognitive frailties—for example, by the provision of visual cues that help residents to find their way around—was related to positive emotion. Two negative relationships were also identified in relation to QOL and buildings that prioritized safety and health. Large homes tended to have high scores for safety and health. Higher scores for the domain safety/health were related to (a) lower scores for enjoyment of activities and (b) lower scores in resident environment control. For example, fire doors were heavy and difficult to open, impeding the free movement of residents. Mary makes clear the importance of communal space ("We play cards in the little room off the corridor"), having access to the garden, and having her own room (her "haven."). Searing and Clemons (2001) explain that there is a relationship between "sense of place" and "sense of self." They also note the symbolism of domestic objects in establishing a sense of place and a sense of self, flagging how "objects in (people's) homes acted as a communication device about themselves to others" (p. 22). This explains the significance for Mary of having her pictures and the "little table" from her home in her room.

Supporting residents to maintain their personal identities is a key task for staff in long-term care settings. Personal identity defines and differentiates us from others (Atchley, 1989; Charmaz, 1994, 2002). Collinson and Hockey (2007, p. 383) explain that while social identities are "those we attribute or impute to others, situating them as social objects . . . ," personal identities refer to the meanings "we attribute to the self." Personal identity, therefore, is about how we view ourselves as unique individuals. Collinson and Hockey (2007, p. 384) also refer to "felt identity," grounded in self-feelings and "largely taken for granted until an event disrupts the routine processes of everyday life and activities." Moving to long-term care involves change and compromise of a magnitude that can significantly impact on the older person's personal, social, and felt identity. Charmaz (1983), focusing on chronically ill housebound adults of all ages, argues that loss of self is a fundamental form of suffering. She identifies four factors that erode the sense of self: (1) restrictions to their daily lives, (2) their sense of social isolation, (3) being devalued, and (4) a belief that they are burdening others. The nature of long-term care has the potential to exacerbate these characteristics; for example, erosion of self is more likely if care is routinized and consequently the person has little "voice" or control. As Charmaz (1983) explains:

> [C]hronically ill persons frequently experience a crumbling away of their former self-images without simultaneous development of *equally valued new ones.* The experiences and meanings upon which these ill persons had built former positive self-images are no longer available to them. . . . Over time, accumulated loss of formerly sustaining self-images without new ones results in a diminished self-concept [emphasis added]. (p. 168)

Older people living in long-term care settings not only have a high incidence of chronic illnesses (such as Mary's osteoarthritis) but also experience the losses associated with moving to a long-term care setting, such as loss of their home, normal routines, and normal social activities, and consequently have a high potential for loss of identity (Bridges, 2007; Cooney, Murphy, & O'Shea, 2009; Tester et al., 2004). However, there is potential for forging "new" self-identities (Charmaz, 1983). Staff have an important role to play in helping the older person to sustain self-images and/or forge new and valued self-images, improving their experience of living in long-term care settings (Bridges, 2007; Cooney et al., 2009; Davies, 2001); for example, Mary has been supported to retain her self-image as a "worker" and "contributor." Other strategies to sustain identity include maintaining personal routines and habits.

Continuity theory (Atchley, 1989) argues that as people grow older, they endeavor to preserve and maintain continuity in their habits, relationships, roles, environments, and values. The move from familiar home surroundings into the strange new environment of a long-term care facility can cause severe discontinuity for residents. Discontinuity "sharply diminish[es] [the individual's] capacity for coherence in some aspect of his or her identity. Discontinuity thus alters identity" (Atchley, 1989, p. 187). Typically, the older person will attempt to maintain continuity by "dealing with a new environment in familiar ways . . . [by] search[ing] for linkages and familiarity" (Atchley, 1989, p. 189). It is important, therefore, that the person has opportunities to continue to do things that he or she valued and enjoyed in the past; for example, it has been made possible for Mary to continue gardening. Having control over day-to-day activities also supports coherence; for example, time of getting up, going to bed, or how one dresses. Cass, Robbins, & Richardson (2009) note that a person's appearance is integral to his or her self-respect. Mary makes this clear when she stresses the importance of having her hair nice and by being fussy about her clothes. However, residents sometimes struggle to maintain their own habits and preferences within the imposed routine of the long-term care setting (Cooney, 2012; Jensen & Cohen-Mansfield, 2006; Murphy, Cooney, O'Shea, & Casey, 2009; Tester et al., 2004). Jensen and Cohen-Mansfield

(2006) found more self-care activities—for example, time of getting up or going to bed and frequency of bathing—changed on admission to long-term care than remained the same. Mimicking self-care routine as closely as possible promotes continuity and control for residents (Cooney, 2012; Jensen & Cohen-Mansfield, 2006). This requires that the inevitable routine of a long-term care setting is sufficiently flexible to meet individual residents' preferences, expectations, and capacities within the routine. Clearly, for Mary there is flexibility; for example, she has choices about staying in bed or going to the dining room for breakfast, what she eats, and how she spends her time.

Connectedness and relationships with others—for example, Mary's friendship with peer residents—is also critical to identity. Charmaz (1983) points out that social isolation fosters loss of self. Similarly, Bradshaw, Playford, and Riaza (2012) conclude that lack of peer friendships in long-term care settings contributes to loneliness and boredom impacting on self-identity. Staff working to enable residents to form peer relationships (as happened in Mary's case) is therefore an important priority for care. Unfortunately, this is sometimes underrecognized, with staff assuming that relationships will happen spontaneously (Murphy, O'Shea, Cooney, Shiel, & Hodgins, 2006). Furthermore, Owen (2006) makes the following argument:

> [F]eelings of helplessness and powerlessness associated with chronic disability affect motivation levels and are compounded if there is a lack of structure and meaning to the day. These feelings can be alleviated by a motivating and challenging environment with opportunities to socialize and become involved in meaningful activity. (p. 46)

The staff have created such an environment for Mary; for example, she feels she is making a meaningful contribution through her "jobs" and has opportunities to socialize. Opportunities to have contact outside of the unit would strengthen this even further. This is an aspect not addressed in Mary's current plan of care. Creating a sense of community within the long-term setting is critical to QOL, but so too is having links with the wider community. Owen (2006) believes engagement with the outside helps residents still feel part of the wider community.

A distinction of note is the difference between "activity" and "meaningful activity" or "occupation." Bambrick and Bonder (2005, p. 78) go so far as to say occupation is an "innate human need." Bambrick and Bonder (2005) interviewed 21 older people living in the community on the importance they attached to engaging in productive work. All engaged in some kind of work, ranging from paid work, child care or other care giving, volunteering, or informally helping others. Three themes describe how participants perceived they benefited from their work: "contribution to self-concept," "giving back to the community," and "staying engaged." Staying productive contributed to their self-concept and allowed them to feel engaged with life. Similarly, Van't Leven and Jonnsson (2002), who interviewed 10 residents on how they perceived the supports and constraints of a nursing home environment on their occupational performance, identified three themes: "continuity of some familiar occupation of personal interest," "self-determination and control in daily activities," and "social contacts with people." Study participants were keen to continue their former hobbies and interests. Many of these were solitary in nature—for example, watching television, needlework, and reading. Most also joined in the group activities on offer. Participants were most positive about activities when they were meaningful to them. These activities gave them a feeling of "having done something" instead of just passing the time. Meaningful activities were described as those that matched their former activities and helped them maintain their identities. The opportunity for contact and conversation with others was also important, and participating in activities was found to help participants become part of the group. Schenk, Meyer, Behr, Kuhlmey, and Holzhausen (2013), who also explored QOL in nursing homes from the perspectives of residents, found participants value activities that give them a feeling of being useful and/or give them pleasure and enjoyment. Staff's focus on identifying "jobs" that Mary enjoys and making it possible for her to interact socially with others adds immeasurably to her QOL.

Mary commented on how she and her friends like to tell stories from their past. Interestingly, storytelling plays a major role in generating valued new self-images. Hockey (1989, p. 151) believes that residents are preoccupied with the "search for coherence, the creation of life history, which transcends the changes and losses of the recent past." It is thought that older people construct their life stories through reinterpreting their experiences, and this helps them to continue to live meaningful and coherent lives (Heliker, 1999; McKee et al., 2005). Storytelling or reminiscence facilitates this process and contributes to identity maintenance, psychological health, and QOL (Bridges, 2007; Cully & LaVoie, 2001; McKee et al., 2005). Opportunities to tell their stories are important to preserving identity.

Another way of preserving self-image is concerned with enabling the person to personalize his or her space, as Mary has done with the help of staff. The importance of a room, somewhere you can close the door, feel at ease, and be free to be yourself—or "have peace and quiet," as Mary terms it—should not be underestimated. Studies have found that the loss of the level of privacy they enjoyed in their own homes is a major issue for older people living in long-term care settings (de Veer & Kerkstra, 2001; Murphy et al., 2009). de Veer and Kerkstra (2001) found that residents who had insufficient opportunity to be alone were less likely to feel at home. Feeling at home is an important contributor to accepting and adapting to life in a long-term care setting (Bradshaw et al., 2012; Cooney, 2012), and there is a strong relationship between the place we call "home" and self-identity (Falk, Wijk, Persson, & Falk , 2012). The move to long-term care strips away what the person associated with home, explaining why opportunities to bring some things from home (Mary has brought her pictures and a table) helps regenerate a sense of home. Ternestedt (2009, p. 164), discussing identity-promoting care in the context of a dignified death, comments that "a nursing home that is experienced as home promotes identity and dignity, but one in which the person does not feel at home constitutes a threat to identity," making clear the importance of generating a feeling of home for the older person. Sherman and Dacher (2005) suggest cherished objects are a "link" to personal identity. Similarly, Kamptner (1989, p. 182) indicates, "(o)ne's belongings may enhance mastery and control in the face of losses . . . [and] may assist individuals in maintaining and preserving their identities in the face of events that erode their sense of self." Sherman and Newman (1977/1978) found a significant positive relationship between residents' life satisfaction scores and having cherished possessions. It is important that care staff understand that residents' personal possessions are not simply a "picture" or a "table," but a repository of residents' memories, a link to their past and to their future. However, having belongings around them is not important for all residents, and some find the associated memories too painful.

What is clear from the literature and Mary's story is that "one size does not fit all." Personal identity and self-esteem are key to a good QOL and can be sustained through giving the person "voice," respecting and acting on his or her choices, knowing the person, and providing opportunities for purposeful living.

Strategies for Changing Practice

While long-term care settings are primarily seen as health care facilities, they also serve the dual role of being the permanent dwelling-place of the majority of their residents. Therefore, long-term care institutions have the potential to influence aspects of residents' lives in areas far more extensive than just health needs. One of the difficulties, as we have seen earlier, is that so little is known about the human needs and preferences of residents; each is seen, in many cases, as just another patient among many others. This can, in turn, exacerbate the powerlessness, hopelessness, and exclusion felt by the resident. Key to helping the person to maintain self-identity is knowing him or her and what is important to each person. Even the most ordinary activities—for example, dressing, grooming, and eating, as well as likes and dislikes—are personally meaningful and critical to strengthening identity and independence. The first part of knowing the resident comes, therefore, at the admission stage and involves being open to learning the person's life story. Knowing the person as an individual takes time, but is critical to helping him or her maintain personal identity. Strategies to support residents to maintain and develop their identity include working in partnership with residents to document their life story, supporting residents to allow them to continue to do things the way they always have (continuity), and generating opportunities for individuals to meet their needs and preferences (for example, Mary's need to work or have a social outlet).

Most governments have put in place legislation and regulations outlining minimum acceptable quality standards for long-term residential care. In addition, many countries have developed and implemented various quality initiatives to ensure that the standards outlined are followed. However, we are much better at generating information on structural and process aspects of care such as buildings, facilities and equipment, staff, safety and hygiene, and licensing and inspections than we are at monitoring whether people's sense of self and identity are being preserved in long-term care. The emphasis on quality of care at the expense of QOL in long-term residential care has been due to the fact that quality of care is easier to measure and assess in view of its more tangible nature. QOL in residential care will, for example, be influenced by people's individual circumstances, personality, and life history, making it imperative that systems are in place within nursing homes to elicit this information from residents at the earliest opportunity. This is particularly important for residents who have dementia or related cognitive impairments.

The move to long-term residential care is a major transition for older people. Older people have to adjust not only to a new home but also to the routine and way of life imposed by the institution. Residents find that their independence and autonomy may be curtailed. Decision making and choice over daily activities as simple as getting up and going to bed, meal times, and dress may be restricted as the care facility imposes its own schedule and routine on the individual. Control over aspects of daily living is essential for residents to be able to express themselves and preserve their sense of self that has been developed over a lifetime. If residents are denied the opportunities for decision making, they may feel useless or ineffective, which, in turn, can undermine personal identity and damage self-esteem. True involvement in decision making in all aspects of their lives promotes the feeling of having a purpose in life, feeling valued, and having a sense of belonging and a feeling of worth. Strategies include giving individuals "voice" to express what they want, building flexibility into routines to accommodate individual needs, giving choices, and sharing decision making.

"Keeping me" also requires that connections to their former self when living at home are preserved to some degree. Allowing people to bring their treasured possessions from home with them may provide comfort and solace to people admitted to long-term care. Contact with family and friends acts as a bridge for residents to their former lives outside residential care and provides an important opportunity for social interaction. Facilities should be proactive in ensuring that these relationships can develop and flourish. For example, social outings to the community where people lived previously are likely to be an important contributor to the QOL and sense of self of residents and should, therefore, form part of the normal care process. A focus on building community links, which both enable older people to engage in community activities and encourage the community to come into the care home and engage with residents, is important for generating connectedness and a sense of community.

Finally, moral philosophy provides a useful set of principles to guide the practice of QOL for older people in long-term residential care, particularly in relation to "keeping me." Rawls (1971) considers the well-being of individuals in terms of "primary goods," which include income, wealth, health, and education, as well as fundamental rights such as freedom of thought and association and self-respect. Primary goods enable individuals to realize their life ambitions and expectations. The most important primary good, according to Rawls, is self-respect. Self-respect incorporates both self-worth and self-confidence, and individuals require these attributes in order to believe that their actions in everyday life are worthwhile and are appreciated by others. Hence, self-respect is largely dependent on the esteem in which we are held by others. We need other members of society to validate our sense of self and confirm our value. For residents of long-term care, their sense of value and self-worth may be challenged as they become increasingly dependent on others. Therefore, it is particularly important that the ethos of the residential care facility is one of empowerment and enablement and that there are regulated structures in place to encourage and promote self-determination for residents.

Clinical Reasoning Questions

1. Analyze the concept of "identity" in the context of aging.
2. What issues or tasks do older people living in long-term care settings need to engage in and/or need support with to preserve their self-identity?
3. Think of an older person you are currently caring for, and consider what strategies you could use to support him or her to preserve self-identity.
4. Examine the relationship between maintaining identity or self-image and person-centered care.
5. Examine the concepts of "functioning" and "capabilities" in the context of planning individualized care for people living in long-term care settings.

References

Atchley, R. C. (1989). A continuity theory of normal aging. *The Gerontologist, 29*(2), 183–190.

Bambrick, P., & Bonder, B. (2005). Older adults' perceptions of work. *Work, 24,* 77–84.

Bernstein, A. B., Hing, E., Moss, A. J., Allen, K. F., Siller, A. B., & Tiggle, R. B. (2003). *Health care in America: Trends in utilization*. Retrieved from http://www.cdu.goV/nchs/date/misc/healthcare.pdf

Bradshaw, S. A., Playford, E. D., & Riazi, A. (2012). Living well in care homes: A systematic review of qualitative studies. *Age and Ageing, 41,* 429–440.

Bridges, J. (2007). Working to help residents maintain their identity. In *My home life: Quality of life in care homes* (pp. 51–64). London, England: Help the Aged/National Care Homes Research and Development Forum. Retrieved from http://myhomelife.org.uk/media/mhl_review.pdf

Cass, E., Robbins, D., & Richardson, A. (2009). *Dignity in care SCIE: Adults' services SCIE guide 15.* Retrieved from http://www.scie.org.uk/publications/guides/guide15/files/myhomelife-litreview.pdf?res=true

Charmaz, K. (1983). Loss of self: A fundamental form of suffering in the chronically ill. *Sociology of Health and Illness, 5*(2), 168–195.

Charmaz, K. (1994). Identity dilemmas of chronically ill men. *The Sociological Quarterly, 35*(2), 269–288.

Charmaz, K. (2002). The self as habit: The reconstruction of self in chronic illness. *OTJR Occupation, Participant and Health, 22* (Suppl. 1), 31S–41S.

Collinson, J. A., & Hockey, J. (2007). "Working out" identity: Distance runners and the management of disrupted identity. *Leisure Studies, 26*(4), 381–398.

Cooney, A. (2012). "Finding home": A grounded theory on how older people "find home" in long-term care settings. *International Journal of Older People Nursing, 7*(3), 188–199.

Cooney, A., Murphy, K., & O'Shea, E. (2009). Resident perspectives of the determinants of quality of life in residential care in Ireland. *Journal of Advanced Nursing, 65*(5), 1029–1038.

Cully, J. A., & LaVoie, D. (2001). Reminiscence, personality and psychological functioning in older adults. *The Gerontologist, 41*(1), 89.

Davies, S. (2001). The care needs of older people and family caregivers in continuing care settings. In M. Nolan, S. Davies, & G. Grant (Eds.), *Working with older people and their families: Key issues in policy and practice* (pp. 75–98). Berkshire, England: Open University Press.

de Veer, A., & Kerkstra, A. (2001). Feeling at home in a nursing home. *Journal of Advanced Nursing, 35*(3), 427–434.

Falk, H., Wijk, H., Persson, L. O., & Falk, K. (2012). A sense of home in residential care. *Scandinavian Journal of Caring Science, 27*, 999–1009.

Gür, H., Cakin, N., Akova, B., Okay, E., & Küçükoğlu, S. (2002). Concentric versus combined concentric–eccentric isokinetic training: Effects on functional capacity and symptoms in patients with osteoarthrosis of the knee. *Archives of Physical Medicine and Rehabilitation*, 83(3), 308–316.

Heliker, D. (1999). Transformation of story to practice: An innovative approach to long-term care. *Issues in Mental Health Nursing, 20*(6), 513–525.

Hockey, J. (1989) *Experiences of death.* Edinburgh, Scotland: Edinburgh University.

Houser, A. (2007). *Fact sheet: Nursing homes*. Retrieved from http://assets.aarp.org/rgcenter/il/fs10r_homes.pdf

Iversen, M. D. (2010) Managing hip and knee osteoarthritis with exercise: What is the best prescription? *Therapeutic Advances in Musculoskeletal Disease, 2*(5), 279–290

Jensen, B., & Cohen-Mansfield, J. (2006). How do self-care routines of nursing home residents compare with past self-care practices? *Geriatric Nursing, 27*(4), 244–251.

Kalunian, K. C., Tugwell, P., & Ramirez, M. (2013). Diagnosis and classification of osteoarthritis. *UpToDate.* Retrieved from http://www.uptodate.com/contents/diagnosis-and-classification-of-osteoarthritis?source=see_link

Kamptner, N. L. (1989). Personal possessions and their meanings in old age. In S. Spacapan & S. Oskamp (Eds.), *The social psychology of aging* (pp. 165–196). Newbury Park, CA: Sage.

Lawton, M. P. (1994) Quality of life in Alzheimer disease. *Alzheimer Disease and Associated Disorders, 8* (Suppl. 3), 138–150.

Logsdon, R. G. & Teri, L. (1997) The Pleasant Events Schedule-AD: Psychometric properties and relationship to depression and cognition in Alzheimer's disease patients. *The Gerontologist.* 37(1), 40–45.

McKee, K., Downs, M., Gilhooly, M., Gilhooly, K., Tester, S., & Wilson, F. (2005). Frailty identity and the quality of later life. In A. Walker (Ed.), *Understanding quality of life in older age* (pp. 117–129). Buckingham, England: Open University Press.

Murphy, K., Cooney, A., O'Shea, E., & Casey, D. (2009). Determinants of quality of life for older people living with a disability in the community. *Journal of Advanced Nursing, 65*(3), 606–615.

Murphy, K., O'Shea, E., Cooney, A., Shiel, A., & Hodgins, M. (2006). *Improving quality of life for older people in long-stay care settings in Ireland.* Retrieved from http://www.ncaop.ie/publications/research/reports/93_Imp_QoL_Long_Stay_Care.pdf

Owen, T. (2006). *My home life: Quality of life in care homes.* Retrieved from http://www.scie.org.uk/publications/guides/guide15/files/myhomelife.pdf

Parker, C., Barnes, S., McKee, K., Morgan, K., Torrington, J., & Tregenza, P. (2004). Quality of life and building design in residential and nursing homes for older people. *Ageing & Society, 24,* 941–962.

Pattie, A. H., & Gillerard, C. J. (1979). *Manual of the Clifton Assessment Procedures for the elderly.* Kent, UK: Hodder and Stoughton.

Rawls, J. (1971). *A theory of justice* (Original ed.). Cambridge, MA: Belknap Press of Harvard University Press.

Rubinstein, R. L. (1990). Personal identity and environmental meaning in later life. *Journal of Aging Studies, 4,* 131–147.

Schenk, L., Meyer, R., Behr, A., Kuhlmey, A., & Holzhausen, M. (2013). Quality of life in nursing homes: Results of a qualitative resident survey. *Quality of Life Research, 22,* 2929–2938.

Searing, E. E., & Clemons, S. (2001). *Perception of sense of place and sense of self through design of the home* [Abstract]. Interior Design Educators Council 2001 Conference, Chicago, IL.

Sherman, E., & Dacher, J. (2005). Cherished objects and the home: Their meaning and roles in later life. In G. D. Rowles & H. Chaudhury (Eds.), *Home and identity in late life: International perspectives* (pp. 63–79). New York, NY: Springer Publishing.

Sherman, E., & Newman, E. S. (1977/1978). The meaning of cherished personal possessions for the elderly. *Journal of Aging and Human Development, 8*, 181–192.

Swift, J. (2002). Osteoarthritis 1: Physiology, risk factors and causes of pain. *Nursing Times, 108*(7). Retrieved from www.nursingtimes.net

Tanaka, R., Ozawa, J., Kito, N., & Moriyama, H. (2013). Efficacy of strengthening or aerobic exercise on pain relief in people with knee osteoarthritis: A systematic review and meta-analysis of randomized controlled trials. *Clinical Rehabilitation, 27*(12), 1059–1071.

Ternestedt, B. M. (2009). A dignified death and identity promoting care. In L. Nordenfelt (Ed.), *Dignity and care for older people* (pp. 146–167). Oxford, England: Blackwell Publishing.

Tester, S., Hubbard, G., Downs, M. MacDonald, D. & Murphy, J. (2004). Frailty and institutional life. In A. Walker, & C. Hagan Hennessy, C. (eds.), *Growing older: Quality of life in old age* (pp. 209–224). Berkshire, England: Open University.

Torrington, J. (2007). Evaluating the quality of life in residential care buildings. *Building Research & Information, 35*(5), 514–528.

United Nations. (2013). *World population prospects: The 2012 revision*. Retrieved from http://esa.un.org/wpp/Documentation/pdf/WPP2012_HIGHLIGHTS.pdf

Van't Leven, N. & Jonsson, J. (2002) Doing and being in the atmosphere of the doing: Environmental influences on occupational performance in a nursing home. *Scandinavian Journal of Occupational Therapy, 9*, 148–155.

Vogel, L. M. (2001). *Identity and the interior environment: Connecting social cognition theory and interior design* [Abstract]. Interior Design Educators Council 2001 Conference, Chicago, IL.

Wren, M. A., Normand, C., O'Reilly, D., Cruise, S. M., Connolly, S., & Murphy, C. (2012). *Toward the development of a predictive model of long-term care demand for Northern Ireland and the Republic of Ireland*. Retrieved from https://medicine.tcd.ie/health_policy_management/assets/pdf/CARDI%20report.pdf

14 SOCIAL ISOLATION

KATHLEEN LOVANIO AND KATHLEEN O'NEIL-MEYERS

Subjective

"Why kill yourself, life will do it for you."

Objective

Nathaniel Nathers is a 96-year-old male who lives alone in a single family home in the community. He presented at the clinic for a geriatric assessment accompanied by his brother Joe, who assists with history. Gathering information about his health over the past year, Mr. Nathers stated his disapproval of having to give up the keys to his car 5 months ago after a police officer stopped him from attempting to enter the highway via the exit ramp. "They took my wheels away. Do you know how long I've been driving a car and never had an accident?" Since he can no longer drive, he had to give up his part-time job making runs to the Motor Vehicle Department to register cars for a local used car dealer. Mr. Nathers has always been an independent and productive person who lived a very satisfying life. He was married 30 years and raised three stepchildren, of whom only one stepson remains alive. However, since this stepson lives in another state, he rarely has contact with him, with the exception of an annual holiday card and phone call. Only two of Mr. Nathers' four siblings are alive today: a sister living in a nursing home with end-stage Alzheimer's disease, and his younger brother Joe, 79 years old, who lives in a neighboring town. After the passing of his wife, Mr. Nathers entered into a 32-year relationship with Josephine, who was 3 years his elder. During the last 6 months of their relationship, Mr. Nathers took on the role of caregiver until Josephine's death from cancer 1 year ago. After Josephine's death, he continued social engagement with a good friend and went to the club daily to play pinochle until he could no longer drive. Always outgoing and sociable, he claims the game is not enjoyable anymore and ignores club members' phone messages offering him transportation to the club.

Joe reported that it became necessary to manage his brother's finances this year because he was not paying his bills on time. Lately, he noted that some days his brother is sharp as a tack and other days confused and depressed. Although independent with basic activities of daily living, a home health aide was hired to bathe Mr. Nathers weekly for safety concerns. A more serious concern was raised when Joe stated that his brother lost his balance and fell twice in the last month. Mr. Nathers refuses to use his cane or walker when in the house. Joe is very concerned about his safety and asked his brother to move in with him and his wife so he would not be alone so much. Mr. Nathers was unyielding about staying in his home and not moving in with his brother and his wife: "This is where I'm going to die, and I'm not going to your house or any other home!" When asked if he ever thought of killing himself, he responded, "Why kill yourself, life will do it for you," and jokingly added, "I couldn't commit suicide if my life depended on it."

Mr. Nathers's medical history includes hypertension and hypercholesterolemia, which are well controlled with Lipitor, 10 mg/daily, and Lisinopril, 10 mg/daily. He also takes a daily multivitamin. There are no known allergies (NKA). He denies the use of alcohol and tobacco products. Advance directives are in place; his brother Joe is his health care durable power of attorney.

Upon physical examination, Mr. Nathers appears alert and is relaxed and cooperative; oriented times two, to person and place, but could not state the day of the week. His vital signs are: BP, supine, 136/78, sitting, 132/76, standing, 128/72; pulse, 72, regular rhythm; respirations 12, unlabored; O_2 sat on room air is 96%; afebrile with a temperature of 97.8°F. He is 65 in. (165 cm) in height and weighs 128 lbs. (58 kg); a recent weight loss of 5 lbs. (2 kg) was noted over the past year. HEENT: normocephalic/atraumatic, pupils equal, round, reactive to light and accommodation (PERRLA), vision grossly intact, hearing impaired, moderate amount of dry brown cerumen bilaterally, oral mucosa is pink and moist, 21 stable natural teeth, and no obvious dental caries. Skin dry, slight abrasion on right forearm, lungs are clear to auscultation bilaterally with no adventitious breath sounds. Cardiac exam reveals a regular heart rate, S1, S2, and no extra heart sounds or murmurs. His abdomen is soft, nontender with bowel sounds present in all four quadrants. Extremities have full range of movement; muscle strength 4/5, some weakness against resistance, positive pedal pulses bilaterally, and trace pedal edema. Timed Up and Go (TUG), less than 20, use of arms getting out of chair, two attempts, wide-base, slightly unsteady, falls into chair, proper use of cane. Patient Health Questionnaire (PHQ)-9: 5; Mini Mental State Examination (MMSE): 23.

Assessment and Plan

Mr. Nathers's sudden decline in functional status and cognitive status is of great concern and will require further follow-up and referrals. Functional status determines whether an older adult has the ability to perform tasks that are required for living independently. Bathing is typically the activity of daily living (ADL) with the highest prevalence of disability and is often the reason why older adults receive home aide services, and continuing weekly bathing by the home health aide was encouraged. The TUG test demonstrated muscle weakness, balance problems, and gait abnormalities that clearly indicate a high risk of falling. In-home physical therapy will be ordered for Mr. Nathers for a comprehensive evaluation and the potential for rehabilitation. In addition, a home hazard evaluation will be conducted by the community home visiting nurse.

The most accepted and frequently used cutoff score for the MMSE is 23. Scores of 23 or lower indicate the presence of some cognitive impairment and the need for further evaluation. It is important to be mindful that cognitive performance varies within populations by age and education (Crum, Anthony, Bassett, & Folstein, 1993). Crum developed population norms by age and education. These norms are useful when one wishes to compare an individual's MMSE scores with those of a population reference group, or when interpreting the scores of individuals that are illiterate, have had minimal schooling (less than 8 years), or are 80 years of age or older. Taking into account Mr. Nathers's age and educational attainment, a normal MMSE score would be 24. The PHQ-9 score of 5 indicates mild depression that will require referral, treatment, and monitoring (PHQ-9, 2014). A positive response to the ninth question ("Do you have thoughts that you would be better off dead, or of hurting yourself in some way?") can provide some foundation for further exploration and risk of suicide; Mr. Nathers answered, "Not at all" to that particular question.

In following up with his chief concern of not being able to drive any longer, the nurse practitioner agreed, for his safety and the safety of others, surrendering his license was the reasonable thing to do. She questioned him further regarding his decision not to relocate to his brother's home, and he stated, "I was never a smart person. I quit school in the fifth grade and worked hard all my life. Owning my home and not having to rely on others for everything is important to me. It makes me feel good—please don't take that away from me, it's all I have left." While living at home is preferable to Mr. Nathers, it can be a hollow victory without intervention, as he faces physical and emotional challenges and difficulties, making meaningful connection with others difficult.

With age, the number of social relationships decreases, as in Mr. Nathers's case—his stepchildren, siblings, wife and significant other, and longtime close friends are no longer part of his once thriving social network. His social network has dwindled down to his brother Joe and a couple of supportive neighbors who drop in occasionally. While Joe is still gainfully employed, he manages to check in on his brother every morning, bringing him breakfast and assisting him in taking his daily medications. Mr. Nathers's limited social networks and increasing functional and cognitive decline are beginning to have detrimental effects on both his quality of life (QOL) and well-being.

For older adults, driving can symbolize independence and freedom by preventing social isolation and allowing them to provide for themselves. Mr. Nathers's social networks continued to deteriorate when he was deemed no longer able to drive safely and was forced to turn in his driver's license. Adjusting now to being homebound, no longer able to do things independently, and having to rely solely on others could be getting just too much for him to bear. He is angry at the fact that he cannot drive and continually apologizing to Joe for being a burden and needing Joe to take time off from work to transport him to medical appointments.

Many community services are available for older adults that are in Mr. Nathers's situation to improve social engagement. As part of his plan of care, a social worker will be assigned to his case to provide information related to community resources and assist with the process. All efforts to coordinate the plan of care will take into consideration Mr. Nathers's dignity and right to free choice. The goal of care at this time is to keep Mr. Nathers living in his home safely and to prevent relocation or institutionalization.

Literature Review

There are a number of population groups vulnerable to social isolation and loneliness, but none as vulnerable as the older adult population. Current prevalence rates of social isolation in older adults have been reported as being as high as 43%, depending on the definition and the outcome measure (Nicholson, 2012). Loneliness and social isolation are two distinct concepts that are often used interchangeably. Social isolation, as defined by Nicholson (2009), "is a state in which the individual lacks a sense of belonging socially, lacks engagement with others, has minimal number of social contacts, and they are deficient in fulfilling and quality relationships." Loneliness, on the other hand, is defined as a subjective concept, resulting from an individual's perceived absence or loss of companionship (Dickens, Richards, Greaves, & Campbell, 2011). While social isolation concerns the lack of structural and functional social support, loneliness relates specifically to one's negative feelings about that situation (de Jong Gierveld, 1998).

Research has shown that several factors contribute to social isolation and loneliness in older adults. For example, studies have shown marital status, number of chronic illnesses, motor and sensory impairments, living alone (Theeke, 2009), greater age, self-report of poorer health, lower socioeconomic status, having no access to transportation, being widowed, low educational attainment (Dickens et al., 2011; Paul & Ribeiro, 2009), incontinence (Yip et al., 2013), participating infrequently in religious activities, and lacking club or organizational affiliations (Pantell et al., 2013) as risk factors for social isolation and loneliness in this age group. Many of these factors can be related to Mr. Nathers's life events.

Health risks associated with social isolation and loneliness have been consistently recognized in the literature, and there is strong evidence that each may have adverse effects on health and well-being (Holt-Lunstad, Smith, & Layton, 2010; Pantell et al., 2013). In a meta-analysis, Holt-Lunstad and colleagues (2010) investigated the association between social relationships and mortality and offered evidence of the damaging effects of the lack of relationships on mortality risk. Pantell et al. (2013) also explored the relationship between social isolation and mortality and provided convincing evidence to support the direct influence of social relationships on mortality. Social isolation and loneliness have been associated with cognitive function. Shankar, Hamer, McMunn, and Steptoe (2013) demonstrated an association between social isolation and loneliness and cognitive function, pointing out that the association is more pronounced in individuals with lower levels of education. Windle, Francis, and Coomber (2011) also reported that loneliness is associated with depression, either as a cause or as a consequence. Recognition of the potential adverse health effects that can be attributed to social isolation and loneliness is critical in the assessment of older adults.

Population aging is taking place in nearly all countries of the world. Globally, the segment of older adults aged 80 (the "oldest old") within the population was 14% in 2013 and is projected to grow to 19% by 2050 (World Population Aging, 2013). The World Health Organization (WHO) has drawn attention to the importance of the relationship between health and social conditions in determining the health of individuals and populations. Social determinants of health are described as conditions in which people are born, live, grow, work, and age, as well as the health system available to them (WHO,

2013). These circumstances are shaped by the distribution of money, power, and resources at the global, national, and local levels. Understanding the underlying determinants of health and inequities among the older adult population is a priority of the WHO. One of the aims of the WHO is to tackle inequities in older adults to both prevent and manage the development of chronic morbidity and to improve survival and well-being across the social gradient (WHO, 2013). A specific aim is to focus on addressing social isolation in this population.

Social isolation and its adverse effects are a global health problem that needs to be addressed to enhance the QOL and well-being in the older adult population. Nurses and advanced practice nurses play a key role in effectively influencing change at the local, systems, national, regional, and international levels to reach these goals. The numerous encounters with older patients allow one to recognize unmet needs of community-dwelling older adults. This knowledge is valuable to draw on in order to impact public policy. Providing cost-effective quality care is important, but it is not the only role a nurse and advanced practice nurse should take on; critical to the role is advocacy for patients and impact on policy.

Strategies for Change in Practice

Social isolation and loneliness is a significant global public health problem leading to numerous harmful outcomes. Health care practices should be made aware of the prevalence and impact of social isolation and loneliness. Prevention is always the best strategy. In primary care, prevention of social isolation in vulnerable groups has the potential to make the biggest difference through early assessment (Nicholson, 2012).

- Primary prevention
  - Influence policy changes to enhance social determinants of health
  - Promote personal health practices and coping skills
  - Link at-risk patients to social programs
  - Provide health education to community groups regarding awareness and impact of social isolation

- Secondary prevention
  - Knowledgeable of risk factors
    - Retirement/poverty
    - Loss of a driver's license/lack of accessible transport
    - Death of a partner or relationship breakdown
    - Relocation to a new community/living alone
    - Sudden disability/poor health
  - High-risk groups
    - Older men living alone
    - Older adults living in remote and rural areas
    - Older migrants
    - Indigenous older people
  - Screen—Lubben Social Network Scale (LSNS-6)
- Tertiary prevention
  - Refer to available community resources
  - Follow-up assessments for those believed to be socially isolated
  - Adult day care

Clinical Reasoning Questions

1. What strategies could you use to tackle isolation of older people living in the community?
2. What social activities programs are available in your area for older people?
3. What if Mr. Nathers had a score of 3 on the PHC-9?
4. What if Mr. Nathers had a score of 20 on the MMSE?
5. Examine the concept of "loneliness" in the context of care planning.

References

Crum, R. M., Anthony, J. C., Bassett, S. S., & Folstein, M. F. (1993). Population-based norms for the Mini-Mental State Examination by age and educational level. *Journal of the American Medical Association, 269*(18), 2386–2391.

de Jong Gierveld, J. (1998). A review of loneliness: Concept and definitions, determinants and consequences. *Reviews in Clinical Gerontology, 8*, 73–80.

Dickens, A. P., Richards, S. H., Greaves, C. J., & Campbell, J. L. (2011). Interventions at targeting social isolation in older people: A systematic review. *BMC Public Health, 11*(647), 2–22. Retrieved from http://www.biomedcentral.com/content/pdf/1471-2458-11-647.pdf

Holt-Lunstad, J., Smith, T. B., & Layton, J. B. (2010). Social relationships and mortality risk: A meta-analytic review. *PLoS Medicine, 7*(7), e1000316. Retrieved from http://www.plosmedicine.org/article/info%3Adoi%2F10.1371%2Fjournal.pmed.1000316

Nicholson, N. R. (2009). Social isolation in older adults. *Journal of Advanced Nursing, 65*(6), 1342–1352.

Nicholson, N. R. (2012). A review of social isolation: An important but underassessed condition in older adults. *Journal of Primary Prevention, 33*(2–3), 137–152.

Pantell, M., Rehkopf, D., Jutte, D., Syme, S. L., Balmes, J., & Adler, N. (2013). Social isolation: A predictor of mortality comparable to traditional clinical risk factors. *American Journal of Public Health, 103*(11), 2056–2062.

Patient Health Questionnaire. (2014). Retrieved from http://www.integration.samhsa.gov/images/res/PHQ%20-%20Questions.pdf

Paul, C., & Ribeiro, O. (2009). Predicting loneliness in old people living in the community. *Reviews in Clinical Gerontology, 19,* 53–60.

Shankar, A., Hamer, M., McMunn, A., & Steptoe, A. (2013). Social isolation and loneliness: Relationships with cognitive function during 4 years of follow-up in the English longitudinal study of ageing. *Psychosomatic Medicine, 75,* 161–170.

Theeke, L. A. (2009). Predictors of loneliness in U.S. adults over age sixty-five. *Archives of Psychiatric Nursing, 23*(5), 387–396.

Windle, K., Francis, J., & Coomber, C. (2011). *SCIE Research Briefing 39: Preventing loneliness and social isolation: Interventions and outcomes.* London, England: Social Care Institute for Excellence.

World Health Organization. (2013). *Social determinants of health.* Retrieved from http://www.who.int/social_determinants/en

World population aging: Economic & social affairs. (2013). Retrieved from http://www.un.org/en/development/desa/population/publications/pdf/ageing/WorldPopulationAgeing2013.pdf

Yip, S. O., Dick, M. A., McPencow, A. M., Martin, D. K., Ciarleglio, M. M., & Erekson, E. A. (2013). The association between urinary and fecal incontinence and social isolation in older women. *American Journal of Obstetrics & Gynecology, 208*(2), 146e1–146e7.

15 STIGMA

Rosemary Ford, Jenneke Footit, Min-Lin Wu, Mary Courtney, David Jackson, and Colleen Doyle

Subjective

"Mr. Ott is just getting old. We don't have mental problems in our family."

Objective

Oscar Ott is a 72-year-old male currently living with a supportive partner in their own residence in an inner city location. He has two adult children from a previous marriage, both of whom he has no regular in-person contact with, as they are both now located overseas. Mr. Ott was an attorney for a prominent law firm, but is now retired. Previously, Mr. Ott participated in a number of sporting pursuits and until very recently walked or jogged on a daily basis.

Mr. Ott has not experienced major health-related problems throughout his life. He is treated with a monotherapy for mild hypertension and takes aspirin as recommended by his cardiologist, whom he visits annually. In the past 12 months Mr. Ott's partner, Jeannette, has noticed that he has become forgetful of friends' and acquaintances' names, often asking for prompts when approaching people in the street or at social gatherings. Jeannette noted that Mr. Ott is aware of this change and exhibits a degree of anxiety when going to functions.

After Mr. Ott's third fall in the past 4 months, Jeannette began to offer him her arm when stepping off a curb or when negotiating wet or slippery surfaces. Understandably,

Jeannette is concerned about Mr. Ott's condition. Mr. Ott too has concerns about his health. Jeannette is afraid that Mr. Ott might be experiencing the early stages of dementia. She is not entirely sure of what dementia is, but thinks that it is a mental illness. She feels that she is responsible. She is afraid that she will lose all her friends, as she is sometimes embarrassed about Mr. Ott's behavior at gatherings.

Mr. Ott is feeling quite upset about his poor memory and falls. He knows that he doesn't think clearly and cannot recall friends' names and place names as he did in the past. Most of the time, he shrugs this off as old age. He mentioned this change to his daughter during one telephone call. She told him to go to his primary health care provider and get checked. His daughter had also noticed Mr. Ott's intermittent irritability and uncharacteristically vague exchanges at times and was fearful that she might be losing her father. She resolved that it was better not spoken about for fear of hastening her father's decline.

At this last visit with the nurse practitioner (NP), Mr. Ott mentioned that he had been feeling lethargic and unsteady on his feet. He also mentioned that he was feeling a bit "down in the dumps." His NP decided to take a routine pathology sample, checked his blood pressure and medications, and told Mr. Ott to get more rest and manage his diet, especially when going out to social events. Mr. Ott was grateful for the NP's verdict and was quite pleased that he was not going insane. Mr. Ott, however, neglected to tell the NP about his anxiety, forgetfulness, and recent falls.

Literature Review

Dementia is becoming a significant health issue and challenge globally, as the incidence and prevalence increase along with the rapidly growing aging population. According to the World Health Organization (WHO, 2012), there were approximately 36 million people worldwide living with dementia in 2010, with expectations of an increase to 65.7 million by 2030 and 115.4 million by 2050. Internationally, the incidence of dementia each year is close to 7.7 million, which equates to one new case every 4 seconds (WHO, 2012). High prevalence is also associated with age. For example, people over 85 years have a twofold higher risk of developing dementia than people in the age range of 60 to 80 years (Alzheimer's Disease International, 2009). This high incidence and prevalence of dementia has a great impact not only on the health care system, such as health care providers and health expenditure, but also on patients and their caregivers.

Globally, the majority of dementia patients live in the community and are cared for by their family members/caregivers, also known as "informal" caregivers or carers (Gallagher-Thompson et al., 2012). In Australia, about 200,000 Australians are carers for people living with dementia in the community (Australian Institute of Health and Welfare, 2012). Similarly, 14.9 million people care for a person with Alzheimer's disease or another form of dementia in the United States (Family Caregiver Alliance, 2011), and there were approximately 670,000 dementia caregivers in the United Kingdom (Alzheimer's Society, n.d.). These numbers are projected to rise in the future as population age profiles change toward a higher proportion of aged people.

Since family caregivers play a crucial role in the quality of life (QOL) of people with dementia, evidence-based practice has emphasized the caregivers' physical, psychological, emotional, social, and spiritual well-being (Brodaty & Donkin, 2009). For example, a recent systematic review was conducted to examine the effectiveness of nonpharmacological interventions for the treatment of both patient and family caregivers (Gallagher-Thompson et al., 2012). Benbow and Jolley (2012) argued that stigma, in terms of stereotypes, prejudices, and discrimination, has resulted in family caregivers delaying recognition and diagnosis, being reluctant to seek help from health care professionals, and being pessimistic about health service responses to dementia. Additionally, other negative effects include social isolation, feelings of shame, and depression (Navab, Negarandeh, Peyrovi, & Navab, 2013; Werner, Goldstein, & Buchbinder, 2010). Stigma continues to have a pronounced impact on the care of people with dementia and their families. As the prevalence and incidence of dementia continue to rise, the issues of stigma affecting family caregivers for family members with dementia cannot be ignored.

Dementia remains a highly feared and misunderstood illness (Dilworth-Anderson, Pierre, & Hilliard, 2012), and as a consequence it is associated with a level of stigma that can prove debilitating for both the individual and his or her family carer. Because of the severity of the condition, people with dementia due to Alzheimer's disease need timely access to a range of care services to enable them and their family carer to achieve the best outcomes. However, the myths of dementia contribute to stigmatization of the individual and the carer (stigma by association), which can inhibit help-seeking outside the family system (Dilworth-Anderson & Gibson, 2002) in the form of dementia screening and diagnosis and access to care and treatment (Benbow & Jolley, 2012).

A particularly damaging misconception held by the general public is that dementia is a "death of the mind." What this label overlooks is the unique illness experience of each individual, including the time and severity of onset and the pattern of cognitive decline. In addition, each individual brings a different set of life skills, values, and beliefs to his or her experience.

Individuals with symptoms of mild Alzheimer's dementia, namely, concentration deficits and decreased ability to manage complex activities, estimate their QOL as good, to fairly good, to a mix of positives and negatives (Katsuno, 2005). This QOL estimate is in fact no different from that of the general adult population. However, amid the enjoyment and quality in their life, these individuals are keenly aware of others' negativity and censure of them. Once their condition is known to be dementia, they find family, friends, and others to act in a way that depersonalizes and devalues them and their contribution to society.

It is estimated that the stage from mild cognitive impairment through to mild Alzheimer's disease is approximately 7 years—it is during this time that early diagnosis and treatment are important. However, a wide gap exists between prevalence estimates and the uptake of diagnosis and treatment (Dilworth-Anderson & Gibson, 2002). Stigma associated with the disease is thought to play a role in keeping the individual and the family carer from seeking diagnosis and help. At this stage, the individual can continue to live his or her life independently, with normal employment and domestic adjustments as required.

Following the slow commencement of the disease, the deterioration from mild to moderate Alzheimer's disease is estimated to be 2 years, with only an 18-month transition through the moderate stage to cognitive impairment of higher severity. Cognitive deficits at this stage prevent independent living, and the family carer steps up to take responsibility for hygiene, nutritional, and shelter needs. It is during this stage that caregivers are keenly aware of the disgust and fear responses of family, friends, and laypeople to the individual with dementia. Fear is fueled by common myths, for example, laypeople fear contagion, the disease, and seeing the ill person (Werner et al., 2010), and believe the ill person to be crazy, dangerous, or incompetent. Now seen through the lens of fear and intolerance, what were previously loved individual traits and characteristics are viewed as evidence of odd behaviors, poor physical and cognitive functioning, and unstable emotions.

The strong negative emotional response of family, friends, and laypeople acts to separate those with dementia from others, to socially distance them, and to marginalize them in society (Behuniak, 2011). Even though family carers remain compassionate, they also experience the emotions of shame, embarrassment, and disgust, resulting in some cases in concealment of the individual, a reduction in contact (Werner et al., 2010), and depression (Montoro-Rodríguez, Kosloski, Kercher, & Montgomery, 2009). In view of the pervasive nature of the stigma, those with Alzheimer's disease adopt the perspective of those who stigmatize them and feel high levels of internalized shame (Burgener & Berger, 2008). Shame felt by the individual and the carer prevents help-seeking from normal health and social amenities.

The notion that dementia is related to laziness or weakness of character was found to be significantly present in Low and Anstey's study (2009). Such findings suggest stigmatization of dementia is still common and widespread. The impact of this showed very clearly in the work of Daly, McCarron, Higgins, and McCallion (2013) when they explored the processes followed by informal carers of persons with dementia to manage their social environments. The concept of "living on the fringes" relates to the carer's efforts to sustain social identity and social situatedness, or place, in the face of stigma-driven alterations in how people respond to them and their person with dementia. Place becomes unsettled as the carer tries to explain away or normalize the behavior in response to the need to avoid the stigmatization. Stigma, normalization of symptoms, and lack of knowledge are significant barriers to early diagnosis (Bunn et al., 2012). When normalization is no longer successful, place becomes threatened as the inevitability of dementia becomes unavoidable and the carer is forced to face the reactions of others to the deteriorating behavior of the person with dementia (Daly et al., 2013).

The third and fourth phases Daly and colleagues identified relate to the need to adapt and build a new support network. Stigmatization drives the behavior of others toward the person with dementia and his or her carer, leading to changes and losses in relationships and the need for carers to create new, safe social environments. This process begins with the fear of losing social recognition and position, followed by disturbances to the carer's sense of where he or she fits and leading to a shrinking of his or her world. Once this point is reached, strategies are developed to protect and nurture personhood for the carers and their person with dementia, as well as establishing a new safe social environment where people respond positively to the person with dementia (Daly et al., 2013).

Addressing stigma in the community would either reduce the sense of place being unsettled and threatened or shorten the period of time the person feels threatened and exposed. With less stigma attached to the diagnosis, the informal carer would be able to develop a new sense of sustained place with supportive networks developing quickly. It is, however, clear from the findings about the increase in caregiver burden by family stigma, or stigma by association (Werner, Mittelman, Goldstein, & Heinik, 2012), that reducing stigma can have a significant impact on the ability of the carer to sustain the caregiving. The emotional cost to the carer of defending the personhood of the person with dementia against the consequences of stigmatization is high and may lead to breakdown in caregiving, with emotional as well as financial implications for the family and carers, as well as financial implications for the health care system. Early recognition of dementia would allow for early interventions with treatments to slow down progression as well as

FIGURE 15.1: The cascading impact of stigmatization on family caregivers and people living with dementia.

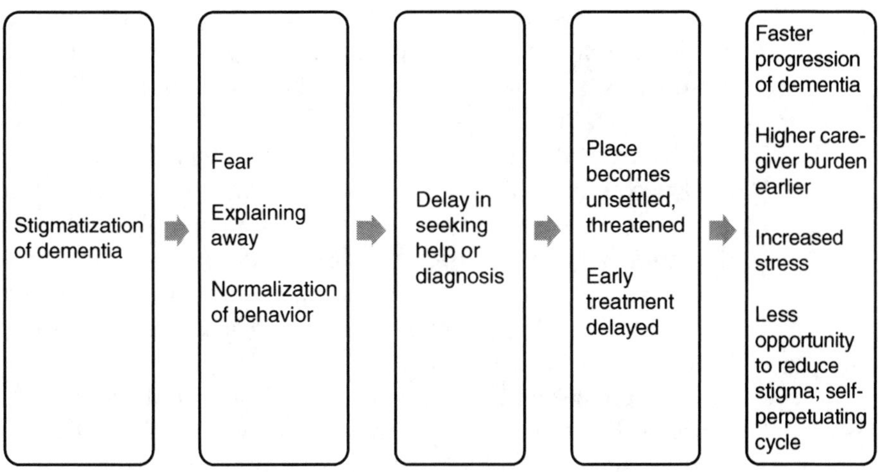

allow families to adapt to the situation and plan carefully for the future (Bradford, Kunik, Schulz, Williams, & Singh, 2009; Chang & Silverman, 2004), but the negative attitude toward dementia is making this difficult for primary health care professionals. Stigmatization would potentially prevent families from benefiting from early diagnosis and intervention with consequent higher risk of breakdown in the caregiving situation. This process can be illustrated in Figure 15.1.

Role Considerations

Finding realistic solutions for supporting people living with dementia in a caring role must be of international importance, and nurses working in all settings can assist with changing attitudes. Solutions should target (a) the nursing workforce, (b) the community at large, and (c) care recipients, carers, and families living with dementia. Programs clearly need to be aimed at providing better support for people in a caring role across cultures and the continuum (Australian Institute of Health and Welfare, 2012).

Primary care providers should be empowered to expand their awareness of available services and be encouraged to take a greater role in early diagnosis and in the creation of a positive environment of support. To this effect, the development and dissemination of best practice guidelines will be an invaluable resource for primary care physicians and other members of the dementia-specific health workforce (Phillips et al., 2012). Health care staff will benefit from both practical and theoretical education regarding negative behavior associated with stigma and stereotyping (Livingston & Mukadam, 2012). Health care organizations may allow people living with dementia greater self-determination and ongoing dignity by participating in and encouraging a combination of person-centered care (Phillips et al., 2012), e-health (Lutz & Young, 2010), and/or consumer-directed care (Ruggiano, 2012).

To effect change at a societal or community level, educational and media campaigns should advocate on behalf of people living with dementia and raise community awareness by opening a dialogue that has the capacity to encompass stigma, stereotyping, and social isolation in the context of ethnicity, religion (Livingston & Mukadam, 2012), and ageism (Radermacher, 2013). Media groups have the opportunity to generate a more accurate representation of people living with dementia, contribute to breaking down stereotypes, facilitate opportunities for contact with people living with dementia, and disseminate and advocate for education that is fair and unbiased (Livingston & Mukadam, 2012).

Individuals and families should be encouraged to actively plan for their future health needs, to support a sense of empowerment, and to maintain self-esteem. For families dealing with the day-to-day reality of dementia, initiatives should allow greater participation in the mainstream community, for example, by encouraging access to community care and leisure programs. QOL and/or well-being should be protected through efforts to allow people living with dementia to maintain social networks. Community involvement and peer support have the potential to prevent and/or reduce the incidence of depression and anxiety (Livingston & Mukadam, 2012; Radermacher, 2013). Funding of supportive programs using cognitive behavioral therapy to challenge negative perceptions and address fear, distress, denial, shame, and blame may assist people toward seeking and accepting early diagnosis and negate the impact of stigma on access to ongoing support services. People living with dementia should be encouraged to be aware of and utilize retained attributes, without focusing on their loss (Livingston & Mukadam, 2012).

Governments must provide an increased range of services in an effort to integrate people living with dementia into the community and decrease separateness (Livingston & Mukadam, 2012). A major shift in how research in this area is funded will be required to encourage and enhance both social and medical research with an intention to transform from a traditionally dominant, medical framework to a more holistic understanding of the impact of stigma and social isolation. Future research may study the effect of antistigma programs and the role of self-stigma and perceived stigma upon depression, self-esteem, and personal control for people living with dementia (Burgener & Berger, 2008; Dalky, 2012; Livingston & Mukadam, 2012).

Cultural Considerations

As the Western world's population profile ages and more people live to advanced age, dementia and cognitive impairment are becoming more common in our communities. Therefore, in the absence of a cure for dementia, we need ways to maintain the QOL of people living with dementia and their families throughout their journey with this disease. Community attitudes and beliefs regarding dementia are vital links in maintaining QOL. This brief review has indicated that the stigma against dementia is still present in many communities, leading to social isolation, delay in seeking diagnosis, and unwillingness to access services even when they are available. There is considerable cultural influence on how dementia is viewed within each community. Awareness campaigns funded by governments would be worthwhile investments as we have shown a link between stigma, isolation, and subsequent reluctance to access services early, leading to poorer outcomes that may eventually lead to greater cost to the health system. Our different cultural communities need to understand more about what dementia is, where it comes from and how it is manifested, and how to manage it—all important health promotion messages. Our review has indicated that stigma stems from fear and misunderstanding about the nature of the disease. However, it is not only the uninformed general public that needs awareness raising—nurses also need targeted interventions that teach them how to model behavior that demonstrates acceptance of people living with dementia, and the value of early diagnosis despite the fact of no cure and few successful drug treatments. Equally, younger generations need education about dementia as they are growing up, as ultimately their attitudes in adulthood will shape the way we live with dementia.

Solutions and Strategies

To address Mr. Ott and Jeannette's case, the NP may formulate and implement the following plan of care:

1. Assessment
   - Undertake a holistic assessment (physical, psychological, emotional, social, spiritual) of both Mr. Ott and Jeannette's situation, taking into account past history and current experience and planning for the future.
   - Review barriers to diagnosis and ongoing health-seeking behavior.
   - Review available support network.
2. Stigma
   - Provide and discuss educational material on cognitive decline, impairment, and dementia.
   - Counsel on stigmatization, perceived stigma, social isolation, embarrassment, and shame. (Resources may include nonconfrontational video material and/or written material from service providers and dementia-specific associations.)
   - Encourage sharing of educational resources and discussion with children, family, and friends.
   - Provide information regarding counseling services available, and assist with referral.
   - Provide resources on safe and supportive environments and facilities.

3. Early diagnosis
   - Highlight the benefits of early diagnosis.
   - Make a referral or encourage a visit with their primary health care provider to assess Mr. Ott's condition, and provide referral to specialist services as necessary.
   - Discuss the benefits of an advanced health care plan.
4. General health and well-being
   - Encourage open communication between Mr. Ott and Jeannette.
   - Encourage maintenance of social activity in supportive environments.
   - Encourage healthy lifestyle choices related to diet, physical activity, spirituality, and adherence to medical therapy.
   - Encourage Jeannette and Mr. Ott to maintain a focus on what good qualities they retain as individuals and in their relationship.

Clinical Reasoning Questions

1. How is dementia viewed in your community? What are the barriers to changing perceptions of dementia in your community? How would you overcome the barriers?
2. What roles can nurses take, and what strategies are available for nurses helping the family caregiver to overcome the effects of stigma and isolation?
3. Which community groups or workforce groups are most important for action in addressing the issue in your area?

References

Alzheimer's Disease International. (2009). *World Alzheimer Report 2009: The Global Prevalence of Dementia*. London, UK: Author.

Alzheimer's Society. (n.d.). *Statistics*. Retrieved from http://www.alzheimers.org.uk/site/scripts/documents_info.php?documentID=341

Australian Institute of Health and Welfare. (2012). *Dementia in Australia* (Vol. Cat. no. AGE 70). Canberra, Australia: AIHW.

Behuniak, S. M. (2011). The living dead? The construction of people with Alzheimer's disease as zombies. *Aging & Society, 31*(Pt. 1), 70–92.

Benbow, S. M., & Jolley, D. (2012). Dementia: Stigma and its effects. *Neurodegenerative Disease Management, 2*(2), 165–172.

Bradford, A., Kunik, M. E., Schulz, P., Williams, S. P., & Singh, H. (2009). Missed and delayed diagnosis of dementia in primary care: Prevalence and contributing factors. *Alzheimer Disease and Associated Disorders, 23*(4), 306.

Brodaty, H., & Donkin, M. (2009). Family caregivers of people with dementia. *Dialogues in Clinical Neuroscience, 11*(2), 217–228.

Bunn, F., Goodman, C., Sworn, K., Rait, G., Brayne, C., Robinson, L., . . . Iliffe, S. (2012). Psychosocial factors that shape patient and carer experiences of dementia diagnosis and treatment: A systematic review of qualitative studies. *PLoS Medicine, 9*(10), 1–12. doi:10.1371/journal.pmed.1001331

Burgener, S. C., & Berger, B. (2008). Measuring perceived stigma in persons with progressive neurological disease: Alzheimer's dementia and Parkinson's disease. *Dementia (14713012), 7*(1), 31–53.

Chang, C. Y., & Silverman, D. H. (2004). Accuracy of early diagnosis and its impact on the management and course of Alzheimer's disease. *Expert Review of Molecular Diagnostics, 4*(1), 63–69.

Dalky, H. F. (2012). Mental illness stigma reduction interventions: Review of intervention trials. *Western Journal of Nursing Research, 43*(4), 520–547.

Daly, L., McCarron, M., Higgins, A., & McCallion, P. (2013). "Sustaining place"—A grounded theory of how informal carers of people with dementia manage alterations to relationships within their social worlds. *Journal of Clinical Nursing, 22*(3/4), 501–512. doi:10.1111/jocn.12003

Dilworth-Anderson, P., & Gibson, B. E. (2002). The cultural influence of values, norms, meanings, and perceptions in understanding dementia in ethnic minorities. *Alzheimer Disease and Associated Disorders, 16*, S56–S63.

Dilworth-Anderson, P., Pierre, G., & Hilliard, T. S. (2012). Social justice, health disparities, and culture in the care of the elderly. *Journal of Law, Medicine & Ethics, 40*(1), 26–32. doi:10.1111/j.1748-720X.2012.00642.x

Family Caregiver Alliance (Producer). (2011). *Fact sheet: Selected caregiver statistics*. Retrieved from http://www.caregiver.org/caregiver/jsp/content_node.jsp?nodeid=439

Gallagher-Thompson, D., Tzuang, Y. M., Au, A., Brodaty, H., Charlesworth, G., Gupta, R., . . . Shyu, Y.-I. (2012). International perspectives on nonpharmacological best practices for dementia family caregivers. *Clinical Gerontologist, 35*(4), 316–355.

Katsuno, T. (2005). Dementia from the inside: How people with early-stage dementia evaluate their quality of life. *Aging and Society, 25*(2), 197–214.

Livingston, G., & Mukadam, N. (2012). Reducing the stigma associated with dementia: Approaches and goals. *Aging Health, 8*(4), 377.

Low, L.-F., & Anstey, K. J. (2009). Dementia literacy: Recognition and beliefs on dementia of the Australian public. *Alzheimer's & Dementia, 5*(1), 43–49. doi:http://dx.doi.org/10.1016/j.jalz.2008.03.011

Lutz, B. J., & Young, M. E. (2010). Rethinking intervention strategies in stroke family caregiving [Report]. *Rehabilitaiton Nursing, 35*(4), 152–160.

Montoro-Rodríguez, J., Kosloski, K., Kercher, K., & Montgomery, R. J. V. (2009). The impact of social embarrassment on caregiving distress in a multicultural sample of caregivers. *Journal of Applied Gerontology, 28*(2), 195–217.

Navab, E., Negarandeh, R., Peyrovi, H., & Navab, P. (2013). Stigma among Iranian family caregivers of patients with Alzheimer's disease: A hermeneutic study. *Nursing & Health Sciences, 15*(2), 201–206. doi:10.1111/nhs.12017

Phillips, J., Pond, C. D., Paterson, N. E., Howell, C., Shell, A., . . . Marley, J. E. (2012). Difficulties in disclosing the diagnosis of dementia: A qualitative study in general practice. *British Journal of General Practice, 62*(601), e546–e553. doi:10.3399/bjgp12X653598

Radermacher, H. (2013). Aging research in community psychology: Where are our elders? *The Australian Community Psychologist, 25*(1), 94–107.

Ruggiano, N. (2012). Consumer direction in long-term policy: Overcoming barriers to promoting older adults' opportunity for self-direction. *Journal of Gerontological Social Work, 55*(2), 146–159. doi:10.1080/01634372.2011.638701

Werner, P., Goldstein, D., & Buchbinder, E. (2010). Subjective experience of family stigma as reported by children of Alzheimer's disease patients. *Qualitative Health Research, 20*(2), 159–169.

Werner, P., Mittelman, M. S., Goldstein, D., & Heinik, J. (2012). Family stigma and caregiver burden in Alzheimer's disease. *Gerontologist, 52*(1), 89–97.

World Health Organization. (2012). *Dementia: A public health priority.* Switzerland, Geneva: Author.

16 STAFF EDUCATION AND PATTERNS TO PROMOTE QUALITY OF LIFE

ALISON KRIS

Subjective

"Get me out of here."

Objective

Mrs. Patricia Parker is an 84-year-old woman who was admitted to Shady Oak Nursing Home following a fall at home in which she sustained a fracture of her right hip approximately 10 days ago. She is status post open reduction and internal fixation (ORIF). While in the hospital, she developed acute delirium postoperatively, for which she was managed with Ativan and Haldol, PRN. During the episodes of delirium, she needed to have her wrists restrained to prevent removal of her IV. After surgery, it was determined that Mrs. Parker was not yet safe to return home, and she was discharged to Shady Oak Nursing Home for subacute rehabilitation with the possibility of long-term placement.

Mrs. Parker was slightly confused prior to her admission to the nursing home. However, since admission, her daughter, Carol, reports a marked increase in her cognitive difficulty. In addition, Carol states that her mother appears to be depressed and withdrawn. Mrs. Parker often does not get out of bed, and seems to have lost weight. Carol reports that she is very upset with the quality of care in the nursing home. While the lobby of the nursing home is beautiful, her mother's room is dark and dirty, and often has a foul smell. The nurses and the nurses' aides rush around and rarely make eye contact, let alone engage in conversation. There is never anyone to talk to at the nurse's station, and she reports it is very difficult to get any information at all about her mother's care. Carol or her sister, Faith, are sure to come to the facility nearly every evening after work because they are concerned that no one would help her mother with dinner if they were not there. Carol, for her part, is stressed and exhausted. She feels guilty that she cannot get her mother the care she deserves, and feels powerless to help.

Mrs. Parker is a petite, thin-appearing woman at 5 ft. 3 in. (160 cm), 110 lbs. (50 kg). She has lost 10 lbs. (5 kg) since her admission to the nursing home approximately 1 week ago. BP is 145/90, pulse 60, respirations 14. She is alert and responsive, yet confused, scoring 19/30 on her Mini Mental State Examination (MMSE). Her eyesight is poor as a result of retinopathy from poorly controlled type 2 diabetes. Her most recent fasting blood sugar (FBS) was 90, her A1C is 8. She also has moderate untreated hearing loss. Prior to her fall, she used a quad cane; however, postsurgery she requires a two-person assist to rise to a standing position. She is able to remain standing with the aid of a walker, but is unable to ambulate. She has had pain in her hip following the surgery 6/10, which responds well to Vicodin. She has a history of untreated osteoporosis, however, and was started on an osteoclast inhibitor while in the hospital. Her lungs are clear to auscultation (CTA). She has a history of atrial fibrillation, for which she had an unsuccessful ablation approximately 20 years ago. Her medications include hydrochlorothiazide (HydroDIURIL) 12.5 mg QD; Coumadin (Warfarin) 5 mg QD; propranolol (Inderal) 80 mg QD; Colace, 100 mg, QD; Micronase (Glyburide) 2.5 mg before meals; Fosamax (Alendronate Sodium) 10 mg, QD; Vicodin, 7.5/750 mg, Q4 PRN, pain; Haldol (Haloperidol) 5 mg, PRN, anxiety; Ativan (lorazepam) 1 mg, PRN, anxiety.

Mrs. Parker spends most of her days in bed. The nursing assistants say that Mrs. Parker is resistant to care, and that she often "refuses" to get washed and dressed in the morning. All of this comes as a surprise to her daughter, who says that it is not that her mother is resistant to care, but she is just in pain and likes things done a certain way. The nursing assistants are rushed, so rather than take the time, for example, to allow her mother to choose her outfit, the certified nursing assistants

(CNAs) rush through the process. "She just needs more time," Carol explains. "When she is rushed, she gets flustered and agitated, especially when she is in pain. She is not trying to be difficult, but the CNAs have a hard time understanding what she is trying to say, and quite honestly, I don't think they really care." Carol also says that when her mom is seen as agitated and resistant to care, she often is given medication to "calm her down." Unfortunately, the medication leaves her even more confused and tired, and she often spends her days in bed. While she was initially admitted for physical therapy, the notes from the physical therapist indicate that she has "refused" physical therapy most days.

Carol also states her mother has been eating very little, and has lost weight. Mrs. Parker needs assistance with meals, but Carol feels that the nursing assistants rush through the meals, and as soon as her mom starts to slow down for even a minute, the meal is over. "I understand that the CNAs are stressed. They have more than one person to feed, and my mom takes a really long time to eat. So I come most days, and my sister comes on the other days. We worry that if we did not come, she would not eat."

Carol expressed that she wants to know what the plan is for her mother, but she has not seen Mrs. Parker's physician in the nursing home. She has asked if the nurses would call him, but they say he makes rounds at a certain time each month and is otherwise not in the facility. "I am concerned that she does not go to physical therapy, even though that is the whole reason for her being here. Where do we go from here?"

Literature Review

This case exemplifies many of the issues associated with quality of care in long-term care facilities. Mrs. Parker is a woman who is particularly at risk from problems with quality of care. For nursing home residents, the quality of care delivered is intrinsically tied to the quality of life (QOL) experienced by nursing home residents. Although there are many ways to understand the meaning of QOL for a nursing home resident, much of the research in this area has operationalized

QOL as a set of defined quality measures such as freedom from pain, freedom from restraints, high-quality nutritional programs, low levels of unnecessary hospitalization, limited use of antipsychotic medications, and the preservation of resident dignity. Each of these quality measures is tied to nurse staffing levels.

Unfortunately, despite increasing levels of resident acuity, the average level of registered nurse (RN) hours per patient day has decreased. Between 1997 and 2007, the levels of registered nurse hours per patient day (RNHPPD) decreased by roughly 20% (Seblega et al., 2010). As Mrs. Parker's daughter describes, when nursing assistants are short of staff, the care is rushed. The rushing is perceived negatively both by patients and by the CNAs themselves (Bowers, Esmond, & Jacobson, 2000). Having more RN hours spent per resident day is linked to improved comfort and enjoyment scores (Shin, 2013).

While the use of physical restraints has declined over the past decade, there has been a significant increase in the use of psychoactive agents to manage episodes of agitation in nursing homes. For residents with dementia, nursing assistants often see pharmaceutical agents as first-line agents in managing agitation (Janzen, Zecevic, Kloseck, & Orange, 2013). Although there is great variability among nursing homes in the use of antipsychotic medication to manage behavioral problems, facilities that use more antipsychotic medications tend to be those with a combination of below average staffing, poor personal care, and a lack of recreational activities.

Mrs. Parker's daughter is concerned about her mother's weight loss. Mrs. Parker has several risk factors that place her at increased risk of weight loss, including her advanced age, the presence of dementia, the possibility of depression, her female gender, and her immobility. Residents need an average of roughly 35 to 40 minutes of feeding assistance in a given meal (Simmons & Schnelle, 2006). However, in a nursing home staffed with a typical ratio of eight residents per CNA, each resident can be given only 7.5 minutes of individualized feeding assistance in an hour mealtime, which includes set-up and removal of feeding trays. Increasing the amount of time spent on feeding, as Mrs. Parker's daughter is doing, can help prevent weight loss.

Role and Cultural Considerations

Research in nursing homes has shown that ethnic and racial minorities are at greater risk of poor-quality care. This risk is twofold. First, minorities are at greater risk of being admitted to a poor-quality nursing home. Second, once admitted, they have a greater risk of receiving poor quality within a given facility. Black residents are more likely to be restrained than White residents (Cassie & Cassie, 2013). In addition, they are more likely to have pressure ulcers, and when they do, the pressure ulcers are usually more severe (Harms et al., 2013). Therefore, issues related to the quality of care are an area of particular concern to minority populations.

As in many other settings, the value of an advanced practice registered nurse (APRN) in improving the quality of care in nursing homes has been demonstrated. Nursing homes that employ nurse practitioners have higher levels of patient satisfaction. In addition, visits from nurse practitioners have been shown to demonstrate improvements across a variety of outcomes. For example, the use of nurse practitioners decreases episodes of urinary incontinence (Ryden et al., 2000). Perhaps more important, however, nurse practitioners have been shown to develop caring, family, and resident-centered relationships with both patients and their families. They are seen as a source of information and support, which is often perceived as lacking in the nursing home setting (Ploeg et al., 2013).

Strategies for Changing Practice

Across hundreds of studies, in nursing homes from countries around the world, the level of nurse staffing in nursing homes remains the largest obstacle to the delivery of high-quality nursing care in nursing homes (Harrington et al., 2012). While the education of nurses in these nursing homes can be improved, educational interventions are wasted if nurses are not empowered with the time necessary to carry out the interventions necessitated by their increased knowledge.

The problems with the quality of care in nursing homes, widely documented by nurse researchers, have led legislators to create laws to improve the quality of care in nursing homes in several countries. In the United States, the legislative mandates requiring higher levels of nurse staffing have led to improvements in the quality of care, which include lower mortality rates and fewer deficiencies (Harrington, Swan, & Carrillo, 2007; Kim, Kovner, Harrington, Greene, & Mezey, 2009, Mueller et al., 2006; Park & Stearns 2009; Tong, 2011). Nurses need to continue to be active in legislative campaigns to improve staffing levels in nursing homes.

1. Refusal of care
   - Examine the causes for refusal of care. Are there different approaches that can be used?
   - Carefully monitor the use of medications. Are pain medications being dosed at appropriate times to ensure adequacy of pain control? In this case, administering pain medications prior to morning care and physical therapy is essential.
   - Inappropriate use of pharmacological therapies to manage resident behavior can lead to apathy and depression. In this case, the use of Haldol should be questioned.
2. Weight loss
   - Adequacy of staffing is essential to ensure proper nutrition, particularly for older adults with cognitive impairment.
   - Slow, careful feeding may be needed. Staffing should be provided to ensure cognitively impaired residents have sufficient staff assistance at each meal.
   - Specialized education as to proper feeding techniques to use with cognitively impaired older adults should be provided to CNAs.
3. Lack of communication
   - Poor communication is a frequently reported problem in nursing homes. The presence of nurse practitioners has been demonstrated to improve patient and family satisfaction with communication.
   - Nurses and other health care providers should check in with family members frequently to ensure their questions have been answered. When physicians are not present at the facility, family members should be provided with information about whom to contact when plans of care change.

Clinical Reasoning Questions

1. During an episode of acute delirium, Mrs. Parker was restrained to prevent removal of her IV lines and was also sedated with Ativan and Haldol. Were these measures appropriate? Why or why not?
2. Mrs. Parker's blood pressure is 145/90, for which she is taking hydrochlorothiazide (HydroDIURIL) 12.5 mg QD. Does this therapy fall within the new guidelines for management of hypertension among older adults? Mrs. Parker also has type 2 diabetes—does this change your answer?
3. Mrs. Parker's case describes many of the common quality of care issues in nursing homes. What is the role of the RN, the APRN, the DNP, and the MD in addressing these quality of care issues? How do these roles differ?

References

Bowers, B. J., Esmond, S., & Jacobson, N. (2000). The relationship between staffing and quality in long-term care facilities: Exploring the views of nurse aides. *Journal of Nursing Care Quality, 14*(4), 55–64; quiz 73–75.

Cassie, K.M., & Cassie, W. (2013). Racial disparities in the use of physical restraints in U.S. nursing homes. *Health and Social Work, 38*(4), 207–213.

Harms, S., Bliss, D. Z., Garrard, J., Cunanan, K., Savik, K., Gurvich, O., . . . Virnig, B. (2013). Prevalence of pressure ulcers by race and ethnicity for older adults admitted to nursing homes. *Journal of Gerontological Nursing, 40*(3), 1–7. doi:10.3928/00989134-20131028-04; 10.3928/00989134-20131028-04

Harrington, C., Choiniere, J., Goldmann, M., Jacobsen, F. F., Lloyd, L., McGregor, M., . . . Szebehely, M. (2012). Nursing home staffing standards and staffing levels in six countries. *Journal of Nursing Scholarship: An Official Publication of Sigma Theta Tau International Honor Society of Nursing/Sigma Theta Tau, 44*(1), 88–98.

Harrington, C., Swan, J. H., & Carrillo, H. (2007). Nurse staffing levels and medicaid reimbursement rates in nursing facilities. *Health Services Research, 42*(3 Pt. 1), 1105–1129.

Janzen, S., Zecevic, A. A., Kloseck, M., & Orange, J. B. (2013). Managing agitation using nonpharmacological interventions for seniors with dementia. *American Journal of Alzheimer's Disease and Other Dementias, 28*(5), 524–532.

Kim, H., Kovner, C., Harrington, C., Greene, W., & Mezey, M. (2009). A panel data analysis of the relationships of nursing home staffing levels and standards to regulatory deficiencies. *Journals of Gerontology Series B: Psychological Sciences & Social Sciences, 64*(2), 269–278.

Mueller, C., Arling, G., Kane, R., Bershadsky, J., Holland, D., & Joy, A. (2006). Nursing home staffing standards: Their relationship to nurse staffing levels. *The Gerontologist, 46*(1), 74–80.

Park, J., & Stearns, S. C. (2009). Effects of state minimum staffing standards on nursing home staffing and quality of care. *Health Services Research, 44*(1), 56–78.

Ploeg, J., Kaasalainen, S., McAiney, C., Martin-Misener, R., Donald, F., Wickson-Griffiths, A., . . . Taniguchi, A. (2013). Resident and family perceptions of the nurse practitioner role in long term care settings: A qualitative descriptive study. *BMC Nursing, 12*(1), 24.

Ryden, M. B., Snyder, M., Gross, C. R., Savik, K., Pearson, V., Krichbaum, K., & Mueller, C. (2000). Value-added outcomes: The use of advanced practice nurses in long-term care facilities. *The Gerontologist, 40*(6), 654–662.

Seblega, B. K., Zhang, N. J., Unruh, L. Y., Breen, G. M., Paek, S. C., & Wan, T. T. (2010). Changes in nursing home staffing levels, 1997 to 2007. *Medical Care Research and Review, 67*(2), 232–246.

Shin, J. H. (2013). Relationship between nursing staffing and quality of life in nursing homes. *Contemporary Nurse, 44*(2), 133–143.

Simmons, S. F., & Schnelle, J. F. (2006). Feeding assistance needs of long-stay nursing home residents and staff time to provide care. *Journal of the American Geriatrics Society, 54*(6), 919–924.

Tong, P. K. (2011). The effects of California minimum nurse staffing laws on nurse labor and patient mortality in skilled nursing facilities. *Health Economics, 20*(7), 802–816.

17 PHYSICIAN–NURSE COMMUNICATION

Toyoaki Yamauchi and Stephanie B. Mostone

Subjective

"Today, let's try eating something."

Objective

Mr. Quentin Quincy is a 75-year-old man who lives at home with his wife, Betty. He had been admitted to the intensive care unit (ICU) after a surgery on his injured right knee. He had been in the ICU for 3 days for postoperative care. He had not eaten anything after the surgery because of his poor appetite.

Upon physical examination, Mr. Quincy appears alert and oriented and lies on his bed. He is 5 feet 10 in. (178 cm) in height, and weighs 140 lbs. (64 kg). His blood pressure is 118/74; his pulse is 70, respirations 16/minute. He is afebrile with a temperature of 98°F. His oxygen saturation is 95%. His lungs are clear bilaterally with no adventitious sounds and good expansion. His cardiac exam reveals a regular heart rate, S1, S2, and no adventitious sounds. His abdomen is soft and nontender, and his bowel sounds are present in all four quadrants. His skin is warm, dry, thin, and intact; his eye examination reveals clear sclera bilaterally and pupils equal, round, reactive to light and accommodation (PERRLA). His ear examination reveals normal tympanic membranes with slightly reduced hearing bilaterally. His oral examination reveals normal moist, pink, mucosa with adequate dentition. Neurological exam reveals 2+ deep tendon reflexes bilaterally and equal strength bilaterally. His knees are fine without pain any more. His current medications include Ibuprofen 200 mg po tid every day.

Hearing his words, the nurse thought this was a good chance to feed him and helped him to sit up. When he was ready to eat, a physician came in to see him to change the dressing. The nurse asked the physician to wait until Mr. Quincy had finished eating. However, the physician replied, "My schedule is full with other patients. The only time I have is now. It won't take long. Let's do it now." The nurse said nothing further, and helped change the dressing. By the time it was completed, Mr. Quincy had lost his appetite and did not start to eat again.

Literature Review

Nurses strive to provide patient-centered care. However, given the need to coordinate views among staff involved and reconcile opposing views and judgments, such patient-oriented nursing care is not always easy to realize. Frequent nurse–physician communication is necessary in the delivery of effective patient care. However, there are many cases in which communication itself is not facilitated. Nurses often believe that their opinions and views are not understood and valued by physicians.

Both nurses and physicians agree that a common goal is to provide patients with better care. However, despite this shared value, the nurse–physician communication does not always work well, which results in a failure of interprofessional collaboration (World Health Organization [WHO], 2010). Communication, particularly between the nurse and the physician, has been directly linked to patient safety and medical outcomes (Friese & Manojlovich, 2012; Interprofessional Education Collaborative Expert Panel, 2011; Manojlovich, Antonakos, & Ronis, 2009). With regard to sentinel events occurring between 1995 and 2004, failures in communication were found to be the root cause in 66% of cases (Smith, 2005). Many governing bodies, including The Joint Commission (2010), the American Nurses Association (2010), the American Medical Association (n.d.), and the Institute of Medicine, have been clear about their expectation that health care professionals communicate between disciplines in order to provide the safest and highest quality care to patients (McCaffrey et al., 2011).

Interprofessional collaboration is an ideal approach to patient care that requires all health care professions within a patient's care to work as a team (Bajnok, Puddester, MacDonalds, Archibald, & Kuhl, 2012; Boykins, 2014). One of the key aspects of interprofessional collaboration is effective communication, without which collaboration cannot occur (McCaffrey et al., 2011). In the case of Mr. Quincy, communication between his nurse and physician was ineffective, and Mr. Quincy's recovery suffered the consequences of this poor interaction. While many health care institutions have begun to adopt the idea of interprofessional collaboration, communication between nurses and physicians continues to be in need of improvement and further training.

Aside from personal attributes (such as personality and confrontation style) that prevent effective communication, there are also well-documented hierarchical and institutional obstacles that impede good nurse–physician communication (Hayers & Collins, 2013; Weller, Barrow, & Gasquoine, 2011). A survey of 78 physicians and 462 nurses completed by Manojlovich and Antonakos (2008) found nurses and physicians might have different definitions of what comprises successful communication. Nurses in this study reported communication as an important part of daily patient care and dissatisfaction with current communication practices with physicians. Physicians, however, reported communication with nurses as less important than nurses' ability to predict physician needs and correctly take down orders. Although this study was completed in only a small portion of the Midwest, it shows the opinions within this study do still exist and there is a need for improved relationships between nurses and physicians. Other studies have found that with proper training and system-level changes implemented by health care institutions, communication can be seen as an important element of the relationship between nurses and physicians by both parties (Bajnok et al., 2012; McCaffrey et al., 2011; Saxton, 2012).

Many institutions have recognized good communication not as an innate ability but rather as a skill that can be learned (Ang, Swain & Gale, 2013; Bajnok et al., 2012; McCaffrey et al., 2011; Saxton, 2012). Training medical staff to communicate efficiently and effectively has become a focus of many hospital education departments (McCaffrey et al., 2011). Nurses and physicians come from many different education backgrounds and may not have learned appropriate ways to communicate with other health care disciplines (Boykins, 2014; Interprofessional Education Collaborative Expert Panel, 2011). Hospitals identify a breakdown in communication as one of the most common causes of sentinel events (Saxton, 2012; Smith, 2005). Not only have hospitals implemented communication training, but many large teaching hospitals have implemented interprofessional training where nurses and physicians are required to practice annual proficiency training together as a team (Bajnok et al., 2012). This educational technique is based in the reality of medical care where the nurse and physician work together every day as a team to care for a patient. Earlier, nurses and physicians were trained for emergency situations in separate sessions, but now, nurses and physicians train together, working to perfect a medical scenario in the team they will communicate with in the future (Interprofessional Education Collaborative Expert Panel, 2011).

The nurse is often the liaison between various medical disciplines including medicine, pharmacy, social work, care coordination, physical and occupational therapy, nutrition, and medical assistants. To create a more efficient method of communication between these disciplines, emphasizing the idea of interprofessional collaboration, many organizations have implemented interprofessional rounds (Johnson & King, 2012; Licata et al., 2013). Rather than each discipline examining the patient at separate times, all disciplines perform rounds for patients as a group to coordinate care more cohesively. This provides patients with a more organized experience in the hospital (Licata et al., 2013). Many hospitals have implemented interprofessional rounds as the standard of communication within their institution, but it is up to each nurse to be an active member of this discussion. In a mixed methods study comparing the relationship of the medical–surgical nurse versus the ICU nurse with their physician counterparts, only 33% of medical–surgical nurses reported participating in interprofessional rounds when compared with 75% of ICU nurses (Johnson & King, 2012). While Johnson and King (2012) could not explain the reasons for this statistically significant (p less than 0.001) difference, qualitative interviews with medical–surgical nurses found a common theme: A greater effort was needed to speak with the physician during interprofessional rounds.

Although interprofessional rounds are meant for collaboration between all health professions, medical–surgical nurses in the Johnson and King (2012) study did not feel comfortable to present their concerns. Recognizing common barriers to effective communication occurring between nurses and physicians can help nurses to be mentally prepared and assertive in their interactions. Past research reveals common barriers to nurse–physician communication including hierarchical intimidation, organizational culture, frequently rotating physicians, approachability of nurse or physician, and time limitations (Bernhofer & Sorrell, 2014; Boykins, 2014; Hayers & Collins, 2013; Saxton, 2012; Tjia et al., 2009; Weller et al., 2011; Williams, Hevelone, & Alban, 2010). Time limitations are a shared barrier for both nurses and physicians. Pertinent information is often left out when communication is rushed, leading to errors in patient care (Tjia et al., 2009). In a study of the perception of 375 long-term-care registered nurses regarding communication barriers with their physician colleagues, 28% reported feeling rushed when reporting concerns to a physician (Tjia et al., 2009). Tjia et al. (2009) found this to be the most consistently reported barrier, followed by difficulty reaching the physician and lack of physician professionalism. In the case study, the nurse was not given time to communicate relevant information to the physician regarding Mr. Quincy's nutrition status. The physician's schedule was of greatest importance, causing communication between the physician and the nurse to be rushed or nonexistent. As a result, Mr. Quincy was unable to complete his meal, further compromising his nutrition status, wound healing, and feeling of autonomy.

Research on communication between nurses and physicians may focus on face-to-face contact; however, communication also occurs through other methods. Telephone or pager communication between nurses and physicians is a very common way of communicating, especially when physicians are caring for patients across multiple nursing units (Weller et al., 2011). Communication through telephone or pager can increase productivity and efficiency in conveying both nonurgent and urgent messages. However, the taking of telephone orders has been found to increase nurse liability, with records showing medication or treatment errors occurring because of incorrect orders (Allinson, Szeinbach, & Schneider, 2005). Consistently reading back verbal orders to the ordering physician, word for word, is one way to improve this method of communication; however, with the advent of computerized charting and ordering systems, many health institutions have banned telephone orders (Koczmara, Jelincic, & Perri, 2006).

The field of health care informatics aims to improve patient care through more seamless patient transitions between primary care provider, specialist, and hospital or health care settings (Lam et al., 2013). With the development of integrated electronic health records (EHRs) in both inpatient and outpatient settings, nurses and physicians have an opportunity to electronically communicate about a patient's progress. Communication in the EHR takes many forms: medical progress notes, nursing notes, physical assessments, and vital signs. The EHR eliminates errors that could occur with written charts such as misinterpretation of medication orders or progress notes (Bridgelal-Ram, Carpenter, & Williams, 2009). Many believe that EHRs have made communication between nurse and physician more efficient than ever (Bridgelal-Ram et al., 2009).

Role and Cultural Considerations

The laws and policies in some countries provide a framework for many communication patterns. For example, in Japan, Article 37 of the Act on Public Health Nurses, Midwives, and Nurses stipulates that without instruction from physicians, nurses are prohibited from using medical equipment, giving a person medicine or instructions about medicine, or taking any other action that carries the risk of harming a person's health if it is not approved by a physician. Therefore, when the nurse carries out these procedures, the physician must provide instruction about medical practices to the nurse. To ensure the physician's instruction is conveyed to the nurse, normally a means of communication regarding instruction is "officially" established. The word "official" here indicates the approval of an organization is required.

Therefore, the official means of communication ensures that all instructions are clearly transmitted, regardless of who is involved or what case it relates to. In principle, instruction is given in writing using an instruction form and receipt of instruction.

Regardless of the setting, communication must be achieved throughout institutions to ensure good patient outcomes. Every nurse must play an important role as an effective communicator for patients and families and foster a culture of good communication throughout the facility. Most nurses are not provided with an adequate amount of education for challenging communication skills where conflicts exist among professionals, especially between nurses and physicians. More education is needed and nurses at both generalist and advanced practice levels must understand the importance of how to resolve such conflicts.

In this chapter, a model for clarifying structures of nurse–physician communication is proposed, but this model is not always appropriate or effective owing to cultural diversity and belief models. Cultural norms and values must also be considered when addressing communication between different professionals. The official and legal society system, including governance, politics, and bureaucratic systems, must be deeply considered.

Strategies for Improvement

In view of the hectic nature of health care, many institutions have implemented the "SBAR" tool to aid all health care professionals in their communication with each other. SBAR stands for situation (a brief explanation of the current situation), background (relevant medical history and information regarding what has brought about the situation), assessment (the best assessment of what could be occurring), and recommendation (what the reporter thinks should happen next) (Boykins, 2014). The nurse caring for Mr. Quincy could have utilized SBAR in the following manner:

- Situation: "Mr. Quincy is currently eating his breakfast."
- Background: "This is the first time since the surgery three days ago that Mr. Quincy has had an appetite."

- Assessment: "With his recent surgery and his need for wound healing, the nursing team has an interest in improving his nutritional status."
- Recommendation: "Perhaps you could look for a time later in the day when you are free for 20 minutes and schedule Mr. Quincy for his dressing change. I think Mr. Quincy would benefit physically and mentally from completing and enjoying his meal."

When compared with the nurse's original response, the SBAR technique allowed the nurse to convey her concern and the medical situation in a clear, concise, professional manner. SBAR has been a successful tool in very simple situations like this as well as in more complex, emergent patient-care situations (Boykins, 2014).

Nurse–physician communication will continue to evolve as more research is completed on the intricacies of interprofessional communication. Styles of communication may always differ between professions, but the goal of communication will never change: to provide safe, patient-centered care. With the patient's best interest as the goal, nurse–physician communication can be a satisfying and constructive experience producing quality medical care. Further analysis of this case may result in the following strategies:

- Competing goals
  - The nurse wants to avoid a missed opportunity to feed the patient.
  - The physician wants to change a dressing for the patient right now.
- How to meet both demands
  - The physician comes to see the patient without notice and makes an unexpected request to the nurse. Then, it is difficult for the nurse to remain calm.
  - The nurse is too confused to find some ways to regain his or her calm (e.g., take a deep breath three times).
  - The nurse feels frustrated by the physician's interruption and so is unable to negotiate. Try to keep a positive attitude when negotiating with the physician.
  - The nurse understands that the physician is busy, and changing the dressing is obviously necessary for the patient.

- The physician says coercively that now is the only chance to change the dressing. On the other hand, the nurse believes that now is the only chance to feed the patient and does not want to bow to pressure from the physician.
- The physician's order of priority is: (1) to change the dressing for the patient; (2) to do it right now.
- The nurse's order of priority is: (1) to feed the patient now; (2) to change the dressing for the patient.
- Both agree to work toward the goal of "recovery" of Mr. Quincy.

Clinical Reasoning Questions

1. What is your plan for follow-up care of Mr. Quincy?
2. What is your plan for follow-up care of this physician?
3. Are there any other standardized guidelines that you could use for this situation?

References

Allinson, T. T., Szeinbach, S. L., & Schneider, P. J. (2005). Perceived accuracy of drug orders transmitted orally by telephone. *American Journal of Health-System Pharmacy, 62*, 78–83.

American Medical Association. (n.d.). *Patient-centered communication.* Retrieved from http://www.ama-assn.org//ama/pub/physician-resources/medical-ethics/the-ethical-force-program/patient-centered-communication.page

American Nurses Association. (2010). *Nursing: Scope and standards of practice* (2nd ed.). Silver Spring, MD: Author.

Ang, W. C., Swain, N., & Gale, C. (2013). Evaluating communication in healthcare: Systematic review and analysis of suitable communication scales. *Journal of Communication in Healthcare, 6*(4), 216–222.

Bajnok, I., Puddester, D., MacDonalds, C. J., Archibald, D., & Kuhl, D. (2012). Building positive relationships in healthcare: Evaluation of the teams of interprofessional staff interprofessional education program. *Contemporary Nurse, 42*(1), 76–89.

Bernhofer, E. I., & Sorrell, J. M. (2014). Nurses managing patients' pain may experience moral distress. *Clinical Nursing Research*, 1–14. doi:10.1177/1054773814533124

Boykins, A. D. (2014). Core communication competencies in patient-centered care. *The ABNF Journal, 25*(2), 40–45.

Bridgelal-Ram, M., Carpenter, I., & Williams, J. (2009). Reducing risk and improving quality of patient care in hospital: The contribution of standardized medical records. *Clinical Risk, 15*(5), 183–187.

Friese, C. R., & Manojlovich, M. (2012). Nurse–physician relationships in ambulatory oncology settings. *Journal of Nursing Scholarship, 44*(3), 258–265.

Hayers, C., & Collins, C. (2013). Organisational contexts of communication in healthcare. *British Journal of Healthcare Assistants, 7*(11), 553–555.

Interprofessional Education Collaborative Expert Panel. (2011). *Core competencies for interprofessional collaborative practice: Report of an expert panel*. Washington, DC: Interprofessional Education Collaborative.

Johnson, S., & King, D. (2012). Nurses' perceptions of nurse–physician relationships: Medical-surgical vs. intensive care. *MEDSURG Nursing, 21*(6), 343–347.

The Joint Commission. (2010). *Advancing effective communication, cultural competence, and patient-and family-centered care: A roadmap for hospitals*. Oakbrook Terrace, IL: Author.

Koczmara, C., Jelincic, V., & Perri, D. (2006). Communication of medication orders by telephone—"Writing it right." *Dynamics, 17*(1), 20–24.

Lam, R., Lin, V. S., Senelick, W. S., Tran, H., Moore, A. A., & Koretz, B. (2013). Older adult consumers' attitudes and preferences on electronic patient–physician messaging. *The American Journal of Managed Care, 19*, eSP7–eSP11.

Licata, J., Aneja, R. K., Kyper, C., Spencer, T., Tharp, M., Scott, M., . . . & Pasek, T. A. (2013). A foundation for patient safety: Phase I implementation of interdisciplinary bedside rounds in the pediatric intensive care unit. *Critical Care Nurse, 33*(3), 89–91.

Manojlovich, M., & Antonakos, C. (2008). Satisfaction of ICU nurses with nurse–physician communication. *Journal of Nursing Administration, 38*(5), 237–243.

Manojlovich, M., Antonakos, C., & Ronis, D. (2009). Intensive care units, communication between nurses and physicians, and patients' care outcomes. *American Journal of Critical Care Nurses, 18*(1), 21–33.

McCaffrey, R., Hayes, R. M., Cassell, A., Miller-Reyes, S., Donaldson, A., & Ferrell, C. (2011). The effect of an educational programme on attitudes of nurses and medical residents towards the benefits or positive communication and collaboration. *Journal of Advanced Nursing, 68*(2), 293–301.

Saxton, R. (2012). Communication skills training to address disruptive physician behavior. *AORN Journal, 95*(5), 602–611.

Smith, I. J. (2005). *The Joint Commission guide to improving staff communication*. Oak Brook, IL: Joint Commission Resources.

Tjia, J., Mazor, K. M., Field, T., Meterko, V., Spendard, A., & Gurwitz, J. H. (2009). Nurse-physician communication in the long-term care setting: Perceived barriers and impact on patient safety. *Journal of Patient Safety, 5*(3), 145–152.

Weller, J. M., Barrow, M., & Gasquoine, S. (2011). Interprofessional collaboration among junior doctors and nurses in the hospital setting. *Medical Education, 45*, 478–487.

Williams, M., Hevelone, N., & Alban, R. F. (2010). Measuring communication in the surgical ICU: Better communication equals better care. *Journal of the American College of Surgeons, 210*(1), 17–22.

World Health Organization. (2010). *Framework for action on interprofessional education and collaborative practice* (WHO/HRH/HPN/10.3). Geneva, Switzerland: Author.

18 ELDER MISTREATMENT

CLAIRE O'TUATHAIL

Subjective

"I never thought anything like this would ever happen. I'm so ashamed. I blame myself because she's my own flesh and blood."

Objective

Roger Reagan is an 80-year-old widowed man who is brought to the hospital emergency department in an ambulance. His neighbor Kathy is with him as she followed the ambulance in her car. Kathy became concerned about Roger as she had noticed the bins still left on the driveway days after they had been emptied by waste disposal. Kathy was also worried because she had not seen Roger puttering around the house with his dog. She rang him several times on the phone, and there was no answer. Roger is physically frail and walks with a walking aid inside and around the outside of the house. He also has a hearing impairment and suffers from chronic obstructive pulmonary disease. Roger has one daughter, on whom he relies for help with activities of daily living—food, washing and dressing, and medication management and administration. Roger's daughter has not been seen for at least a week. Kathy called for an ambulance when she found the back door unlocked and Roger lying on the floor of the utility room.

Roger was examined in the emergency department, and a chest x-ray and right hip x-ray were ordered. The chest x-ray showed consolidation in the right lung, characteristic of bacterial pneumonia. The hip x-ray confirmed a femoral fracture occurring in the proximal end of the femur. Roger was also found to be hypotensive, dehydrated, and malnourished. His clothes were dirty, and there was a strong smell of urine; he had not had a proper wash in several weeks. He was found to have numerous 1-cm circular bluish-red bruises on the upper aspect of both arms, and bruising on his posterior torso and on both legs.

Roger explained to the nurse that he was not able to care for himself very well at home and that his daughter was his main caregiver. On further assessment and questioning, he admitted that he was embarrassed to say that his daughter had not been to the house for at least a week. He said he was able to walk around the furniture to get to the toilet in the utility room, but he was not really able to do much else by way of looking after himself. He fell on the way to the toilet yesterday and was not able to get up from the floor. He also said he could not remember when he last took his medication.

He said that his daughter had always tried to do her best but she had problems of her own. She was in a new relationship with a man who was a drug addict. He said his daughter would occasionally go off to her boyfriend's house when she needed to get respite from the intensity of caring for him. Roger gives his daughter money, but he fears it is funding the drug habit of the daughter's boyfriend.

Roger is alert and slightly disoriented. He is breathless on exertion. His oxygen saturation level is 92% on admission and drops to between 86% and 92% on exertion. He appears ungroomed and disheveled. His clothes are dirty and smell of urine. His vital signs are BP: 90/60 mmHg, P: 110, respirations: 28 per minute. His temperature is within normal range, 98.1°F. There is hyperinflation of the chest, coarse crepitation on inspiration, and an audible wheeze on expiration. His abdomen is normal on examination, and bowel sounds are present.

Roger appears dehydrated and undernourished, his skin is dry with decreased turgor consistent with dehydration, and he appears to have muscle wasting. His right leg is externally rotated and shorter than the left leg, and his leg pain assessment score is 5/10 on a visual analog scale. He has 5 bluish-red 1-cm bruises on the medial aspect of his left arm and 7 bluish-red bruises on the medial aspect of his right arm. There are five 2-cm by 4-cm bruises on his posterior torso at different stages of healing, and they range from blue-red to green to yellow. The bruising on both legs is to the back of the calf, 1 cm by 2 cm in size and at different stages of healing. The nurse carefully asks Roger if he can explain the bruising, and he denies that his daughter has ever intentionally hurt him. Following written consent from Roger, all the bruises have been photographed and a copy placed in the medical record.

Literature Review

Older people have been the victims of abuse for centuries, but it is only in the last 40 years that elder abuse has been recognized as a social problem occurring within social relationships. Evidence suggests that the prevalence of elder abuse in community-dwelling older people may be anywhere between 2% and 5% (Cooper, Selwood, & Livingston, 2008; Naughton et al., 2012), depending on the definition used and methodology applied. Estimates of prevalence are likely to be an underestimate, since a number of factors such as fear, stigma, and lack of trust prevent older people from reporting incidents of abuse (Mayda, Magnus, Duggan, & Taylor-Butts, 2012). Figures on prevalence are therefore likely to be just the tip of the iceberg (Acierno et al., 2010). The most widely accepted definition of elder abuse is "A single or repeated act or lack of appropriate action, occurring within any relationship where there is an expectation of trust, which causes harm or distress to an older person" (World Health Organization [WHO], 2002, p. 3). There are a broad range of theories of elder abuse that include psychological, sociological, and cultural factors. There are six frequently referred to theories of elder abuse in the literature: psychopathology of the abuser; transgenerational violence; the web of dependency; caregiver stress; caregiving context; and sociocultural climate. The six frequently cited theories are summarized in Table 18.1.

What is common across all theories of abuse is that it occurs in the context of a relationship of trust and involves

TABLE 18.1: Theories of Elder Abuse

Theory	Major Assumptions
Psychopathology of the abuser	Alcohol or drug abuse by the abuser and/or mental illness among family members are risk factors for abuse
Transgenerational violence	Children who are victims of abuse or who witness abuse between their parents are more likely to become perpetrators of violence when they reach adulthood
The web of dependency	Caretaker is dependent on the older person for housing and money; the older person is dependent on the caregiver for daily activities due to ill health
Caregiver stress	Increasing care needs or problematic behavior, combined with the caregiver feeling forced to care for an unwanted older person or external stress for caregiver contribute to abuse
Caregiving context	Factors such as social isolation, shared living arrangement, lack of close family ties, and lack of community support or access to resources contribute to abuse
Sociocultural climate	Factors such as inadequate housing, recent relocation and adaptation to culture, loss of support systems, and the decline of stature within the family create a climate that supports abuse

Adapted from Jones, Holstege, and Holstege (1997).

behavior by someone and the effect that this behavior has on the other person. The five most commonly cited types of elder abuse are:

1. Physical abuse
2. Psychological abuse
3. Financial abuse
4. Sexual abuse
5. Neglect

Elder abuse is a multifaceted issue complicated by social and biological influences such as ageism, individual social circumstances, and normal aging processes, and McCreadie (2002) states that in order to understand elder abuse, a considerable amount of deconstruction has to occur.

Johannesen and LoGiudice (2013) undertook a systematic review of risk factors for elder abuse to identify which risk factors are consistently identified in elder abuse literature.

Their findings suggest risk factors for the older person include cognitive impairment, behavioral problems, psychiatric or psychological problems, functional dependency, poor physical health or frailty, low income or wealth, trauma, or past abuse (Johannesen & LoGiudice, 2013). Perpetrator risk factors included caregiver burden or stress and psychiatric or psychological problems (Johannesen & LoGiudice, 2013). Family disharmony and poor or conflictual relationships were identified as relationship risk factors, and low social support and living with others were identified as environmental risk factors (Johannesen & LoGiudice, 2013). In identifying elder abuse in the domestic dwelling setting, health professionals are in a crucial position to respond appropriately. However, evidence suggests that they underrecognize and underrespond appropriately to abuse (Fulmer et al., 2005; Manthorpe et al., 2007).

Role and Cultural Considerations

Recognition of elder abuse with appropriate and timely response by health care professionals is important to ensure the safety and well-being of older people in the hospital or in a community setting. In addition to the normal nursing assessment of Roger, the nurse can use a screening tool to identify the risk of or potential for abuse. The Elder Abuse Suspicion Index (EASI) is a useful six-item questionnaire for screening for elder abuse in the clinical setting (Yaffe, Wolfson, Lithwick, & Weiss, 2008). If suspicions are raised, the tool prompts the physician or nurse to refer the older person to adult protective services for further evaluation. To address the issue of abuse, the nurse will need to ask some initial questions. Interviewing an older person about abuse requires skill and patience, and it is important to build a rapport with the older person. A useful strategy is to ask some general questions, followed by some more specific ones. It is important that any conversation about the possibility of abuse takes place with Roger in the absence of his daughter. Questions might include:

- Has anyone at home ever hurt you?
- Has anyone at home ever touched you without your consent?

- Has anyone at home ever made you do things you did not want to do?
- Has anyone at home ever scolded or threatened you?
- Are you afraid of anyone at home?
- Are you often left alone at home?
- Has anyone at home ever failed to help you take care of yourself when you needed help?

(Adapted from Aravanis and American Medical Association [1992].)

Follow-up questions should focus on exploring the abuse—what, how, when, how often? Who is the perpetrator? How does the patient cope? Assess safety issues in the patient's living situation; if the patient is in immediate danger, call law enforcement/police. When elder abuse is suspected or detected, the nurse should report concerns to his or her line manager and/or adult protective services, sometimes referred to as elder abuse response teams or case workers for elder abuse. It is important that every nurse caring for older people, regardless of the clinical setting, is aware of the local policies relating to the identification and management of elder abuse. Where a nurse suspects abuse and the patient is in immediate danger, it is necessary to inform law enforcement and subsequently ensure protection of the older person.

In Roger's case, the nurse will need to know what he can do for himself and what activities of daily living (ADL) he needs assistance with from his daughter. The nurse will establish what the daughter's caregiving role is and whether she is a legal guardian for Roger. In the course of the physical assessment, the nurse will ask about how the bruising occurred and document the exact size, shape, and color of each of the bruises. A body chart can be used to complete this documentation. The nurse could discuss prevention strategies with Roger and allow him to explore his options for the possibility of another caregiver to be involved in his care, in addition to having his daughter live with him. Alternatively, he may want his daughter to find another place to live. Developing a plan for safety is an important role for the nurse to consider with Roger. He could carry a mobile phone around the house to ensure that if he fell or needed help, he could call someone. Also, a medical alert alarm could be worn by Roger; when activated, the call would go straight to emergency services.

Nurses are on the front line of services to older people both in the hospital and community health services and are therefore in a prime position to identify and respond appropriately to elder abuse. Some countries (e.g., Canada, Israel, and the United States) have mandatory reporting legislation that ensures that practitioners respond appropriately when there are concerns. Nurses have an ethical and professional responsibility to ensure appropriate treatment and protection of patients in their care, especially older people. The nurse's role in the comprehensive nursing assessment of the older person in his or her care is crucial to the identification and management of abuse. When assessing the older person, the nurse must undertake a review of the issues relating to family relationships and dynamics and, in particular, any family member caring for the older person and living at home. Family functioning and history of family violence are also important issues for the nurse to consider. Nurses need to understand variations in the cultural and ethnic background of the older person in order to fully understand the context of elder abuse within the family. Indeed, general population understanding of abuse in one country may differ from understandings of abuse in another country. For example, the most significant form of elder abuse in Kenya is considered to be abandonment of an older person in a hospital (WHO, 2002), and this is witnessed as a seasonal problem with higher incidences in times of drought, poor crop yield, and loss of livestock. In India, lack of caring by a daughter-in-law is considered abusive, and in Hong Kong, "dumping" an older person in a nursing home is perceived as abusive (Kwan, 1995).

Assessment and Strategy

Roger's case study highlights many of the issues relating to abuse of older people in domestic settings. Risk factors in Roger's case are that he is old and vulnerable, and his assessment reveals that he has diminished ability to care for himself. Roger has been admitted to hospital following a crisis at home. In this case, Roger is subjected to neglect and abandonment by his daughter, and because she is taking money from him to fund a drug habit, he is being financially abused as well. He says he feels he is giving her the money under undue pressure. During the assessment, Roger reveals that his daughter has been absent for over a week and that this has happened several times in the past. Roger explains that his daughter normally provides him with physical assistance, and a lack of recent help from her has led to his poor state of hygiene and, subsequently, the chest infection and fracture. He has unexplained bruising to his arms, torso, and legs, and on further questioning he states that "she sometimes gets a bit rough with me." He says she is always in a rush to get him washed and dressed, and she sometimes pokes him in the back and grabs him by the arm to get him in and out of the chair. Roger says that when he cannot move his legs quickly, she gives his legs a prod with her foot. This assessment reveals that he is being subjected to physical abuse by his daughter. Roger is found to have mild cognitive impairment using the Mini Mental State Exam, his score is 20 points out of 30, and this would explain why he is unable to care for himself, prepare meals, or remember when he has last taken his medication.

Strategies to prevent further abuse in Roger's case might include discussing the option to have another home caregiver in addition to the daughter living at home. An alternative might be to suggest that the daughter will need to find alternative accommodation. Roger should carry a mobile phone or alarm system when he is mobilizing around the house and outside. Kathy, his neighbor, could also have a key so she can call in to see him regularly. Following an assessment of Roger's needs, the nurse should make a referral to community support services so that Roger can be assessed for supports needed to be able to remain at home for as long as possible.

When an older person is admitted to the hospital, the nurse may suspect elder abuse in the course of his or her assessment of the patient. The term *elder abuse* describes intentional acts or omissions by a caregiver or trusted other that causes harm or distress to an older person. In this case, Roger is a vulnerable older adult and has a diminished capacity for self-care. Vulnerable older adults are often easy targets for perpetrators of elder abuse. The abuse in this case may be relatively recent, or it may be happening over a long period of time and surfaces only when Roger is admitted to the hospital.

The types of abuse in this case are neglect, abandonment, financial exploitation, and physical abuse of Roger by his daughter. Roger's daughter has not provided help with activities of living for at least 1 week, and this has happened in the past. His injuries, worsening medical condition, and poor hygiene are all related to his lack of care by his daughter. He has bruises, and it is uncertain whether they were inflicted intentionally by his daughter.

Distinguishing elder abuse from problems due to the normal progression of aging can sometimes be challenging. In Roger's case, he has a fractured neck of femur as a result of his fall. This type of injury is not uncommon in physically frail older people with visual and physical impairments. In addition, bruising can be the result of furniture-walking around the house and can occur easily when the patient has long-term use of steroids. He has a mild cognitive impairment, which may influence his ability to remember where he put his medication and if and when he last took a dose.

Older people are often reluctant to disclose that they have experienced abuse for a number of hypothesized reasons. One of the suggested reasons for this lack of disclosure is that the older person feels responsible. In this case, Roger states, "I blame myself because she's my own flesh and blood." Another explanation is that the older person is embarrassed about being abused by an adult child and feels powerless to stop it. In this case, Roger says, "I never thought anything like this would ever happen. I'm so ashamed." Pride may prevent acknowledgment of this powerlessness, and there may be a reluctance to admit to physical or cognitive decline associated with the aging process. The older person may fear retribution by the caregiver if he or she discloses abuse, which may lead to more severe forms of physical and psychological abuse, and there is the fear that reporting the abuser may lead to institutionalizing the older person.

Conclusion

As the global population of older people is increasing, the issue of elder abuse will continue to be a concern for nurses in all practice settings. This case study challenges nurses and advanced practitioners to reflect on the crucial aspects of their role in cases of elder abuse. It is important that nurses are able to effectively identify and recognize abusive situations and take appropriate action. This discussion has briefly outlined issues, challenges, and responses within the area of elder abuse in the domestic setting; however, the issues apply to all care settings for older people.

Clinical Reasoning Questions

1. What are the physical, psychosocial, and environmental risk factors that need to be considered in cases of elder abuse?
2. What are the key assessment instruments for use with older people that would contribute to the assessment of an older person at risk of elder abuse?
3. What impact does the family unit have on the existence of elder abuse?
4. What is the role of the nurse in record keeping/documentation in cases of elder abuse?
5. What do you need to change in your practice to ensure you are able to recognize and respond appropriately to elder abuse?

References

Acierno, R., Hernandez, M. A., Amstadter, A. B., Resnick, H. S., Steve, K., Muzzy, W., & KilRoger, D. G. (2010). Prevalence and correlates of emotional, physical, sexual, and financial abuse and potential neglect in the United States: The National Elder Mistreatment Study. *Journal Information*, *100*(2), 292–297.

Aravanis, S. C., & American Medical Association. (1992). *Diagnostic and treatment guidelines on elder abuse and neglect*. Chicago, IL: American Medical Association.

Cooper, C., Selwood, A., & Livingston, G. (2008). The prevalence of elder abuse and neglect: A systematic review. *Age and Aging, 37*(2), 151–160.

Fulmer, T., Paveza, G., Vandeweerd, C., Guadagno, L., Fairchild, S., Norman, R., . . . Bolton-Blatt, M. (2005). Neglect assessment in urban emergency departments and confirmation by an expert clinical team. *Journals of Gerontology. Series A, Biological Sciences and Medical Sciences, 60*(8), 1002–1006.

Johannesen, M., & LoGiudice, D. (2013, January 1). Elder abuse: A systematic review of risk factors in community-dwelling elders. *Age and Aging, 42*(3), 292–298.

Jones, J. S., Holstege, C., & Holstege, H. (1997, October). Elder abuse and neglect: Understanding the causes and potential risk factors. *American Journal of Emergency Medicine, 15*(6), 579–583.

Kwan, A. Y. (1995, June 22). Elder abuse in Hong Kong. *Journal of Elder Abuse & Neglect, 6*, 65–80.

Manthorpe, J., Biggs, S., McCreadie, C., Tinker, A., Hills, A., O'Keefe, M., . . . Erens, B. (2007). The UK national study of abuse and neglect among older people. *Nursing Older People, 19*(8), 24–26.

Mayda, J., Magnus, B., Duggan, J., & Taylor-Butts, A. (2012). Feasibility study for a survey measuring abuse and neglect of older adults. *Journal of Elder Abuse & Neglect, 24*(2), 161–178.

McCreadie, C. (2002). A review of research outcomes in elder abuse. *Journal of Adult Protection, 4*, 3–8.

Naughton, C., Drennan, J., Lyons, I., Lafferty, A., Treacy, M., Phelan, A., O'Loughlin, A., Delaney, L. (2012). Elder abuse and neglect in Ireland: Results from a national prevalence survey. *Age and ageing, 41*(1), 98–103. doi: 10.1093/ageing/afr107.

World Health Organization. (2002). *The Toronto declaration on the global prevention of elder abuse*. Geneva, Switzerland: Author.

Yaffe, M. J., Wolfson, C., Lithwick, M., & Weiss, D. (2008). Development and validation of a tool to improve physician identification of elder abuse: The Elder Abuse Suspicion Index (EASI). *Journal of Elder Abuse & Neglect, 20*(3), 276–300.

19 CONNECTED ENVIRONMENTS FOR HEALTHY AGING

HELEN BARTLETT AND MATTHEW CARROLL

Subjective

"It's so hard for me to get around."

Objective

Susan Samuels lives on her own in the family home. Since her husband died 2 years ago, she has lost interest in leisure activities and socializing and only goes out occasionally to a neighborhood general store, which is about a 20-minute walk away. Her driver's license has lapsed, and she has lost the confidence to resume driving. While Susan receives periodic phone calls from her adult children overseas and sister-in-law, she complains that she rarely has anyone to talk to for days. She feels lonely and isolated and that life is not worth living.

Susan is 78 years old. She nursed her husband at home for 3 years after his stroke, and after he died, contact with health and social services ceased. Her siblings are no longer alive, and her two adult children and grandchildren live overseas. She lives on the edge of a rural town, where she and her husband moved on retirement to enjoy more rural pursuits. Susan worked for a few years as a primary school teacher until she had her family and subsequently volunteered from time to time with a local children's charity. Susan owns her own home and is a self-funded retiree, receiving a small teacher's pension and drawing on modest savings to supplement her income.

Susan visits the general practitioner (GP) occasionally and is on medication (Metoprol 25 mg twice daily) for high blood pressure, which was 140/80 at her last visit. She is quite mobile, but suffers from arthritis, for which she takes paracetamol as pain relief. During her last visit, she completed the Geriatric Depression Scale (Yesavage & Sheikh, 1986), receiving a score of 6/15, which is suggestive of depression and warrants further follow-up. Her home is a single-story family residence, with a small garden at the front and back. It has not been renovated for many years and is very damp in winter because there is no proper heating. She used to be very active and enjoyed walking, gardening, and cooking. However, she now finds the garden overwhelming and worries about its upkeep. Her diet consists mainly of processed foods and is low in protein, fresh fruit, and vegetables. She likes to read and follow current affairs, but no longer buys a newspaper or visits the library. Her main stimulation is provided by the TV, which Susan has on most of the day. Her neighbors are working couples or busy young families who have little interaction with Susan, and she does not like to bother them. She has found it difficult to maintain contact with friends as she does not drive any longer.

Susan's assessment will need to take into account many factors impacting on her situation, including her geographical location, driving capacity, financial status, social and family networks, health status (including nutrition), and the availability of formal and informal support locally. Although immediate measures to improve her health outcomes can be taken, many of these broader factors are likely to remain as barriers to aging well, and longer term solutions such as a change in her living arrangements may be needed.

An assessment of Susan's home and community care needs would help address a number of issues highlighted in the case study, including the health and social isolation concerns, as well as home maintenance issues. The aim of home and community care services (also known as domiciliary, nonmedical home care, or social care) is to provide continuity of environment, maintain independence and social connections, and reduce admission to acute or long-term care (Low, Yap, & Brodaty, 2011). Nurses, as part of multidisciplinary teams, play a key role in the assessment and delivery of home and community care services, with need for case management to ensure access and uptake of appropriate services (Low et al., 2011; Ryan, McCann, & McKenna, 2009).

Home and community care assessment would include an assessment of mobility limitations, which are a key predictor of adverse health outcomes including disability, cognitive impairment, institutionalization, and falls (Van Kan et al., 2009). Gait speed of walking at the usual pace over 4 m has been found to be a quick and reliable marker of functional health status, with people taking more than 5 seconds to complete the course likely to be in need of further assessment and support (Van Kan et al., 2009). Given Susan's minimal engagement with the health system since her husband's death, it is also likely that the assessment will identify other unrecognized chronic conditions, including depression, which will require the development of a coordinated care plan, including home and center-based supports.

Literature Review

The case study highlights the complexity of the aging experience, with Susan presenting with an array of health and social care needs, as well as issues concerning access to services arising from her rural location and driving cessation. There is a growing recognition of the need for a coordinated response that simplifies access to services, connecting the disparate environments of aging. This was identified in a recent review of the Australian aged care system (Productivity Commission, 2011), which found that clients, carers, and service providers had difficulty navigating the system. One of the outcomes of this review has been the establishment of a single online gateway for aged care services aimed at giving people more choice, control, and access to a wider range of aged care services (see www.myagedcare.gov.au).

One of the key issues highlighted in the case study is the experience of social isolation, with the prevalence of severe isolation estimated to be around 7% of all older people, and around one third reporting being sometimes lonely (Bartlett, Warburton, Lui, Peach, & Carroll, 2012). Social isolation has been repeatedly associated with increased morbidity and mortality and reduced psychological health and well-being (Bartlett et al., 2012). Widowhood is often a trigger of social isolation, and is again associated with increased mortality and morbidity, in part because of the loss of a confidante and health advocate, which may reduce the likelihood of health-seeking behaviors (Stroebe, Schut, & Stroebe, 2007).

Involvement in later life learning activities has been highlighted as playing a critical role in addressing social isolation by reconnecting older people to their communities, as well as building confidence and self-worth and helping to maintain health and well-being (Townsend & Delves, 2009). Similarly, the Internet has been shown to be a powerful tool for older people to build and maintain social connections (Hogeboom, McDermott, Perrin, Osman, & Bell-Ellison, 2010), and has also been associated with reduced risk of depression (Cotten, Ford, Ford, & Hale, 2012) and increased independence through access to online services such as banking, shopping, or health care management (Wagner, Hassanein, & Head, 2010).

Taking technology further, recent developments in smart home technologies provide an array of unobtrusive devices such as sensors, tele-health, and communications systems that can create a safer home environment. A recent review found that such devices are generally acceptable to older people and that the limited research to date suggests that they can help maintain functional and cognitive status and support aging in place (Morris, Adair, Miller, OzSusan, & Hansen, 2013).

Another important factor influencing both health and social outcomes as people age is involvement in physical activity. The benefits of physical activity in maintaining health and well-being are well documented, including reducing the risk of developing chronic diseases, increased independence, and improving quality of life and well-being, with health benefits found in people increasing their physical activity levels relatively late in life (Hamer, Lavoie, & Bacon, 2014). Moreover, for those older adults who already present with one or more diseases, commencing a regular exercise program reduces disease symptoms and medication needs (Opdenacker, Delecluse, & Boen, 2011). To achieve these benefits, international guidelines recommend a minimum of 150 minutes a week of moderate-intensity activity, broken down to 30 minute sessions each day, preferably on all days of the week. In addition, activities should challenge the individual's strength, fitness, balance, and flexibility (Sims et al., 2006).

One factor closely associated with social isolation and access to services is driving cessation, with older women likely to cease driving earlier than men (Adler & Rottunda, 2006).

Driving cessation is associated with accelerated declines in health and depression (Edwards, Lunsman, Perkins, Rebok, & Roth, 2009), in part because driving plays an important instrumental role in accessing services and maintaining health and well-being. While public transport is often touted as the alternative to private vehicle use, the mobility issues that led to driving cessation are also likely to impact on the ability to use public transport (Adler & Rottunda, 2006). More effort is needed to look at ways to maintain driving as long as possible, including through physical and cognitive interventions (Edwards et al., 2009) as well as restricted driving regimes such as staying within a limited geographical area and driving during the daytime. In addition, there is a need to provide greater support to people as they approach the point of ceasing driving to ensure a smooth transition and reduce the likelihood of adverse outcomes (Liddle, McKenna, & Bartlett, 2007).

Geographic location can also play a pivotal role in access to services and networks as well as opportunities to engage in learning and physical activity groups. In the current case, Susan and her husband moved to a rural setting postretirement to enjoy the pastoral lifestyle. Known as counterurbanization or tree and sea changing, the experience of living in a rural or coastal community may be initially positive, but with declining health and reduced access to services and facilities and often geographic separation from family and social networks, life can become increasingly challenging (Morton & Weng, 2013). Although the research is scarce, there is evidence to suggest that rural communities face greater challenges because of the combined effects of accelerated aging of the population (due to the out-migration of younger people seeking greater work opportunities as well as the in-migration of older people referred to previously), reduced access, environmental exposures (including the need to drive extended distances), and lifestyle risk factors such as greater rates of smoking and drinking and reduced likelihood of health service utilization (Australian Institute of Health and Welfare, 2012; Davis & Bartlett, 2008).

Finally, the evidence also points to the increased risk of malnutrition or undernutrition in later life, particularly for those who are experiencing social isolation. A recent study of community-living older adults receiving nursing home care in Victoria, Australia, found that just over 40% of participants were either malnourished or at risk of malnutrition (Rist, Miles, & Karimi, 2012). Another study, also undertaken in Victoria, found that one in six older adults visiting a GP for annual health assessment was at nutritional risk (Winter, Flanagan, McNaughton, & Nowson, 2013). These studies highlight the nutritional issues and risk factors for older people living in the community and point to the need for preventive health strategies that incorporate routine nutrition screening and intervention programs with a focus on meal preparation and opportunities for eating in social settings.

Solutions and Strategies

A multifaceted approach is needed to address the challenges experienced by Susan. The community nurse practitioner has an important role in working as part of the health and social care team to facilitate support and provide preventive services. The evidence suggests that a collaborative approach between agencies is important to ensure those in need are identified and receive care and support that is coordinated and effective (Everingham, Cuthill, Warburton, & Bartlett, 2012).

The research evidence outlined previously supports a range of strategies and solutions to address Susan's situation. She would benefit from improved networks to increase social engagement; learning opportunities to provide mental stimulation; increased physical activity levels to reduce health risks associated with inactivity; help with her home and garden to enable her to live independently for as long as possible; support to renew her driving license and/or regular transport assistance; and health screening to assess nutritional status and monitor and prevent chronic diseases, including depression.

The following support options should be explored:

- Regular contact with primary health care services for screening and referrals as necessary. GPs and community nurses can mobilize the necessary resources.
- Participation in social gatherings, for example, a local luncheon club or activity group, where Susan could make new contacts and increase her connections.

- Improved access to information and communication with her family overseas through a home computer. Good broadband coverage would be necessary, which can also be a challenge in rural areas.
- Volunteer schemes to assist Susan with transport, provide companionship, and help with gardening. Given her previous interest in volunteering, Susan might also be assisted to find ways to make a contribution to volunteering in her community.
- Local physical activity/exercise classes and walking groups to ensure that Susan increases her physical activity to at least 30 minutes a day on 5 days of the week. The possibility of finding her an exercise buddy should be explored.
- Learning resources to access could include University of the Third Age (U3A), seniors' associations, computer clubs, book clubs, and mobile library services.
- Social welfare services to assist Susan to remain independent in her home for as long as possible might include home help and gardening/home maintenance.
- Assessment of future housing options, including potential plans for assisted living/retirement accommodation. While aging in place should be supported as far as possible, in Susan's case future housing options may need to be explored given the condition of her house and garden, along with the rural location, which limits her access to services and opportunities for social connection.

Clinical Reasoning Questions

1. What other health and social services should be involved in the multidisciplinary review of Susan's home and community care needs?
2. Are there any issues that can be quickly and easily addressed?
3. Is the rural setting impacting on Susan's access to services? If so, are there tele-health options or other ways to ensure that she has access to the services that she needs?
4. What specific role might a community nurse play in the multidisciplinary assessment of this individual?

References

Adler, G., & Rottunda, S. (2006). Older adults' perspectives on driving cessation. *Journal of Aging Studies, 20*(3), 227–235. doi:http://dx.doi.org/10.1016/j.jaging.2005.09.003

Australian Institute of Health and Welfare. (2012). *Impact of rurality on health status.* Retrieved from http://www.aihw.gov.au/rural-health-impact-of-rurality/

Bartlett, H., Warburton, J., Lui, C., Peach, L., & Carroll, M. (2012). Preventing social isolation in later life: Findings and insights from a pilot Queensland intervention study. *Aging and Society, 33*(7), 1167–1189.

Cotten, S. R., Ford, G., Ford, S., & Hale, T. M. (2012). Internet use and depression among older adults. *Computers in Human Behavior, 28*(2), 496–499. doi:http://dx.doi.org/10.1016/j.chb.2011.10.021

Davis, S., & Bartlett, H. (2008). Healthy aging in rural Australia: Issues and challenges. *Australasian Journal on Aging, 27*(2), 56–60. doi:10.1111/j.1741-6612.2008.00296.x

Edwards, J. D., Lunsman, M., Perkins, M., Rebok, G. W., & Roth, D. L. (2009). Driving cessation and health trajectories in older adults. *The Journals of Gerontology Series A: Biological Sciences and Medical Sciences, 64A*(12), 1290–1295. doi:10.1093/gerona/glp114

Everingham, J., Cuthill, M., Warburton, J., & Bartlett, H. (2012). Collaborative governance of ageing: Challenges for local government in partnering with the seniors' sector. *Local Government Studies, 38*(2), 161–181.

Hamer, M., Lavoie, K. L., & Bacon, S. L. (2014). Taking up physical activity in later life and healthy aging: The English longitudinal study of aging. *British Journal of Sports Medicine, 48*(3), 239–243.

Hogeboom, D. L., McDermott, R. J., Perrin, K. M., Osman, H., & Bell-Ellison, B. A. (2010). Internet use and social networking among middle aged and older adults. *Educational Gerontology, 36*(2), 93–111. doi:10.1080/03601270903058507

Liddle, J., McKenna, K., & Bartlett, H. (2007). Improving outcomes for older retired drivers: The UQDRIVE program. *Australian Occupational Therapy Journal, 54*(4), 303–306. doi:10.1111/j.1440-1630.2006.00614.x

Low, L.-F., Yap, M., & Brodaty, H. (2011). A systematic review of different models of home and community care services for older persons. *BMC Health Services Research, 11*(1), 93.

Morris, M., Adair, B., Miller, K., OzSusan, E., & Hansen, R. (2013). Smart-home technologies to assist older people to live well at home. *Journal of Aging Science, 1*(101), 2.

Morton, L. W., & Weng, C.-Y. (2013). Health and healthcare among the rural aging. In N. Glasgow & E. H. Berry (Eds.), *Rural aging in 21st century America*. Dodrecht, Netherlands: Springer.

Opdenacker, J., Delecluse, C., & Boen, F. (2011). A 2-year follow-up of a lifestyle physical activity versus a structured exercise intervention in older adults. *Journal of the American Geriatrics Society*. doi:10.1111/j.1532-5415.2011.03551.x

Productivity Commission. (2011). *Caring for older Australians: Overview* (Report No. 53, Final Inquiry Report). Canberra, Australia: Author. Retrieved from http://www.pc.gov.au/__data/assets/pdf_file/0016/110932/aged-care-overview-booklet.pdf

Rist, G., Miles, G., & Karimi, L. (2012). The presence of malnutrition in community-living older adults receiving home nursing services. *Nutrition & Dietetics, 69*(1), 46–50.

Ryan, A. A., McCann, S., & McKenna, H. (2009). Impact of community care in enabling older people with complex needs to remain at home. *International Journal of Older People Nursing, 4*(1), 22–32. doi:10.1111/j.1748-3743.2008.00152.x

Sims, J., Hill, K., Hunt, S., Haralambous, B., Brown, A., Engel, L., . . . Ory, M. (2006). *National physical activity recommendations for older Australians: Discussion document*. Retrieved from http://www.health.gov.au/internet/main/publishing.nsf/Content/B656FF3728F48860CA257BF0001B09D9/$File/pa-guide-older-disc.pdf

Stroebe, M., Schut, H., & Stroebe, W. (2007). Health outcomes of bereavement. *The Lancet, 370*(9603), 1960–1973.

Townsend, R., & Delves, M. (2009). Tree changes or wholesale changes: The role of adult education in transitions in regional life. *Rural Society, 19*(2), 96–105.

Van Kan, G. A., Rolland, Y., Andrieu, S., Bauer, J., Beauchet, O., Bonnefoy, M., . . . Inzitari, M. (2009). Gait speed at usual pace as a predictor of adverse outcomes in community-dwelling older people: An International Academy on Nutrition and Aging (IANA) Task Force. *Journal of Nutrition, Health & Aging, 13*(10), 881–889.

Wagner, N., Hassanein, K., & Head, M. (2010). Computer use by older adults: A multi-disciplinary review. *Computers in Human Behavior, 26*(5), 870–882. doi:http://dx.doi.org/10.1016/j.chb.2010.03.029

Winter, J., Flanagan, D., McNaughton, S., & Nowson, C. (2013). Nutrition screening of older people in a community general practice, using the MNA-SF. *Journal of Nutrition, Health & Aging, 17*(4), 322–325.

Yesavage, J. A., & Sheikh, J. I. (1986). 9/Geriatric Depression Scale (GDS) recent evidence and development of a shorter violence. *Clinical Gerontologist, 5*(1–2), 165–173.

20 POSITIVE RELATIONSHIPS IN RESIDENTIAL DEMENTIA CARE

ANDREW HUNTER

Subjective

"Yes I like to talk to people but the staff are very busy. I don't like to bother them—they don't have much time to chat."

Objective

Mr. Thomas Trent is a 77-year-old man who lives in a nursing home. He moved there 2 years ago following the death of his wife and after receiving a diagnosis of Alzheimer's disease. Thomas has a Mini Mental State Score of 10, which indicates severe cognitive impairment (NICE-SCIE, 2011). He is being treated for high blood pressure, which is well controlled. Otherwise, Thomas enjoys good physical health. Until recently, he has attended to his own personal care. But over the last 2 months, Thomas required encouragement to dress and wash himself, resulting in his shouting at staff members and, on one occasion, slapping a member of the staff. This incident left Thomas tearful, and he continues to express his regret and upset.

Until recently, Thomas has participated in activities within the nursing home. He usually enjoys music and exercise groups and has enjoyed spending time with the nursing staff, when they are available. Over the past 2 months, Thomas has spent more time in his single room. When not there, he can be found at the nurses' station or nursing home reception area. Thomas indicates that he wants to spend more time in the company of staff as he does not want to be with the "old ones," referring to the other residents. The nursing home staff are growing increasingly frustrated at Thomas's "interference" at the nurses' station and in the reception area. There was one incident where Thomas shouted at the receptionist and relatives of another resident when they did not include him in their discussion.

Thomas has a nephew who visits once a month. He enjoys these visits and spends long periods talking about the past, about relatives, and experiences with his nephew. Thomas's nephew used to take him out for the day. But recently he told the nursing staff that he does not feel comfortable taking Thomas away from the nursing home alone, as he is concerned he will not be able to persuade Thomas to return with him. The nephew disclosed to the nursing staff that he thinks Thomas is "getting worse" and that Thomas tells him he hates the nursing home and wants to go home. The nursing team is now considering how to respond to the changes in Thomas's behavior and have discussed a number of options including antipsychotic medication.

Literature Review

Much of the research and theoretical literature produced around dementia care in the last 20 years has attempted to understand how relationships with others, specifically staff, impacts on the lives of people with dementia. The future care that Thomas receives is dependent on the staff's understanding of dementia, their attitude to dementia, and, crucially, their relationship with Thomas. The changes in Thomas's behavior could be viewed by staff as inevitable symptoms of dementia, his response to his social circumstances, or even simply as an older man being difficult. Regardless of their interpretation, the response of the staff at this time will impact upon the care received and the quality of life experienced by Thomas in the coming months and years.

There is a growing understanding in national and international literature that current dementia care provision is not meeting the needs of people with dementia. Reports considering dementia provision in the United States and internationally (O'Shea, 2007; Thies & Bleiler, 2012) make the general observation that both inpatient and community-based services are not rising to the challenge. With specific reference to residential care, *2012 Alzheimer's Disease Facts and Figures* (Thies & Bleiler, 2012) and *Implementing Policy for Dementia Care in Ireland* (O'Shea, 2007) are clear regarding the nature of change required and the complex nature of care delivery for residents with dementia. More resources are required to delay the point at which people are required to enter residential care, and their quality of life should be supported at home for as long as possible. When residential care is required, service providers need to acknowledge that quality of life for people with dementia is a complex issue, influenced by many things other than conventional nursing and medical care. The need to improve communication skills of people caring for dementia patients at all levels has been demonstrated in the literature (Thies & Bleiler, 2012; O'Shea, 2007). The need for these improved communication skills is further evidenced by the fact that 90% of people with dementia experience behavioral and psychological symptoms of dementia. These include agitation, aggression, loss of inhibitions, and psychosis. These symptoms cause great distress for both the individuals with dementia and those caring for them (NICE-SCIE, 2011).

Although it is commonly believed that people with dementia cannot learn new things and develop relationships, there is a growing body of research affirming that positive change is possible and that the nature of staff–resident relationships is fundamental to residents' quality of life (QOL). Cahill and Diaz-Ponce (2011), in their qualitative study, undertook 55 face-to-face interviews considering QOL with residents with dementia. They identified four key themes: social contact, attachment, pleasurable activities, and affect. This study identified that residents with dementia, specifically those with severe dementia, were seeking human contact in response to feelings of isolation and loneliness. The human contact sought by residents with dementia is best understood in the context of positive staff–patient relationships whereby psychosocial interventions (PSIs) are undertaken in an effective and purposeful manner.

Bates, Boote, and Beverley (2004) define *psychosocial interventions* (PSIs) as therapeutic endeavors involving human interactive behavior between therapist(s) and client(s) throughout the course of the intervention (Bates et al., 2004,

p. e2). In application to the case involving Thomas and his need for human contact with the nursing home staff, PSIs may focus on practical and timely approaches to communication and care. A PSI used in the context of a staff–resident relationship with Thomas may be as simple as staff taking the time to discuss something that is pleasurable to him or asking him what he wishes to do rather than directing them.

In a more recent research study, Smebye and Kirkevold (2013) considered the impact of relationships on personhood in dementia care. They researched 10 cases (each comprising a person with dementia, a family caregiver, and a professional caregiver), undertaking semi-structured interviews to explore the definition and impact of the relationships. This research identified a range of relationship types that served to diminish or sustain the personhood of the people with dementia. Smebye and Kirkevold (2013) noted that when staff attempted to collaborate with and engage residents with dementia, staff could move beyond a focus on physical needs using their improved relationship and enhanced knowledge as a basis to address residents' psychosocial needs.

Mutuality between residents with dementia and their caregivers has long been viewed as contributing to the nature of care. In seminal work that developed the concept of personhood in dementia, Kitwood and Bredin (1992) undertook research using observation to empirically develop 12 indicators of relative well-being for people with dementia, noting that the experiences, outcomes, and pressures felt by residents with dementia are not unique to them. This research found that residents with dementia are dependent on staff who are also subject to personal pressures such as ill health and financial worries. This work and the work of Kitwood (1997) introduce the concept that staff must address their own needs before being able to effectively work with residents with dementia, identifying a process of interdependence among residents with dementia, staff, and the institution. The understanding that how caregivers and society at large think about people with dementia impacts their well-being is an important concept that has been further developed by contemporary dementia writers and researchers. Bartlett and O'Connor (2007) argue that the concept of personhood must be extended into the realms of citizenship and discrimination. In the case of Thomas, such an understanding on the part of nursing home staff could help them reframe Thomas's needs. This understanding offers hope that the difficulties the caregivers are experiencing trying to care for Thomas will be addressed in a manner that is mutually beneficial.

In an effort to understand how the personhood of residents with dementia is affected by staff experience of caring, Edberg et al. (2008) undertook content analysis of focus group data from 35 nurse interviews. Analysis considered the staff's capacity to deliver the care they wanted to and the strain on staff and reduced job satisfaction when their capacity was reduced in response to factors such as limited education and managerial support. The researchers identified that care delivery, including staff–resident relationships, is defined by the interaction of the needs of residents with dementia, staff needs, other residents' needs, and the needs of the institution. This research concludes that the interaction between these factors creates a conflict between staff values, the staff's urge to do the best for residents with dementia, and the many practical constraints that prevent them from doing so, including staffing levels, lack of education, and limited time. This understanding shows that staff strain is caused by limited personal ability to undertake the nursing care the staff wish to perform, including developing meaningful relationships. The impact of failing to deliver the care staff wanted to, as well as staff strain, was found to be a personal consequence of their powerlessness (Edberg et al., 2008).

Ward, Vass, Neeru, Cydonie, and Beau (2008) offer an alternative view to those researchers who view staff ability to deliver as being influenced by levels of individual empowerment. They developed a conceptual understanding based on interviews and videos of care interactions with 32 staff and 28 residents with dementia. Their qualitative study considered communication between staff and residents with dementia, identifying a mismatch between the tasks staff prioritize and the social needs of residents with dementia. Ward et al. (2008) recorded low levels of communication between residents with dementia and staff. This was attributed to lack of resources and a workplace cultural focus on completing achievable physical tasks. Ward et al. (2008) conclude that staff are too willing to label residents with dementia as unable to communicate. This results in staff failing to view residents with dementia as complete human beings with physical, psychological, and social needs.

Although much of the literature that promotes the importance of staff–resident relationships is qualitative, Fossey et al. (2006) provide cluster randomized control trial data showing that training to support for care home staff communication offers viable alternatives to antipsychotic medication for the management of challenging behavior. Similarly, Bird, Jones, Korten, and Smithers (2007), in their randomized control trial of psychological approaches toward behavioral and psychological symptoms of dementia, note the importance of staff variables such as attitude when determining outcomes. Bird et al. (2007) conclude that resident outcomes are impacted by staff decisions about what tasks to undertake. This process balances building relationships with residents with dementia against tasks such as routine physical care. These authors conclude that the tasks decided upon are defined by the priorities of the workplace in interaction with the staff's own skills and sense of empowerment.

Scholl and Sabat (2008) reviewed the research pertaining to staff–resident relationships relative to care. They identified that the negative attitudes of staff tend to reduce opportunities to maximize the capacity of residents with dementia. This results in residents with dementia indicating frustration and embarrassment at their own deterioration while stressing that staff had limited time for social interaction. The nursing staff's lack of knowledge about residents with dementia and failure to engage with them result in further frustration and self-depreciation on the part of residents. The authors theorize that this lack of engagement may stem from the view that there is no point in engaging in relationships with residents because dementia is progressive and deterioration inevitable. Such attitudes risk compounding communication challenges faced by the nursing staff. Consequently, nurses and other staff members avoid social engagement with residents, which is shown to be the fundamental level at which PSIs can impact upon care. Scholl and Sabat (2008) offer an understanding that PSIs can comprise basic communication and recognition skills as well as formal techniques. In Thomas's case, the application of such knowledge would enhance staff's ability to recognize distress and reduce his social isolation by the considered use of basic day-to-day communication. In this case, the lack of such PSIs results in Thomas's unmet needs growing and the amplification of behaviors that confirm staff attitudes, which then leads to diminished staff–resident relationships, recourse to medication, and further isolation.

Role and Cultural Considerations

In considering the need for change in the manner in which nursing home care is delivered, specifically in relation to care of people with dementia, the impact of general social attitudes to dementia must be considered. A pilot study by Alzheimer's Australia (2012) sought the views of 614 adults between 40 and 65 years of age, 89.9% of whom knew a person with dementia and 21.8% of whom were the primary carers for someone who had dementia. They found that 34% of the sample admitted to finding people with dementia irritating. Over 50% felt they could not have a meaningful conversation with a person with dementia. In case study research, Sabat, Napolitano, and Fath (2004) found that malignant social positioning of people with dementia will take place in residential settings influenced by contextual factors as well as by general social attitudes to dementia. In Thomas's case, efforts to improve care must include staff accepting that some of the behaviors they identify as frustrating are in fact Thomas attempting to assert himself and assume control of his life.

Much of the literature that elucidates staff–patient relationships considers what staff actually do with and for residents with dementia and what influences staff decisions. A staff's ability to challenge the culture of negative values and attitudes relative to dementia care is central to this understanding. Brodaty, Draper, and Low (2003) undertook a self-completion questionnaire survey of 253 nursing home staff considering strain and satisfaction. The data were subject to cross-sectional analysis against behavioral assessments of 647 residents with dementia. The researchers argued that there is a link between staff reflection and action. This study suggests that lack of education, workplace pressures, and personal concerns result in poor understanding of care, subsequent negative attitudes to residents with dementia, and resultant lack of PSI utilization (Brodaty et al., 2003).

There are resources available to staff targeted at changing the culture of nursing homes who care for people with dementia and enhancing person-centered care (Alzheimer's Society, 2011a, 2011b). These resources promote individualized care planning and acknowledge the centrality of staff–resident relationships to the use of PSIs. Cohen-Mansfield (2003) highlighted the need to develop an etiology-based approach to psychosis in dementia to replace diagnostic approaches that result in overuse of medication. This research is applicable to Thomas's case as identification of causation followed by an etiology-based response could alleviate some of Thomas's need. In Thomas's case, the lack of an etiology-based approach can be seen as arising from the pressures described by Cohen-Mansfield (2003). If staff are struggling to meet their own needs, physically and psychologically, and are working in rigid, poorly resourced care settings, they may take the easiest option—recommending antipsychotic medication when faced with behavioral and psychological symptoms of dementia rather than building relationships, identifying the cause of distress, and applying PSIs.

The literature clearly demonstrates that where education is not ongoing and is not supported by managerial approaches that focus on refreshing staff values and attitudes to care, there is a tendency for staff to resort to less positive communication and more limited interaction. Positive culture change will not occur where staff are not able to challenge their negative attitudes of residents with dementia. Where staff have no alternative view, care will continue to be delivered uncritically, with limited scope for change.

Solutions and Strategies

The way Thomas relates to his environment and the people around him has changed as his disease has progressed. Accordingly, his behaviors have changed, and the manner in which staff adjust to these changes will define the nature of his care. The relationships between Thomas, his nephew, and staff are central to how his future care will develop. In order to address Thomas's changing needs, the nursing staff need to attend to the following areas:

- Staff education
  - Promote enhanced understanding of and implementation of person-centered care
  - Practice enhancing staff communication skills
  - Challenge staff to become aware of behavioral and psychological symptoms of dementia
  - Provide information on the risks and benefits of antipsychotic drugs
  - Explore short-term alternatives to antipsychotic medication
- Collaboration and engagement
  - Involve Thomas and his nephew in decision making regarding care, treatment, and activities
  - Provide ongoing assessment and identification of the changes in Thomas's unmet need
  - Build on training to develop a more in-depth understanding of Thomas (behavioral etiology, history, interests, personality, and culture)
  - Encourage continued social interaction between Thomas's nephew, Thomas, and staff

Clinical Reasoning Questions

1. How would you go about identifying Thomas's unmet needs?
2. What expertise or resources could you call on to address the solutions and strategies?
3. How could you utilize Thomas's nephew to enhance the staff's relationship with Thomas?
4. How would you ensure your practice is collaborative and engaging/partnership working?
5. Is there any local practice guidance that you could use to achieve the solutions and strategies?

References

Alzheimer's Australia. (2012). *Exploring dementia and stigma beliefs: A pilot study of Australian adults aged 40 to 65 years*. Australia: University of Wollongong.

Alzheimer's Society. (2011a). *Optimising treatment and care for people with behavioural and psychological symptoms of dementia: A best practice guide for health and social care professionals*. London, England: Alzheimer's Society.

Alzheimer's Society. (2011b). *Reducing the use of antipsychotic drugs: A guide to the treatment and care of behavioural and psychological symptoms of dementia*. London, England: Alzheimer's Society.

Bartlett, R., & O'Connor, D. (2007). From personhood to citizenship: Broadening the lens for dementia practice and research. *Journal of Aging Studies, 21*, 107–118.

Bates, J., Boote, J., & Beverley, C. (2004). Psychosocial interventions for people with a milder dementing illness: A systematic review. *Journal of Advanced Nursing, 45*(6), 1–15.

Bird, M., Jones, R. H., Korten, A., & Smithers, H. (2007). A controlled trial of a predominantly psychosocial approach to BPSD: Treating causality. *International Psychogeriatrics, 19*(5), 874–891.

Brodaty, H., Draper, B., & Low, L. F. (2003). Nursing home staff attitudes towards residents with dementia: Strain and satisfaction with work. *Journal of Advanced Nursing, 44*(6), 583–590.

Cahill, S., & Diaz-Ponce, A. M. (2011). I hate having nobody here, I'd like to know where they all are: Can qualitative research detect differences in quality of life among nursing home residents with different levels of cognitive impairment? *Ageing and Mental Health, 15*(5), 562–572.

Cohen-Mansfield, J. (2003). Nonpharmacologic interventions for psychotic symptoms in dementia. *Journal of Geriatric Psychiatry and Neurology, 16*, 219.

Edberg, A. K., Bird, M., Richards, D. A., Woods, B., Keeley, P., & Davis-Quarrell, V. (2008). Strain in nursing care of people with dementia: Nurses' experience in Australia, Sweden and United Kingdom. *Aging & Mental Health, 12*(2), 236–243.

Fossey, J., Ballard, C., Juszczak, E., James, I., Alder, N., Jacoby, R., & Howard, R. (2006). Effect of enhanced psychosocial care on antipsychotic use in nursing home residents with severe dementia: Cluster randomized trial. *British Medical Journal, 332*, 756–761.

Kitwood, T. (1997). *Dementia reconsidered.* Buckingham, England: Open University Press.

Kitwood, T., & Bredin, K. (1992). Towards a theory of dementia care: Personhood and well-being. *Ageing and Society, 12,* 269–287.

NICE-SCIE. (2011). *Dementia: The NICE-SCIE guideline on supporting people with dementia and their carers in health and social care.* London, England: The British Psychological Society and the Royal College of Psychiatrists.

O'Shea, E. (2007). *Implementing policy for dementia care in Ireland: The time for action is now.* Galway, Ireland: NUI Galway Irish Centre for Social Gerontology.

Sabat, S. R., Napolitano, L., & Fath, H. (2004). Barriers to the construction of a valued social identity: A case study of Alzheimer's disease. *American Journal of Alzheimer's Disease and Other Dementias, 19*(3), 177–185.

Scholl, J. M., & Sabat, S. R. (2008). Stereotypes, stereotype threat and ageing: Implications for the understanding and treatment of people with Alzheimer's disease. *Ageing and Society, 28*(1), 103–130.

Smebye, K. L., & Kirkevold, M. (2013). The influence of relationships on personhood in dementia care: A qualitative, hermeneutic study. *BMC Nursing, 12,* 29.

Thies, W., & Bleiler, L. (2012). 2012 Alzheimer's disease facts and figures. *Alzheimer's and Dementia, 8,* 131–168.

Ward, R., Vass, A., Neeru, A., Cydonie, G., & Beau, C. (2008). A different story: Exploring patterns of communication in residential dementia care. *Ageing & Society, 28*(5), 629–651.

21 FOSTERING RESIDENT-TO-RESIDENT RELATIONSHIPS

Mary Gannon

Subjective

"Just the thought of coming to live here made me lonely!"

Objective

Ursula Unger has been a resident in a long-term care setting for the last 8 months. Ursula had lived alone in rural Ireland for many years following the death of her parents in the late 1990s. Although she never married, Ursula has a large extended family and friends with whom she is in constant contact. Her whole life changed last winter when she slipped on ice while feeding her cat, "Fluffy," sustaining a fractured hip. She had been unable to move or call for help and was found by a visiting neighbor a short while later.

"I thought no one would ever find me. . ., I thought I was a goner. I've never been so cold or afraid in all my life."

While Ursula's physical injuries healed, the emotional impact of her fall shattered her confidence and, not wanting to be a burden on any family members, she decided that admission to a care setting would be the best and safest option.

"They have enough to do besides minding me."

For many years she had attended the day center attached to her local nursing home. Its location in close proximity to her home, together with knowing both the staff and the layout of the care setting, were the main reasons she chose St. Agatha's. Although Ursula knew the center well, she had concerns about her ability to maintain independence and continue to enjoy some of the social interests she had fostered for many years. Ursula is strong willed, opinionated, and used to doing things her way. Although this had served her well all her life, she feared it might not be as endearing in a community setting. As a very social person and used to her own space, the thought of living with so many people did not appeal to her.

"Would she fit in? Would she be able to find a quiet space in what appeared to be a very hectic and noisy environment?"

These questions she feared would appear trivial to staff, but they were really important to her. *How would she listen to her beloved TV soaps?* Monday, Wednesday, and Friday nights would never be the same again. Over the years, these actors had become her constant companions, adjusting to her reduced hearing at the twist of a button. From the comfort of her armchair she had attended weddings, births, deaths, extramarital affairs, and so much more that had added color to her dark, empty nights.

"I know it must seem silly to you but I love my soaps."

Ms. Unger is an 83-year-old lady who was admitted to a long-stay care facility from an acute care setting following a total hip arthroplasty. Having sustained a fall in the last number of months, evidence would suggest that Ursula is at a higher risk of falling again (Gulanick & Myers, 2014; Health Service Executive, Department of Health and Children, & the National Council for Aging & Older People, 2008); therefore, it is essential to conduct a comprehensive falls risk assessment that explores the intrinsic, extrinsic, and environmental factors in order to determine Ursula's specific needs prior to the development and implementation of an appropriate falls prevention care plan/strategy. In Ursula's case, it will be necessary to complete a physical assessment to identify any age-related physical changes that could affect posture or mobility, and assess sensory deficits (vision and hearing tests).

Literature Review

The number of people aged 65 and over in the Republic of Ireland has been increasing steadily over the past number of years, from 11.3% of the population in 2010 to an estimated 15.3% in 2021 (Central Statistics Office [CSO], 2011). This phenomenon is replicated globally with the American population of older people 65 years+ expected to increase over the decade 2010 to 2020 by an estimated 36%, or 55 million (U.S. Department of Health and Human Services, 2011). Germany has the highest recorded population proportion of older people in the European Union (EU) at 20.7%, with the EU average at 17.4%. Globally, the population of people 80 years and older has increased from 7% in the 1950s to a current level of 14%. (United Nations Department of Economic and Social Affairs Population Division, 2013). Therefore, as the number of older people increase, they will require improved support, resources, and expertise to meet their needs (Bowers et al., 2012).

For many older people, aging at home among family and friends is their preferred choice, with life in a residential care setting being their least preferred option (Bradshaw, Playford, & Riazi, 2012). In Ireland, 27% of people over 65, mainly female, live alone (CSO, 2011). This is reflected globally, with the United States reporting approximately 29% of noninstitutionalized older people living alone and 47% of older women age 75+ living alone (U.S. Department of Health and Human Services, 2011). Similarly, in the United Kingdom, 17% of people over 60 years live alone (Office for National Statistics [ONS], 2011). Living alone was identified as a significant factor for admission into a care facility (McCann, Donnelly, & O'Reilly, 2011). By the year 2021, the number of older people using residential care facilities in the Republic of Ireland will rise by 59% and by an estimated increase of 45% in Northern Ireland (Wren et al., 2012).

The decision to move to a nursing home is multifaceted, and it typically unearths many challenges for older people, including the task of "learning to live in a nursing home"

(Anderberg & Berglund, 2010). Bury (1982) termed the phrase "biographical disruption" to explain a person's life-world adaption in dealing with the impact of chronic illness. Chronic illness can impact all areas of life and may not be the sole determinant of a change in location; they do, however, challenge the balance between nurturing abilities while aiding with disabilities. For many older adults, these changes can ultimately result in relocation to long-term care. Although Ursula had independently made the decision to move into residential care, it resulted from a change in her life-world and the impact injury had on her ability to cope independently and feel secure doing so.

Kahn and Antonucci (1980) identified the changes that occur in social networks and connections over the life course. The Convoy Model of Social Relations built on the works of the anthropologist David Plath (1980), who constructed the Convoy Theory, describes the various relationships developed through life that both shape identity and add to the unique individuality of each person. Convoys, seen as dynamic in nature, are composed of individuals who help to shape and positively impact the aging experience (Phillips, Ajrouch, & Hillcoat-Nallétamby, 2010). Although many factors impact on social networks, relocation can reduce the size and accessibility of an individual's interactions (Wrzus et al., 2013), heightening the need to develop and nurture connectedness within the care setting (Cooney, Dowling, Gannon, Dempsey, & Murphy, 2013). In a systematic review of qualitative studies that focused on quality of life (QOL) in care homes, connectedness and involvement with others emerged as one of four key themes (Bradshaw, Playford, & Riazi, 2012). Social connections with peers had the ability to reinforce acceptance, establish friendships, and positively contribute to the ultimate sense of belonging (Bradshaw, Playford, & Riazi, 2012).

Connectedness to others, whether staff, family, or peer relationship/friendships, contributes to a sense of belonging and facilitates acceptance to a new home (Bradshaw, Playford, & Riazi, 2012; Brown Wilson, 2009). Munn et al. (2008) identified open and honest communication as fundamental to staff and family relationships, with many studies describing the relationship between older people and staff as "like family"

(Gannon & Dowling, 2012; Phillips et al., 2006; Touhy, Brown, & Smith, 2005). Allied with resident choice, independence, and the preservation of autonomy, the older person integrates into the "ward family" (Gannon & Dowling, 2012) and directly contributes to negotiated care (McCormack, 2003) in the process of making this his or her "home" (Cooney, 2012). Ursula was encouraged to personalize her single room as she wanted. She had done so by adding some of her favorite photos and pictures from home. The cushion she had made in school took a place of pride on the armchair, and her mother's quilt lay across the foot of her bed. Her radio and alarm clock sit on the locker by her bed.

A key component in adapting to a new "home" for many older people is their ability to develop relationships within the nursing home while maintaining contact with existing friends and family. Older people today are part of the global technological community that regularly link and use Internet technology in their daily lives (Gatto & Tak, 2008). While e-mail and Skype connect older people to family and friends outside the nursing home, it can also be used to link those within the care setting. Connectedness in Ursula's case was not limited by or dependent upon others. Ursula's extrovert personality enabled her use of social technology (mobile phone, etc.) to the benefit of all. Ursula organized events and accidentally became the event manager for the unit who provided social opportunities for other residents that had not previously been explored. Extroverts, by their sheer natural instinct, seek out the company of others and tend to be happier (Gaffney, 2011). Wilkinson, Kiata, Peri, Robinson, & Kerse (2012) found that happiness can be contagious and positively affects the emotional response of coresidents. Happiness is an emotion that we have control over, and we can "learn" to become happier by practicing the attitudes and behavior of happy people (Gaffney, 2011, p. 107). Hubbard, Tester, and Downs (2003) conducted an ethnographic observational study in four nursing homes in Scotland that found that humor and slapstick comedy were used in both verbal and nonverbal interactions to both entertain and facilitate the development of relationships. Ursula had a contagious laugh and a bubbly personality that people liked to be around. She could make even the most mundane act fun and could see the bright side in every situation.

It is important to acknowledge the impact that culture of the nursing home can play in relationships. Since the introduction of the National Quality Standards for Residential Care Settings for Older People in Ireland (Health Information and Quality Authority [HIQA], 2009), nursing homes have embraced the concept of person-centered/relationship-centered care delivery within "home-like" environments (McCormack, 2003; McCormack et al., 2010; Nolan, Brown, Davies, Nolan, & Keady, 2006). Organizational leadership that values the importance of relationships and fosters the inclusion of residents' and families' opinions can directly influence a relationship-centered approach to care delivery (Wilson, 2009). Valuing the opinions of staff, resident, and family is a significant factor in the development of an "enriched environment" that nurtures, supports, and acknowledges all members equally (Hubbard et al., 2003; Nolan, Davies, & Brown, 2006). The role of staff is crucial in the transition of older people into a care setting through the development of a warm, friendly, and comfortable environment that values their individuality (Coyle, McCormack, Carragher, & Bond, 2011). Replicating the home from home is not without challenges. McConnell, Brown, Shoda, Stayton, & Martin (2011) expound the positive physical and psychological consequences of pet ownership. The center's resident cat, "Purdy," became Ursula's constant companion. Unknowingly, Purdy had helped Ursula to feel at home in St. Agatha's.

Physical space and environmental layout can have an impact on how relationships are shaped (Hubbard et al., 2003; Wilson, 2009). Shared spaces that are homey, with furniture reflective of a resident's home, portrays and heightens the sense of comfort and intimacy, aiding the social relationships present within (Wilson, 2009). Single bedrooms allow older people to style their rooms to suit their needs and decorative preferences (Anderberg & Berglund, 2010). Ursula claimed ownership of her space through the introduction of a few sentimental treasures from home; however, what gave her the most pleasure was her television. She would be able to laugh at Jack and monitor the newlyweds all she wanted. The volume could be as high as she wanted, and a pair of headphones supplied by the nurse ensured she would not disturb any of her neighbors. She was in TV soap heaven.

Individual spaces can offer privacy and dignity while respecting personal autonomy, thus affording the older person the opportunity and self-determination to socialize and mix with others as and when they please. A comparative study conducted by Oishi, Kurtz, Maio, Park, and Whitchurch (2011) identified that Korean retirees were happier when interacting with familiar people, unlike their American counterparts, who were no happier interacting with familiar than with unfamiliar people. For many older people, it may take time to become familiar with people and place. It had taken time for Ursula to feel at home with the other residents in the ward. She had attended bingo at the invitation of the lady in the next room, but she did not enjoy it. "It was boring and nobody talked to me," she explained to the nurse. The nurse introduced her to someone who played cards, and things started to look up. Some of her friends from the day care center came to visit, and when Ursula asked if they would like to play cards, the regular ward card game commenced. The ward sitting room had a table big enough for the six players, and the daily card game took place at 2 p.m. This did not interfere with the game at the day care center, but forged links with older people that had not happened before. The membership changed daily as new respite clients joined in, and even some staff were deemed to be "okay" at cards. The stakes remained unchanged, and the laughs and jokes depicted the great "craic" enjoyed by all. Ursula looks forward to 2 o'clock every day.

In conclusion, the decision to relocate to long-term care for older people and their families is complex and not to be taken lightly. Although for many people emphasis is placed on location, size, and the ability of the care home to meet the health care needs of the older person, it is essential that the social areas and events provided for and with the older person are explored prior to admission. Staff must be aware of their role in creating environments that are welcoming and jovial. It is important to recognize the importance of laughter and fun in everyday life, for if laughter is contagious (Wilkinson et al., 2012), nursing homes or their staffs must not become the vaccine to kill it—better to be the carrier that spreads the epidemic.

Role and Cultural Considerations

Maintaining connections/connectedness is inextricably linked to an older person's QOL (Cooney, Murphy, & O'Shea, 2009; Murphy, O'Shea, Cooney, Shiel, & Hodgins, 2006; Register & Scharer, 2010). Empowering the older people to claim ownership of his or her space, respect for his or her personal identity (calling people by name), and valuing his or her opinions are central tenets in the development of meaningful relationships (Cloutier-Fisher & Harvey, 2009).

Cultural influences impact on the care we provide to older people, and an awareness of them is essential to effective care delivery (Jarvis, 2008). Ursula's religious beliefs have always played a large role in her life, and it is paramount to acknowledge the impact they have on her care. As a Roman Catholic, Ursula retains her wish to fast for 1 hour prior to the receipt of communion, abstain from eating meat on Fridays, and abstain totally from certain foods during the 7 weeks of Lent. Although these are no longer an obligation of her faith, she has chosen to retain these cultures. Allowing Ursula to practice her faith her way is an important aspect of who Ursula is.

For some older people, moving into residential care can result in a loss of privacy. Having moved from a rural home, where space and quietness were prevalent, into a busy ward filled with people and noise can be a daunting event. Individual rooms offer the older person an opportunity to retain a sense of personhood and autonomy, which can positively impact on his or her QOL (Anderberg & Berglund, 2010; Murphy et al., 2006); however, for those with high dependency or who are social introverts, this can result in isolation and loneliness. It is essential for health care professionals to give consideration to the components necessary for the development of relationships for and with older people. Providing opportunities for social interaction through introductions of people of the same ethnicity, from the same area, or with the same hobbies or interests can assist in the development of relationships. Group activities can link like-minded individuals in a social context; however, care must be taken to ensure such interests are guided by resident choice (HIQA, 2009) and are not a paper exercise to meet legislative or regulatory requirements.

Older people are autonomous beings in control of their own lives—lives that are unique, special, and are woven into the fabric of our communities. Baars (2012, p. 161) proposes that "the concept of 'life-worlds' refers not only to the domain of personal relationships, family life, or friendship, but extends into the daily interactions, efforts, creativity of those people who work in systematic worlds where decisions are taken with major implications for the daily reality of aging people all over the world." As nurse practitioners, we must recognize the importance of the older person's ability to live fully in time, embracing the person as a whole—his or her past, present, and hopes for the future. Capturing the past is not just a method of reminiscence; it acknowledges the value of this person and recognizes what is important to him or her. The adoption of a collaborative approach that involves the person, his or her family, and professional carers is a central tenet of the provision of quality care built on therapeutic relationships, and one that fosters connectedness. Nursing documentation that captures the biological, psychological, social, spiritual, cultural, and personal lives of older people allows us to identify and address the individual needs of the most important person in our care.

Solutions and Strategies

Referrals will be required to the medical team to complete a medication review, physiotherapy, and occupational therapy, as well as to the dietitian for a nutritional review. Ursula's hearing impairment is minimal and does not impact her ability to communicate her needs clearly and effectively. It is mainly due to a build-up of wax, which she controls through the use of aural drops instilled each night. Ursula wears prescription glasses (for both reading and everyday use), and she underwent a complete optical review 3 months ago. Her name has been imprinted on the inside of the side arms of her glasses to avoid loss or error.

A nutritional assessment was completed with the Malnutrition Universal Screening Tool (MUST). Ursula's height at 167 cm (65 in.) and weighing 177.8 lbs. (81 kg) resulted in a BMI of 29, which places her in the overweight category. The prevalence of obesity has increased globally and is a common focus of dietary concern in all aspects of society today. Older people are not immune to this problem, and there are many contributory factors at play that may need to be addressed in conjunction with food intake. Successful weight management is multifaceted, including lifestyle changes, healthy eating, exercise, and, above all else, the willpower to maintain a healthy approach to weight control. While Ursula acknowledged her dietary problem (she freely admits her love of sweets, candies, desserts, etc.) and she has lost weight in the past, she had always gained it back with more. Aided by the dietitian, Ursula was placed on a weight-reducing calorie-controlled diet, which would include weekly weigh-ins and the development of a menu that Ursula felt she could adhere to. Ursula was encouraged to increase her fruit, vegetable, and water intake, and family were encouraged to bring fruit when visiting. A food diary would be maintained by Ursula and reviewed weekly. As an added incentive, Ursula decided to put €2 in her money box each week, to be doubled if weight was lost. This would be used to purchase a new purse for Christmas.

Ursula's obesity directly impacted her ability to mobilize with her Zimmer frame. Having suffered from osteoarthritis for many years, she had been using a Zimmer frame prior to her fall; however, increased episodes of arthritic pain and fear of falling had meant she would not attempt to walk without a person in attendance. Functional assessment (manual handling risk assessment and the Waterlow pressure ulcer prevention score of 16) revealed impaired ability to mobilize independently without aids, impaired ability to move in bed, and difficulty in sitting in and standing up from a chair.

Occupational therapist review ensured that Ursula's equipment needs were adequately addressed through the use of the following aids:

- Ursula's Zimmer frame was replaced with a lighter model complete with wheels to the front and a seat that could be used should she feel weak or tired while ambulating. It was hoped that this would provide Ursula with the ability to ambulate independently and would offer the ability to rest at periods on her journey. The basket at the front gave her the ability to carry her purse, playing cards, reading glasses, and newspaper.

- Ursula's ability to independently sit or stand from the seated position, identified in the manual handling risk assessment, was maintained with the provision of
  - a high seated chair with adjustable legs and
  - a raised toilet seat with extra support bars.
- To promote Ursula's tissue oxygenation and thus prevent pressure ulcer development, a nimbus pressure relieving mattress was used.

The physiotherapist review resulted in the adoption of a low-intensity aerobic exercise regime. Ursula was encouraged to

- Walk the length of the corridor and back three times per day, increasing to once an hour within 6 weeks
- Use the exercise bike initially on low intensity and minimum gradient for 10 minutes/day, gradually increasing (speed and gradient) to 30 minutes/day over a 6-week period
- Actively participate in the ward exercise program each morning

In the older population, falls result in a higher risk of mortality and require a comprehensive assessment of risk in order to identify and address issues of concern (Talley & O'Connor, 2014). Completing a multifactorial comprehensive falls risk assessment that includes intrinsic, extrinsic, and environmental factors aids the effective falls management strategy (Health Service Executive, Department of Health and Children, & the National Council for Aging & Older People [2008]). Ursula's falls risk was assessed with the use of the Cannard Falls Risk Assessment Tool (National Health Service, 2010), and having scored 12 (+13 = high risk), a falls prevention program was commenced. Ursula's pain was monitored by the use of the Abbey Pain Scale (Royal College of Physicians, British Geriatrics Society, and British Pain Society, 2007) and varies between

3 and 6 (mild). Ursula is encouraged to report pain at early onset and analgesia is administered every 6 hours according to need, with its effectiveness monitored and documented.

Ursula's social history, captured in her life story, had identified her love of cards, TV soaps, and cats. Her admitting nurse had recognized Ursula from the day center and noted the change in Ursula's demeanor. She remembered Ursula as a bubbly personality, jovial and full of life. She also recalled how Ursula, being an avid card player, was the main instigator of the daily card games in the day center. Stakes were not high at 10 c/game, but the honor of winning or at least not cheating or playing the wrong card was profound. During the time Ursula was in the acute setting, she had not been able to enjoy many of her hobbies and had become quiet and withdrawn.

The main focus of Ursula's social plan of care was to support and encourage involvement in the ward's social events, introduce Ursula to other residents (particularly those with similar interests or from her home-place), and reestablish links with her friends from the day center. Ursula was invited to dine in the communal dining room with the other residents. Sitting rooms afforded scenic views and quiet areas where she could either mix with others or sit quietly. Ursula would also be introduced to the home's resident cat, Purdy.

Clinical Reasoning Questions

1. What strategies do I have in place to identify and address the social interests of my residents?
2. Are residents and families in my care encouraged to personalize and claim ownership of their care/space?
3. As a nurse practitioner, how can I ensure that residents in single rooms maintain and develop relationships?
4. What changes can I make in my practice to encourage social interactions for the residents, staff, and families in my care setting?
5. Would I like to live in the nursing home where I work?

References

Anderberg, P., & Berglund, A. L. (2010). Elderly persons' experience of striving to receive care on their own terms in nursing homes. *International Journal of Nursing Practice, 16*, 64–68.

Baars, J. (2012). Critical turns of aging narrative and time. *International Journal of Aging and Later Life, 7*(2), 143–165.

Bowers, H. , Clark, A., Crosby, G., Easterbrook, L., Macadam, A., MacDonald, R., . . . & Smith, C. (2009). *Older peoples' vision for long term care.* Retrieved from http://www.jrf.org.uk/sites/files/jrf/older-people-vision-for-care-full.pdf

Bradshaw, S. A., Playford, E. D., & Riazi, A. (2012). Living well in care homes: A systematic review of qualitative studies. *Age and Aging, 41*, 429–440.

Brown Wilson, C. (2009). Developing community in care homes through a relationship-centered approach. *Health and Social Care in the Community, 17*(2), 177–186.

Bury, M. (1982). Chronic illness as biographical disruption. *Sociology of Health and Illness, 4*(2), 167–182.

Central Statistics Office. (2011). *Household survey*. Retrieved from http://www.cso.ie/en/statistics/population

Cloutier-Fisher, D., & Harvey, J. (2009). Home beyond house: Experiences of place in an evolving retirement community. *Journal of Environmental Psychology, 29*, 246–255.

Cooney, A. (2012). "Finding home": A grounded theory on how older people "find home" in long-term care settings. *International Journal of Older People, 7*, 188–199.

Cooney, A., Dowling, M., Gannon, M. E., Dempsey, L., & Murphy, K. (2013). Exploration of the meaning of connectedness for older people in long-term care in context of their quality of life: A review and commentary. *International Journal of Older People Nursing, 9*(3), 192–199. Retrieved from http://www.ncbi.nlm.nih.gov/pubmed/23437765

Cooney, A., Murphy, K., & O'Shea, E. (2009). Resident perspectives of the determinants of quality of life in residential care in Ireland. *Journal of Advanced Nursing, 65*(5), 1029–1038.

Coyle, A., McCormack, B., Carragher, L., & Bond, R. (2011). *Places to flourish—A pattern based approach to foster change in residential care*. Nursing Homes Ireland, Health Service Executive, Atlantic Philanthropies,

University of Ulster, Dundalk Institute of Technology. Retrieved from http://lenus.ie/hse/handle/10147/190291?mode=simple

Department of Health & Children. (2010). *Long-stay activities statistics 2010*. Dublin, Ireland: Government Publications.

Gaffney, M. (2011). *Flourishing*. Dublin, Ireland: The Penguin Group.

Gannon, M., & Dowling, M. (2012). Nurses' experience of loss on the death of older persons in long-term residential care: Findings from an interpretive phenomenological study. *International Journal of Older People, 7*(4), 243–252.

Gatto, S. L., & Tak, S. H. (2008). Computer, Internet, and e-mail use among older adults: Benefits and barriers. *Educational Gerontology, 34*, 800–811.

Gulanick, M., & Myers, J. L. (2014). *Nursing care plans: Diagnoses, interventions, and outcomes* (8th ed.). Philadelphia, PA: Elsevier.

Health Information and Quality Authority. (2009). *National quality standards for residential care settings for older people in Ireland*. Dublin, Ireland: Author.

Health Service Executive, Department of Health and Children, & the National Council for Aging & Older People. (2008). *Strategy to prevent falls and fractures in Ireland's aging*. Retrieved from http://www.lenus.ie/hse/bitstream/10147/46105/4/HSEStrategyFalls.pdf

Hubbard, G., Tester, S., & Downs, M. G. (2003). Meaningful social interactions between older people in institutional care settings. *Aging & Society, 23*, 99–114.

Jarvis, C. (2008). *Pocket companion: Physical examination & health assessment* (5th ed.). St. Louis, MO: Saunders Elsevier.

Kahn, R. L., & Antonucci, T. C. (1980). Convoys over the life course: Attachment, roles and social support. In P. B. Baltes & O. G. Brim (Eds.), *Life-span development and behavior* (Vol. 3, pp. 253–286). New York, NY: Academic Press.

McCann, M., Donnelly, M., & O'Reilly, D. (2011). Living arrangements, relationship to people in the household and admission to care homes for older people. *Age & Aging, 40*, 358–363.

McConnell, A. R., Brown, C. M., Shoda, T. M., Stayton, L. E., & Martin, C. E. (2011). Friends with benefits: On the positive consequences of pet ownership. *Journal of Personality and Social Psychology, 101*(6), 1239–1252.

McCormack, B. (2003). A conceptual framework for person centered care practice with older people. *International Journal of Nursing Practice, 9*, 202–209.

McCormack, B., Dewing, J., Breslin, L., Coyne-Nevin, A., Kennedy, K., Manning, M., . . . Slater, P. (2010). Developing person-centered practice: Nursing outcomes arising from changes to the care environment in residential settings for older people. *International Journal of Older People Nursing, 5*, 93–107.

Munn, J. C., Dobbs, D., Meier, A., Williams, C. S., Biola, H., & Zimmerman, S. (2008). The end-of-life experience in long-term care: Five themes identified from focus groups with residents, family members, and staff. *The Gerontologist, 48*(4), 485–494.

Murphy, K., O'Shea, E., Cooney, A., Shiel, A., & Hodgins, M. (2006). *Improving quality of life for older people in long-stay care settings in Ireland* (Report No. 93). Dublin, Ireland: National Council on Aging and Older People.

National Health Service. (2010). *Cannard falls risk assessment pack*. Retrieved from http://library.nhsggc.org.uk/mediaAssets/OFPS/213665%20Cannard%20Falls-%20Generic%200910.pdf

Nolan, M. R., Davies, S., & Brown, J. (2006). Transitions in care homes: Towards relationship-centered care using the "Senses Framework." *Quality in Aging and Older Adults, 7*(3), 5–14.

Nolan, M. R., Brown, J., Davies, S., Nolan, J., & Keady, J. (2006). *The senses framework: Improving care for older people through a relationship-centred approach. Getting research into practice (GRiP) report no.* 2. University of Sheffield. Retrieved from http://shura.shu.ac.uk/280

Office for National Statistics. (2011). *General lifestyle survey*. Retrieved from www.ons.gov.uk

Oishi, S., Kurtz, J. L., Maio, F. F., Park, J., & Whitchurch, E. (2011). The role of familiarity in daily well-being: Developmental and cultural variation. *Developmental Psychology, 47*(6), 1750–1756.

Phillips, J., Ajrouch, K., & Hillcoat-Nallétamby, S. (2010). *Key concepts in social gerontology*. London, England: Sage.

Phillips, J., Davidson, P. M., Jackson, D., Kristjanson, L., Daly, J., & Curran, J. (2006). Residential aged care: The last frontier for palliative care. *Journal of Advanced Nursing, 55*(4), 416–424.

Plath, D. (1980). *Long engagements*. Stanford, CA: Stanford University Press.

Register, M. E., & Scharer, K. M. (2010). Connectedness in community-dwelling older adults. *Western Journal of Nursing Research, 32*(4), 462–479.

Royal College of Physicians, British Geriatrics Society and British Pain Society. (2007). *The assessment of pain in older people: National guidelines* (Concise guidance to good practice series, No. 8). London, England: Author.

Talley, N. J., & O'Connor, S. (2014). *Clinical examination: A systematic guide to physical diagnosis* (7th ed.). Australia: Elsevier.

Touhy, T. A., Brown, C., & Smith, C. J. (2005). Spiritual caring: End of life in a nursing home. *Journal of Gerontological Nursing, 31*(9), 27–35.

U.S. Department of Health and Human Services. (2011). *A profile of older Americans: Administration on Aging (AoA)*. Author. Retrieved from http://www.aoa.gov/Aging_Statistics/Profile/2011/docs/2011profile.pdf

United Nations Department of Economic and Social Affairs Population Division. (2013). *World population ageing 2013*. Retrieved February 17, 2015, from http://www.un.org/en/development/desa/population/publications/pdf/ageing/WorldPopulationAgeing2013.pdf

Wilkinson, T. J., Kiata, L. J., Peri, K., Robinson, E. M., & Kerse, N. M. (2012, March). Quality of life for older people in residential care is related to connectedness, willingness to enter care and co-residents. *Australasian Journal on Aging, 31*(1), 52–55.

Wrzus, C., Hänel, M., Wagner, J. & Nayer, F. J. (2013). Social changes and life events across the life span: A meta-analysis. *Psychological Bulletin, 139*(1), 53–80.

Wren, M., Normand, C., O'Reilly, D., Cruise, S., Connolly, S., & Murphy, C. (2012). *Towards the development of a predictive model of long-term care demand for Northern Ireland and the Republic of Ireland*. Belfast, Ireland: Trinity College Dublin.

22 PROMOTING FAMILY CONNECTIONS

ASSUMPTA RYAN

Subjective

"I've known for some time that I would probably need to go into a long-term care facility, but it all happened so quickly after I fell at home. I was taken to hospital and then moved to this nursing home. I was devastated! I never wanted to leave home as I had lived in that small community all my married life, and I was surrounded by family and friends who called regularly. I don't think that I will ever settle in here . . . it's just not home!"

Objective

Mrs. Vivian Velvet is an 80-year-old woman who recently moved into a local nursing home after a fall at home. Upon physical examination, she appears alert and oriented. She is 65 in. (165 cm) in height and weighs 110 lbs. (50 kg). She is afebrile with a temperature of 97.8°F. Her BP is 160/80, pulse 118, and respirations 16/minute. Her cardiac and abdominal exam reveals nothing of note. Her oxygen saturation is 95%, and both her lungs are clear. Her skin is dry and thin but intact. She has bruising on her arms and legs from her recent fall. She wears a hearing aid and uses spectacles for reading. Her gait is unsteady, and she has been advised to use a walker since her admission to the nursing home. She has been assessed as a high risk of falls with a score of 60 on the Morse Falls Scale, and she is also at a medium risk of malnutrition (Malnutrition Universal Screening Tool). She obtained a score of 11 on the

30-item Geriatric Depression Scale. Her current medications include Lipitor 20 mgs OD, Naproxen 250 mg BD, Sinemet 100 mg TID, and Paracetamol PRN. Mrs. Velvet had been living alone since her husband died 18 months ago. She suffers from Parkinson's disease and osteoarthritis, and her mobility has been getting worse, particularly in the last year. Despite this, Mrs. Velvet insisted that she was able to manage at home with the help of her daughter, Laura, and the community care assistants who called three times a day. As Mrs. Velvet became increasingly dependent, her daughter found it very difficult to continue her caregiving role, as she had young children and worked full time.

Mrs. Velvet was deeply attached to her home. Her daughter was her primary caregiver and called her every morning and evening; she also helped out at mealtimes. They both dressed up every Sunday and went for a drive in the local village, stopping for coffee and a chat with passers-by. Although no longer in her own home, Mrs. Velvet would like Laura to remain involved in her care, but Laura, although keen to do so, is reluctant to "rock the boat." The staff in the nursing home are all very kind, and Mrs. Velvet does not want to appear too demanding.

After Mrs. Velvet fell, her daughter realized that long-term care was the only option. However, she felt very guilty about this decision as she knew that it would not be her mother's choice. The situation was not helped by circumstances surrounding the move. Resigned to the inevitability of the move, Mrs. Velvet had indicated a preference for Flowerfield, a nursing home close to where she lived and where some of her friends resided and visited. However, this nursing home had no vacancies, so Mrs. Velvet was moved to another nursing home in the area in the hope that a bed would become available at Flowerfield. The trauma of the fall and the move has taken its toll on Mrs. Velvet. She appears sad and withdrawn since her admission to the nursing home and shows little interest in getting to know the residents or staff. She tells the nurses that she feels disconnected from family and friends and displaced from her home just like "a fish out of water." She would like her daughter to be more involved in her care in the nursing home and to continue to do some of the things she had done before the move, but she does not know how to make this happen without upsetting the staff.

Literature Review

Across the developed world, current policy is to support older people to live independently in their own homes for as long as possible. However, an increase in the number of people with chronic illness and dementia, along with the costs associated with providing around-the-clock care to older people at home, means that nursing and residential homes will continue to play an important role in the care and support system. This is borne out by the fact that there are currently over 18,000 care homes across the United Kingdom, supporting approximately 400,000 older people, most of whom are over 80 years of age (Owen & Meyer, 2012).

Aging in place is a broad term for a concept, which recognizes the deep attachments that older people have to their homes. Andrews et al. (2005) acknowledged that the philosophy of aging in place recognizes that the movement of older people between care settings and from homes to institutional environments is often to the detriment of their health and against their wishes. Mrs. Velvet's reluctance to move into long-term care confirms the importance of home for older people. Home, for many older people, is a powerful symbol of autonomy and independence, whereas institutions are associated symbolically with the loss of autonomy and independence (Wiles, 2005).

The relationship between place of residence and sense of self can explain Mrs. Velvet's response to the move. If one's sense of self is inextricably linked to one's place of residence, then it follows that entry to care will be a huge upheaval for older people. This is borne out in other studies (Keefe & Fancey, 2000; McCann, Ryan, & McKenna, 2005) that showed that most older people wished to remain at home and by their profound sense of loss at not being able to do so. When this is no longer an option, the choice of nursing home becomes a crucial decision and reflects the importance of aging in place. Even though Mrs. Velvet was not able to remain in her own home, moving to Flowerfield would, as she perceived it, enable her to remain part of her own community. Mrs. Velvet's story highlights the importance of familiarity, continuity, and stability in the lives of older people, a recurrent theme in the literature on entry to long-term care (Ryan & Mc Kenna, 2013).

Admission to a nursing home is a stressful experience for older people and their families. For families, the experience is associated with conflicting emotions such as guilt, anger, sadness, and relief, and there is a general consensus that residents and relatives are largely unprepared for the realities of nursing home life. Such realities include the actual and potential losses associated with entry to care from the perspective of residents. These include loss of role, lifestyle, freedom, autonomy, and privacy, in addition to the loss of home, personal belongings, and potentially the social loss of family and friends. From the families' perspective, relief from the demands of their caregiving role may be replaced by feelings of guilt and anxiety, especially if their older relative is unhappy in the nursing home. In an attempt to cope with this and to maintain contact with their relatives, many carers wish to remain involved in aspects of their relative's care and, as is the case with Mrs. Velvet, this can also be the expressed wishes of the older person. However, communicating this request to nursing home staff can be problematic; as a result, there can be a degree of misunderstanding about each other's role. On the contrary, admission to a nursing home can mark the beginning of a new role, a role that, if properly negotiated, has the potential to benefit all three parties—the relative, the resident, and the nursing home staff.

Mrs. Velvet's case study highlights a recurrent theme in the literature that suggests that care home staff are unaware of the importance of family and friends in the lives of care home residents. A number of studies have focused on the role of families in care homes, and it is widely accepted that moving to a nursing home does not end family involvement or responsibility (Bauer, 2006; Robinson, Reid, & Cooke, 2010). On the contrary, a nursing home placement provides a new set of challenges for families such as how much help to provide, how to initiate relationships with staff, how to sustain their relationship with their relative, and how to redefine their own identity and role (Brown-Wilson, 2009; Ryan, Mc Kenna, & Slevin, 2011).

Mrs. Velvet is not unusual in wishing for her daughter to remain involved in her care after the placement. Davies and Nolan (2006) described three discrete roles for family members in care homes: *maintaining continuity* through the continuation of loving family relationships and by helping staff to get to know the residents as individuals; *keeping an eye* by monitoring and participating in care provision within the home; and *contributing to community* by interacting with other residents, relatives, and staff, and providing a link with the outside world. Despite this, there is evidence to suggest that the activities of staff in care homes are still primarily geared toward the provision of physical care, with the psychosocial needs of residents and families a secondary concern (Nakrem, Vinsnes, Harkless, Paulsen, & Seim, 2012), prompting the authors to recommend a new model of practice that views collaboration with families as a legitimate and necessary part of the role of care home staff.

There is evidence to suggest that families who provide direct care prior to the placement continue to play a major role in direct caregiving after the nursing home placement (Davies, 2001). Families also have a key role to play in individualizing and personalizing care, often going to extraordinary lengths to maximize the resident's quality of life (QOL) and maintain links to his or her past. In fulfilling these roles, family members provide a kind of support that nursing home staff have neither the time nor the knowledge of the resident's life and personality to provide. Families provide a lifeline of special care for their relative following placement, and this role is sustaining for both caregiver and care-receiver alike. They also play a key role in educating staff about their relatives' idiosyncrasies, and in doing so impart helpful information that could be gleaned from no other source but nonetheless provides a sense of personal identity while at the same time explaining seemingly incongruous behavior.

The important role of family members in long-term care settings such as nursing homes has been well documented. Family involvement is linked to residents' QOL (Kellett, 2000) and decreased family stress (Gaugler, Anderson, Zarit, &

Pearlin, 2004). However, the quality of staff–family relations has been shown to influence family involvement (Sandberg, Nolan, & Lind, 2002). There is also evidence of confusion on the issue of family involvement, with some studies reporting instances where both family members and staff assumed primary responsibility for the same tasks (Gaugler et al., 2004). Tension between families and nursing home staff with respect to each other's role in providing care is a recurrent theme in the literature (Davies & Nolan, 2004; Nolan & Dellasega, 2000). Ryan and Scullion (2000) reported that families felt that the biographical expertise that they had developed over their long years of caring was neither requested nor valued by nursing staff. Nursing staff in turn reported difficulties with families' preoccupation with their own relative, whereas the staff were responsible for the welfare of all the residents. Consistent with the findings of other studies (Gaugler et al., 2004; Kellett, 2000), Mrs. Velvet's case study revealed some evidence of blurred role boundaries and lack of clarity about who does what.

Brown-Wilson (2009) used a constructivist approach to undertake case studies of three care homes with the overall aim of exploring relationships between residents, families, and staff. On the basis of data from interviews, participant observation, and focus groups, the author concluded that the key factors influencing relationships were leadership, continuity of staff, personal philosophy of staff, and contribution of residents and families. However, it is important to note that even though there is strong evidence to suggest that family involvement positively affects the care of residents and the emotional health of residents and family members (Gaugler & Teaster, 2006; Robison et al., 2007), others (Andershed, 2006; Reid, Chappell, & Gish, 2007) caution that staff need to be sensitive in determining why, how, and how much family caregivers want to be involved. Whether they are providing care to residents because of a personal desire to do so or on the basis of their perceptions of the quality of care in the nursing home are key issues in terms of caregivers' emotional and physical health outcomes.

Various studies have recommended the need for change in the relationship between care home staff and relatives. These include clarifying the roles and responsibilities of groups

(Brown-Wilson, 2009; Lee, 2010), valuing and accessing caregiver knowledge and biographical expertise (Davies & Nolan, 2003; Robinson et al., 2010), and helping carers to perceive the transition in a more positive light (Davies & Nolan, 2004; Ryan et al., 2011). Weman, Kihlgren, and Fagerberg (2004) acknowledged that families were a resource in the care of older people. In the United States, Gaugler and Ewan (2005) conducted a study to identify predictors of staff attitudes toward family members and found that staff who reported greater quality in their relationships with residents also demonstrated more positive attitudes to family members. These findings emphasize the need to consider family, residents, and staff relationships in concert when designing and implementing nursing interventions to improve the quality of life and care in residential settings.

The literature reviewed so far suggests that families are more willing to help in nursing home care than what is acknowledged by staff and that there is a degree of misunderstanding of each other's role. This gives rise to a situation where many families are underused as a resource within the nursing home setting, often to the detriment of residents, relatives, and staff.

Role and Cultural Considerations

With a worldwide aging population, rise in emergency admissions, and shorter lengths of hospital stays, there is often limited time for acute nurses to discuss long-term care options with older people and their families. However, nurses in the acute care setting have around-the-clock input into patient care. More than any other professional group, they have opportunities to get to know their patients in a range of contexts. They are therefore ideally placed to offer practical and emotional support to older people and their families as they grapple with decisions about entry to long-term care. However, nurses in acute settings must also recognize the pressure they may be placing on families as they attempt to free up acute beds. Families need time to consider all their options, and nurses need to recognize the importance for many families of aging in place when assisting with the selection of a care home. Having time to choose the right home and having their choice respected is essential for a successful transition to long-term care. This is especially important in rural communities where nurses play a key role in advocating for older people and their families (Ryan et al., 2011).

Caring for older people in long-term care settings is a very different type of nursing than that which is required in more acute environments. Although older residents have psychological and social needs, these often remain unmet as a result of nurses' preoccupation with the physical aspects of care. Nurses and other care home staff may benefit from educational opportunities designed to facilitate a shift in thinking from an overconcentration on the "nursing" element of their day-to-day activity to a greater emphasis on ways of making residents and their families feel at home. For their part, nursing home owners need to recognize the importance of investing in the education of their staff as many have a weak track record in this area.

There is a need for change in the relationship between care home staff and relatives. These include the creation of a more welcoming environment, clarifying the roles and responsibilities of groups, valuing and accessing family knowledge and biographical expertise, and helping families and residents to perceive the transition in a more positive light. Other areas for improvement include more informal meetings between residents, relatives, and staff; introducing mechanisms for two-way feedback about matters concerning relatives and staff; and encouraging staff to consider relatives as expert partners in care unless this is contrary to the wishes of the relative or the older person.

Care home staff has a key role to play in taking a more proactive role in supporting residents to forge relationships with other residents and their families. This necessitates the collection of biographical information from residents so that this can be used to make connections with other residents. Even very tenuous connections pertaining to residents' education or employment history can be used effectively to construct familiarity, and in doing so to facilitate a wider social intercourse than would otherwise be possible. However, residents' willingness to engage with fellow residents cannot be taken for granted, and nurses have a role in identifying the parameters of new relationships. Care plans, which reflect the expressed wishes of residents and families, should be developed as a way of ensuring that the social and cultural aspects of care are not overlooked. As studies on group dynamics suggest that some group members assume or are given a leadership role, there is no reason to suggest that this should be any different in care home settings. Therefore, more established residents and families, if they so wish, could assume a mentoring role for new residents and their families.

Nurses in long-term care settings need to understand the needs of families to continue caregiving and its therapeutic effects on the older person and the family. Collaborative relationships are not just about sharing roles and responsibilities but also about sharing perspectives. An understanding of each other's perspective is an important precursor to more open communication about roles and responsibilities.

Solutions and Strategies

Clearly, many families wish to continue providing care to their relatives after the placement. In failing to recognize the actual and potential contribution of families, nursing homes run the risk of alienating the very people who need a sense of belonging and attachment to the nursing home community. Developing caring partnerships is crucial if the resources of nurses and families are to be maximized for the benefit of nursing home residents. However, it seems unlikely that this will occur unless both parties recognize each other's unique contribution to the care of the older person and work in partnership to maximize this. Families have biographical expertise, which they should be encouraged to share with nurses with the aim of providing high-quality holistic care to residents. Nurses have technical expertise and a wider range of experience caring for older people, and this can be shared with families to enable them to make a more complete contribution to the care of their older relative.

However, it must be recognized that a more collaborative approach to working will not be achieved unless changes are introduced at a very practical level. These changes could include more regular and informal meetings between care home staff and families. These meetings should augment the informal chats that both parties have and concentrate on a holistic review of the older person and the family, particularly the primary caregiver. Roles and responsibilities could be discussed and clarified at the outset and again as the need arises.

Clearly, good communication must underpin any staff–family relationship. Good-quality care is best delivered by nurses who have gained a deep understanding of the resident and a good working relationship with the family. For families to play as full a role as possible, they need to be involved in the assessment, planning, implementation, and evaluation of care. They need encouragement, information, and perhaps some training to continue their participation in care. Time, for the resident and the family, is the most important contribution the nurse can make in building and maintaining a caring relationship. This time can be used to discuss problems, thoughts, and feelings and to provide stimulating activities for the resident. However, the availability of more time has major implications for staffing levels. Relatives require patience and understanding from staff in nursing homes. Their actual and potential contribution should be recognized and valued. However, families also need to demonstrate sensitivity to staff difficulties and concerns. Improved communication and sharing of information between family carers and staff has the potential for an improved working relationship that can only prove beneficial to all concerned.

Strategies, such as the use of narratives and life stories, are also effective means of enhancing relationships in care homes. Incorporating biographical information from residents and families into care plans is essential for the delivery of person-centered care. Equally important, workshops for staff and relatives to improve communication have been shown to be effective in providing insights into each other's actual and potential roles. However, initiatives such as these require commitment on the part of residents, relatives, and nursing home staff and can have major resource implications.

Clinical Reasoning Questions

1. How would you facilitate a more positive transition to long-term care for Mrs. Velvet and her daughter?
2. What are the barriers to Mrs. Velvet's daughter's continued involvement in her care?
3. What would you do if a situation arose where residents requested a degree of family involvement that was not tenable from the perspective of the family member?
4. What do you understand by the terms *relationship-centered care* and *person-centered care*?
5. What measures can nurses take to promote family connections in long-term care settings?

References

Andershed, B. (2006). Relatives in end of life care, Part 1: A systematic review of the literature the five last years, January 1999–February 2004. *Journal of Clinical Nursing, 15,* 1158–1169.

Andrews, G. J., Holmes, D., Poland, B., Lehoux, P., Miller, K. L., Pringle, D., & McGilton, K. S. (2005). "Airplanes are flying nursing homes": Geographies in the concepts and locales of gerontological nursing practice. *International Journal of Older People Nursing, 14*(8b), 109–120.

Bauer, M. (2006). Collaboration and control: Nurses' constructions of the role of family in nursing home care. *Journal of Advanced Nursing, 54*(1), 45–52.

Brown-Wilson, C. (2009). Developing community in care homes through a relationship-centered approach. *Health & Social Care in the Community, 17,* 177–186.

Davies, S. (2001). *Wanting what's best for them. Relatives' experience of nursing home entry: A constructivist inquiry* (Unpublished doctoral dissertation). Faculty of Medicine, School of Nursing and Midwifery, University of Sheffield, England.

Davies, S., & Nolan, M. (2003). "Making the best of things": Relatives' experiences of decisions about care home entry. *Aging and Society, 23,* 429–450.

Davies, S., & Nolan, M. (2004). "Making the move": Relatives' experiences of the transition to a care home. *Health and Social Care in the Community, 12*(6), 517–526.

Davies, S., & Nolan, M. (2006). "Making it better": Self-perceived roles of family caregivers of older people living in care homes: A qualitative study. *International Journal of Nursing Studies, 43*, 281–291.

Gaugler, J. E., Anderson, K. A., Zarit, S. H., & Pearlin, L. I. (2004). Family involvement in the nursing home: Effects on stress and well-being. *Aging and Mental Health, 8*, 65–75.

Gaugler, J. E., & Ewan, H. H. (2005). Building relationships in residential long-term care. *Journal of Gerontological Nursing, 31*(9), 19–26.

Gaugler, J. E., & Teaster, P. (2006). The family caregiving career: Implications for community-based long-term care practice and policy. *Journal of Aging & Social Policy, 18*, 141–154.

Keefe, J., & Fancey, P. (2000). The care continues: Responsibility for elderly relatives before and after admission to a long-term care facility. *Family Relations, 49*(3), 235–244.

Kellett, U. M. (2000). Bound within the limits: Facing constraints to family caring in nursing homes. *International Journal of Nursing Practice, 6*(6), 317–323.

Lee, G. E. (2010). Predictors of adjustment to nursing home life of elderly residents: A cross-sectional study. *International Journal of Nursing Studies, 47*(8), 957–964.

McCann, S., Ryan, A. A., & McKenna, H. P. (2005). The challenges associated with providing community care for people with complex needs in rural areas: A qualitative investigation. *Health and Social Care in the Community, 13*(5), 462–469.

Nakrem, S., Vinsnes, A. G., Harkless, G. E., Paulsen, B., & Seim, A. (2012). Ambiguities: Residents' experience of "nursing home as my home." *International Journal of Older People Nursing, 8*(3), 216–225. doi:10.1111/j.1748-3743.2012.00320.x

Nolan, M., & Dellasega, C. (2000). "I really feel I've let him down": Supporting family carers during long-term care placement for elders. *Journal of Advanced Nursing, 31*(4), 759–767.

Owen, T., & Meyer, J. (2012). *My home life: Promoting quality of life in care homes*. London, England: Joseph Rowntree Foundation.

Reid, R. C., Chappell, N. L., & Gish, J. A. (2007). Measuring family perceived involvement in individualized long-term care. *Dementia, 6*, 89–104.

Robison, J., Curry, L., Gruman, C., Porter, M., Henderson, C. R., Jr., & Pillemer, K. (2007). Partners in caregiving in a special care environment: Cooperative communication between staff and families on dementia units. *The Gerontologist, 47*, 504–515.

Robinson, C. A., Reid, R. C., & Cooke, H. A. (2010). A home away from home: The meaning of home according to families of residents with dementia. *Dementia, 9*(4), 490–508.

Ryan, A. A., & Mc Kenna, H. P. (2013). Familiarity as a key factor influencing rural family carers' experience of the nursing home placement of an older relative: A qualitative study. *BMC Health Services Research, 13*, 252. doi:10.1186/1472-6963-13-252

Ryan, A. A., Mc Kenna, H. P., & Slevin, O. (2011). Family caregiving and decisions about entry to care: A rural perspective. *Aging and Society, 32*(1), 1–18.

Ryan, A. A., & Scullion, H.F. (2000). Family and staff perceptions of the role of families in nursing homes. *Journal of Advanced Nursing,* 32(3), 626–634.

Sandberg, J., Nolan, M. R., & Lind, U. (2002). Entering a new world: Empathic awareness as a key to positive family/staff relationships in care homes. *International Journal of Nursing Studies, 39*, 507–515.

Weman, K., Kihlgren, M., & Fagerberg, I. (2004). Older people living in nursing homes or other community care facilities: Registered nurses' views of their working situation and cooperation with family members. *Journal of Clinical Nursing, 13*, 617–626.

Wiles, J. (2005). Conceptualizing place in the care of older people: The contribution of geographical gerontology. *International Journal of Older People Nursing, 14*(8b), 100–108.

23 FAMILY CAREGIVER SUPPORT

COLLEEN DOYLE, CECILY HUNTER,
AND VANESSA M. WHITE

Subjective

"I know he'd do it for me if things were the other way round."

Objective

Mrs. Wilma Widener is an 85-year-old family caregiver living in the outer suburbs of Brisbane, Queensland, who has been looking after her 87-year-old husband, James. James received a diagnosis of vascular dementia 2 years ago. His condition has been slowly deteriorating with some periods of stability, but typically episodes of deterioration associated with transient ischemic attacks for the past 5 years. His most recent assessment of cognitive functioning on examination was in the moderate dementia range, with a Mini Mental State Examination score of 14. On a daily basis, he is now unable to remember when to take medication, and needs some assistance with showering, dressing, eating, and drinking. He is no longer able to drive a car, having relinquished his driver's license 2 years ago at the request of his family physician—a difficult decision as he had been the driver for the couple. The couple had no children and no relatives nearby. Wilma had never learned to drive, and hence the couple are now isolated and have difficulty accessing local shopping services because public transport is difficult and taxi services are expensive and unreliable. James spends much of the day passively watching television and sleeping. Wilma is able to cook for the couple, but needs assistance with getting James out of bed, dressing him, and showering him as he is a big man. James requires regular visits from a physiotherapist to maintain his walking ability as he is very inactive. An occupational therapist has advised on the layout of the home and placement of activities such as simple board games and everyday tasks such as folding clothes to assist James in cognitive stimulation. The couple are supported in the community by a suite of community services coordinated by their case manager, a community nurse with experience in dementia care.

James is often disoriented when he wakes from his afternoon nap, and experiences sundowning agitation late some afternoons when he thinks he is late for work. He also regularly spends nighttimes wandering inside the house, disturbing Wilma's sleep. His community nurse manager was able to provide advice to Wilma on how to manage his behavior and how to improve their sleep patterns. She also provides regular emotional support for Wilma, who is socially isolated.

Literature Review

There is a large literature on caregiving and dementia. Family caregivers of people living with dementia experience high levels of depression and anxiety (Pinquart & Sorensen, 2004). The literature provides some evidence that community service support and the services of a case manager to coordinate services leads to better outcomes for people living with dementia and their family caregiver (You, Dunt, Doyle, & Hsueh, 2012). Schoenmakers, Buntinx, and DeLepeleire (2010) reviewed the literature on home care interventions and well-being and found that family caregivers did receive some benefit from formal support, although the benefits could only be described as small. The emotional support provided by community service networks may be an important component of community services.

Doyle et al. (2009) investigated the meaning of caregiving for family caregivers of people living with dementia as part of a national evaluation of dementia care in Australia, and previously unpublished results are provided here. We conducted interviews with 70 family caregivers who were receiving community services designed to assist people living with dementia to stay in their own home rather than be admitted to residential aged care. The difference between this study and those previously published was that the program of services (called the Extended Aged Care at Home Dementia program) that our participants were receiving was designed to meet the specific needs of people living with dementia, and recipients were otherwise eligible for admission to residential care, so they were highly dependent. We asked family caregivers about their expectations for receiving community services, and the effect on their quality of life. The semistructured interviews were undertaken over the phone by the authors (CH and VW), and ethics approval was obtained from the La Trobe University Human Research Ethics Committee. We undertook a qualitative analysis of themes raised in the interviews. The interviews provided a family caregiver perspective on receiving community services and support from a case manager for people who are very frail and living with dementia.

Men and women in this study who were caring for a spouse/partner all emphasized the importance of community support in helping them in a caring role that often consumed all their time and energy but that was an integral component of a long life together. Community services supported the more able person in keeping a longstanding agreement between spouses that each one would care for the other if, and when, the need arose. In the words of one carer who saw her situation in this light, "I know he'd do it for me if things were the other way round."

The attitudes to caring were different for male and female study participants. Some men found it difficult to take on the role of carer with all its attendant domestic duties, but, as more than one said, having "settled down, [I am] now adjusted to it." Another husband carer, looking after his physically well wife whose severe dementia was associated with constant activity day and night, said, "It is a difficult job and takes some adjusting to—you have to plan and observe to avoid problems." An elderly wife carer had promised her husband that she would do all she could to look after him when it was necessary. A carer whose youngest child was still at school said she had adjusted to the task of caring for her highly dependent husband and accepted that her life was largely confined to her home, because if he went into care "it would be the end of him."

Family caregivers interviewed for this study experienced 24/7 demands on their care, while community services and supports are rarely able to satisfy the total needs of individuals. Carers' need for support arises out of their particular position in life, their individual interests and inclinations, and how the person they are caring for experiences dementia. For example, getting a break from care appears to be important for all carers. However, the literature on one need that appears to be met with variable success is the need for relief from care during the night. The carers of people whose dementia causes them to be very active at night may rarely get a full night's sleep. A husband carer in this situation managed his need for sleep by locking himself in the bedroom, leaving his wife to move about the house as it suited her, having taken every precaution to ensure that she could come to no harm. Another carer found emergency respite met her need for a night's sleep from time to time, but her husband's continual activity at night combined with his tendency to fall was a continuing source of worry throughout the time community services were in place.

Research findings indicated that, overall, carer satisfaction with community service supports seems to be shaped by the capacity of their case manager to assemble, from the available resources, what appears to the carer as a reasonable balance of support to assist her or him in addressing the particular issues she or he faces in the caring role and in relation to other responsibilities. A small number of carers had no clear idea of their needs. In a few instances, the discharge of the care recipient from the hospital into the carer's custody was reported by the carer to be conditional upon the carer's acceptance of community services. For one husband, whose wife experienced the sudden onset of dementia following an operation, the important thing was to bring his wife home from the hospital rather than take the advice of hospital staff and admit her to residential care. In his view, his principal need was to have the time to do the shopping, but he subsequently realized, with the help of his case manager, that his needs were much wider.

Most carers found that health professionals did perceive their needs. Many carers needed assistance with activities of daily living such as showering. Some wives/partners required this because of the increasing infirmity of the person they were caring for. For men caring for their wives or mothers, showering and hair washing were important needs also. Some husband carers needed assistance with meal preparation and housework. Other husband/partner carers prided themselves on being able to meet all their wife's/partner's care needs and did not use all the services they were entitled to because, as one carer put it, "if he'd let the service provider do all they wanted to, he'd just be sitting about and he doesn't want that." Another husband carer was happy with community supports; he enjoyed "his day off to play golf" and thought that "professionals" tended to see problems. He felt his approach was more positive because he focused on "working out solutions." Another husband found that the assistance provided with showering and dressing his wife each day was essential to his managing to care for her at all. She had spent some time in residential care, but because of "the running around" he had to do, and because they both found separation stressful, she came home again. However, as his own health declined and additional needs arose, he was not able to have these met because of his wife's opposition. He could have had assistance in getting his wife to bed, but she would not accept this because of her dislike of having strangers in the house. Despite this, her husband believed that she enjoyed the stimulation of having different people around. Both she and her husband were quite isolated at home, and he also enjoyed the change of having workers in the house.

As a result of the study findings, one need that appears to be more likely to be identified retrospectively is the need for female company experienced by women who are largely confined to their homes and who are cared for by their husbands/sons. Male carers in this situation were inclined to identify the female company provided by service provider workers as contributing to the improvement in the quality of life of their mother/wife that they perceived following the introduction of community supports. For women caring for highly dependent husbands, the constancy of care may not be a problem because "they have always done things together." On the other hand, getting a break from 24-hour care can be vital in contributing to a carer's capacity to continue looking after a highly dependent spouse, even if only to have a break to "do some thinking." Help with heavy outside work can be a pressing need for women caring for husbands/partners who may have previously assumed all responsibility for such work. The principal need for one carer was that her husband should have the opportunity to get the exercise he needed. He had always been an energetic, sports-loving man, and his energy persisted despite his deterioration in mental capacity. Her increasing frailty meant she was unable to meet this need, but her service provider was successful in doing so because it was able to secure at least one worker who was able to play golf with this man. A carer, who initially did not think community services had much to offer, found that her needs became much clearer as her husband's condition deteriorated suddenly to the point where he was confined to bed. This carer found community services "satisfactory in every way." With the deterioration in her husband's condition, this carer got very little relief from care. Where previously she was able to go out when the worker was there, she now had to remain at home to assist the worker. At her 3-month review interview, she reported that the community services were vital because it made it possible for her to care for her husband at home rather than admit him to residential care. The other need that was mentioned more often by wives caring for husbands was the need to know that if and when further help was required, it would be available, indicating that they appreciated the emotional support provided by community supports.

The literature on respite care shows that it is greatly valued by carers, especially if it is flexible and can provide a range of options to suit the specific needs of individual caregivers (O'Connell, Hawkins, Ostaszkiewicz, & Millar, 2012). Not all carers are willing to use respite care. One study found that one quarter of family carers of people with dementia did not access respite care (Bruen & Howe, 2009). Getting a break from care was important to almost all carers we interviewed, but what this meant for individual carers varied greatly according to their particular circumstances. Factors that appear to be particularly important are whether the carer shared the same residence as the care recipient and the severity of the dementia. For carers living under the same roof with someone who could not be left alone at all, getting a break from caring meant having a few hours each week to go to appointments and do the shopping. Some carers in this group were able to play a game of golf or pursue some other form of recreational interest. In cases where the care recipient is fit enough to get around, carers often get the best break from care by being able to remain at home while the care recipient is taken out. For one carer whose mother was particularly enthusiastic about going out, having a worker to do this at times was a great relief.

Many carers are constrained in what they can do during a break from care by lack of energy, even when the time is available. For those whose sleep was frequently interrupted, getting a break from care meant being able to go to sleep for a few hours without any disturbance. A carer who used her respite in this manner described it as a mixed blessing. Her husband wanted to go out with her rather than remain with the worker, and she did not like to tell him he could not come. Another carer felt very isolated in her home caring for a highly dependent husband. On occasions when she did not feel well, she used the time when a worker was in the house to go to bed. However, this carer also used other respite time to continue doing volunteer work for a few hours each week.

Carers receiving services are in the position of having to take strangers into their homes and into their lives to an extent that they may never have encountered previously. For some this requires a significant degree of adjustment. However, carers' comments suggest that despite this, the relationships they form with workers and case managers are very important to them. For an elderly woman caring for her husband who suffered from a brain tumor, the backup she was given in her caring role, from the case manager and workers, was one of the most useful aspects of community services. She noted that her case manager seemed to go out of her way to help. When the husband was admitted to the hospital and discharged soon after, the case manager, knowing that the carer did not drive, took him home. This carer was not alone in finding the support of the case manager invaluable. Another carer commented that her case manager had "given her more help in understanding her husband's condition than any organization had done." This case manager also supported the nondriving carer by dropping her off at the shops or at appointments. Even in cases where the service provider did not altogether meet a carer's needs, the carer was likely to identify the moral support he or she received from the case manager as useful. Another carer described her case manager as "on the ball," responding immediately to new concerns. Carers have identified frequent changes in case manager—and some might experience this change three or four times over a period of 6 months or so—as extremely frustrating.

Workers are, as might be expected, a vital component in the provision of services. Many carers expressed great satisfaction with the workers they encountered, commenting that they "were a nice class of person" and "able to coax" a reluctant care recipient into an activity that might be in his or her best interests—such as showering or changing soiled clothing—but one he or she may have been reluctant to embark upon. Carers valued the interaction with workers, with one noting that she can "discuss her father with them," and they listen to her, which gives her an outlet for worries she is unwilling to burden her friends with. Another carer valued the worker as "another adult" in the house to share the caring responsibility. In cases where the care recipient is very frail and confined to the house and, as a consequence, the carer is as well, carers note that "a change of face" in the house is beneficial for them both. It has already been noted that where carers report a positive change in the quality of life of the care recipient they are likely to link this improvement with the presence of workers in the house. A few carers report that workers go out of their way to help, often in ways that are beyond the stipulated services. A husband who had 5 hours respite in 1 day to enable him to get in a game of golf reported that workers would often use this time to cook meals for the following days.

One element in community services that carers are universally unhappy with is the number of workers who are used to provide the services and changes in workers, especially when the carer is not notified of a change. This is so even in cases where the carer will express overall satisfaction with the services they are receiving. Having up to four workers providing services can be a source of anxiety for carers and care recipients. Having these workers change frequently because of holiday replacements and illness is a further cause of anxiety.

Carers find themselves in the tiresome position of having to make frequent explanations concerning what is done for the person they are caring for, where everything is, and the care recipient's likes and dislikes. In some cases, the carer will give up the idea of going out during the worker's attendance when a new worker arrives unexpectedly because he or she wants to make sure that the person he or she is caring for is comfortable with this individual. In such cases, the provision of a respite service is made useless because of the conditions in which the service is provided. The effect of a worker's late arrival or failure to turn up at all on carers who are combining employment and caring can be demoralizing. In these cases, the role of the case manager is vital in providing a stable point of call.

Role and Cultural Considerations

Nurses working in the community have many roles to juggle, especially when managing community support services for their clients. In the area of dementia care, nurses need extra training in assessment and management issues as the field is evolving rapidly. Tools that are helpful for a nurse in community care include those assessing cognitive function as well as those useful for monitoring change in behavioral and psychological symptoms of dementia. For family caregivers, emotional needs may be as important to support as instrumental needs, and the community nurse should be aware of the increased risk of mood disorders, such as depression and anxiety, in family caregivers as well as in the person living with dementia. Short assessment tools such as the Geriatric Depression Scale can be useful to screen for depression in family carers. For many carers, an empathic caring nurse willing to listen may be just the emotional support that is required.

Cultural attitudes to community services will have an impact on the relationship that the community nurse develops with his or her clients. Some families expect more than is able to be provided by scarce community services and will need counseling. Interpreter services may not be available to assist with medical interviews, in which case the community nurse may rely on family members to interpret, requiring extra sensitivity on the part of the nurse to family dynamics. For the generation who lived through world wars and the Great Depression, accepting help from community services may be difficult and resisted out of a sense of pride or duty. The stigma of mental illness in this generation may make discussing dementia and mood disorders painful for the clients.

Solutions and Strategies

Wilma's community case manager will increase her regular review assessments to be sensitive to the couple's changing needs as James's condition deteriorates.

1. The nurse will consider referring Wilma to a psychologist or therapist with skills in cognitive behavior therapy and counseling older people to assist with emotional support.
2. The nurse will arrange for Wilma to attend a dementia support group that meets in the local area and has respite care facilities for people with dementia—this will help Wilma get a break from caring and at the same time provide a social outlet.
3. If funds allow, the nurse can assist Wilma to arrange purchase of a "smart" television that will allow a more interactive experience for both James and Wilma by linking in with patient support groups on the TV, including those provided by the local Alzheimer's association.
4. The nurse case manager can organize a fitness program delivered under the guidance of the physiotherapist, which will help both James and Wilma to maintain physical fitness. A gentle exercise program for Wilma will help her to prevent anxiety and depression and keep her well enough to manage the physical demands of caring.

Clinical Reasoning Questions

1. What social services would you recommend to support Wilma and James in your area?
2. What clinical guidelines would you refer to in monitoring Wilma and James's needs?

3. What issues would be covered in an advance care planning conversation with Wilma?
4. What would you recommend for sundowning behavior?

References

Bruen, W., & Howe, A. (2009, May). *Respite care for people living with dementia. "It's more than just a short break"* (Discussion paper 17). Retrieved from http://www.fightdementia.org.au/common/files/NAT/20090500_Nat_NP_17RespCarePplLivDem.pdf

Doyle, C., Day, S., Dunt, D., McKenzie, R., Dort, P.V., Yates, K., & White, V. (2009). *Dementia initiative national evaluation: National evaluation of EACHD program.* Melbourne, Australia: LAMA Consortium, The University of Melbourne.

O'Connell, B., Hawkins, M., Ostaszkiewicz, J., & Millar, L. (2012). Carers' perspectives of respite care in Australia: An evaluative study. *Contemporary Nurse, 41*(1), 111–119.

Pinquart, M., & Sorensen, S. (2004). A systematic review of the effectiveness of psychosocial interventions for carers of people with dementia. *Aging & Mental Health, 5*, 107–119.

Schoenmakers, B., Buntinx, F., & DeLepeleire, J. (2010). Support the dementia family caregiver: The effect of home care intervention on general well-being. *Aging & Mental Health, 14*(1), 44–56.

You, E., Dunt, D., Doyle, C., & Hsueh, A. (2012). Effects of case management in community aged care on client and carer outcomes: A systematic review of randomized trials and comparative observational studies. *BMC Health Services Research, 12*, 395.

III

ASSESSING AND MANAGING COMMON CLINICAL CHALLENGES

MEREDITH WALLACE KAZER

Older adults are populating the world in unprecedented numbers. The Administration on Aging (2013) reports that there were approximately 43.1 million older adults living in the United States in 2012. This number reflects a 21% increase over the past decade for a total of 13.7% of the total population. The number of older adults in the United States is projected to rise to 79.7 million by the year 2040. Currently, 1 in 7 individuals in the United States is an older adult. The past 3 decades have also borne witness to a 93% growth in the number of centenarians, or those who live to the age of 100. Currently, there are 61,985 centenarians living in the United States.

As seen throughout this book, the rising population of older adults brings many challenges to health care services and environments that seek to provide older adults with the highest quality of life (QOL). One additional area that challenges QOL for older adults is centered on personal health. The Administration on Aging (2013) reports that older adults have at least one chronic health condition, and many report multiple chronic conditions. The most commonly occurring medical illnesses among older adults include arthritis, which is experienced by 50% of the population, followed by heart disease (30%), cancer (24%), and diabetes (20%).

The final section of this book was developed as a clinical resource to guide clinicians through strategies to maintain QOL amid several medical conditions that are experienced among older adults. Using real cases, the section provides meaningful clinical cases through which clinicians may enhance clinical reasoning and improve understanding of issues older adults encounter in preventing and managing these illnesses throughout environments of care. The cases in this section were chosen to enhance understanding of both commonly occurring medical issues and some less commonly occurring conditions. Using the case study approach, readers are able to develop a broad understanding of the impact of these health issues on the QOL of older adults, learn their role in managing these issues, and develop strategies for improving QOL through improved disease prevention and management.

This section of the book is organized around 11 chapters that draw attention to several medical conditions that impact older adults. The first two chapters of this section provide an opportunity to improve understanding of one of the increasing concerns among older adults worldwide, dementia. Dementia is a broad term used to refer to a group of approximately 26 specific diagnoses, including Alzheimer's disease. As Dr. Cooney reports in Chapter 25, there are an estimated 44.35 million individuals worldwide who have dementia. This number is projected to rise to 75.62 million in 2030 and 135.46 million in 2050 (Alzheimer's Disease International, 2013). Dementia brings about a number of physical problems, such as difficulty eating, drinking, and speaking. In addition, caregivers are often troubled by the behavioral issues associated with this disease.

The first three chapters of Section III of this book attempt to manage many of the physical and behavioral challenges associated with dementia through creative strategies and solutions. In Chapter 24, Dr. Casey reports that there are systematic reviews focused on the impact of physical activity programs on people with dementia. Various types and intensities of exercises were examined in these studies, including aerobic strengthening, flexibility, and balance elements. In Chapter 25, "Knowing Me," Dr. Cooney suggests biographical approaches to managing the behavioral issues associated with dementia. While biographical methods, such as reminiscence, have been supported in the literature for many years, the author of this chapter provides compelling new evidence for the use of these approaches to improve QOL. Using life story work (LSW), older adults with dementia are provided with a framework for discussing their life experiences. This provides an approach to care that is both meaningful and productive for older adults living at home or in institutional settings. In Chapter 26, Keady and Burrow discuss the challenges of clients managing dementia and multiple chronic illnesses in the United Kingdom. The authors provide strategies to help older adults with dementia and caregivers to improve QOL.

The third section of this book focuses more on the treatment of illness among older adults rather than the illness itself. Many older adults take a variety of prescription and nonprescription medications for their illnesses. Although these medications often improve QOL, there are a number of concerns with medication usage among the older population. Urinary incontinence is not a normal aging change; however, owing to many physical changes of aging, it occurs frequently among older adults. There are several different types of urinary incontinence, often occurring concurrently. This case, discussed in Chapter 28, "Continence Care," details the social implications of a widowed woman who fears leaving her house because of the possibility of an accident. Authors Moore and Kelly provide a thorough review of the occurrence of stress urinary incontinence and provide strategies for getting the client in this case back to the senior center. Moreover, the strategies are applicable to clients throughout care settings.

The third section of the book continues to address commonly occurring physical challenges among older adults. Because respiratory, mental health, and cardiac conditions are significant challenges as clients age, the section includes case studies that focus on each of these issues. Within this section, Dr. Casey addresses the needs of clients with COPD in Chapter 29, and Drs. O'Connor and Cauffield explore the complex issues of depression and suicide in Chapter 30. There is a common myth that health promotion activities are not beneficial to older adults in their later years. However, Drs. Lacey and Madara make the case in Chapter 31 that older adults are never "too old" to take care of their hearts.

As Section III continues, readers will also become familiar with issues associated with men and their families diagnosed with prostate cancer. Dr. Casey discusses the primary prevention of type 2 diabetes, and Dr. Lovanio explores the greatly needed strategies associated with developing good sleep hygiene in Chapter 34. Finally, Dr. Kris provides a case study in Chapter 35 on end-of-life care, in which she challenges providers to work toward the goal of helping older adults experience a "good death."

As readers work through this book, they will be captivated by the case studies contained within and developed by the literature that supports the issues discussed. The goal of this book is to increase both the depth and breadth of gerontological nursing among readers. Each chapter focuses on a different physical or mental health issue common to older adults and uses a case study approach to illustrate the issue in a manner that enhances understanding. The end goal is to improve nursing care to achieve the highest possible QOL for older adults.

References

Administration on Aging. (2013). *Profile of older Americans*. Washington, DC: Author. Retrieved from http://www.aoa.gov/Aging_Statistics/Profile/2013/docs/2013_Profile.pdf

Alzheimer's Disease International. (2013). *Policy brief for heads of government: The global impact of dementia 2013–2050.* London, England: Author. Retrieved from http://www.alz.co.uk/research/GlobalImpactDementia2013.pdf

24 PHYSICAL ACTIVITY FOR PEOPLE WITH DEMENTIA

DYMPNA CASEY AND CATHERINE HOUGHTON

Subjective

"I just loved to dance, but it's all over now . . . I can't seem to remember how. . . . When John, my husband, and I took to the floor, he was a great dancer, you know, we just floated around the room. . . . I miss him . . . I miss my dancing . . . I miss being active."

Objective

Xena Xemacs is a 70-year-old woman with moderate Alzheimer's disease who lives at home with her daughter Joan, her main caregiver. Xena was admitted to the respite center while her daughter Joan has a 2-week holiday. It's the first holiday that Joan has had in 2 years. Xena is 5 feet 5 in. (65 cm) and weighs 110 lbs. (50 kg). Her temperature is normal at 98°F, blood pressure is 130/78, and pulse 78, and her respirations are 16/minute. Her lung sounds are clear bilaterally, and her cardiac assessment indicates a regular heartbeat. Her balance is good and her gait is normal. Her skin, although pale, is warm, dry, and intact; her abdomen is soft and nontender; and bowel sounds are present in all four quadrants. Her Mini Mental State Examination (MMSE) score is 21 (mild dementia). The remainder of her physical assessment is unremarkable, and there is no evidence of pain. She requires some assistance with personal hygiene, but overall, if given cues, she can manage well. For instance, when handed her face cloth she will wash her face; when given her toothbrush with the toothpaste on, she can brush her teeth. She is fully continent, and despite some speech difficulties, when she cannot find the words, she is able to express when she needs to go to the toilet and her choices in food and drink. Xena was diagnosed with dementia 3 years ago, at the age of 67, by the consultant psychogeriatrician. That visit was prompted by Joan due to the family history of dementia and the fact that she had noticed that her mother was beginning to show signs of memory problems. She noticed that her mother, who loved the *Miss Maple* detective television series, was less able to follow the plot lines and remember the characters. Then she began to call Joan a few times a day, telling her the same information or task to complete, having no recollection that she had already phoned her. In addition, Joan slowly noticed that her Mom had less and less food in the refrigerator despite each week having a full grocery list for shopping; it became clear that her mother was not remembering to buy the food for the week.

Over the past few months, Xena has become even more forgetful and seems to talk more about her childhood and the distant past. She gets annoyed and upset more often when she cannot remember the names of her friends. Xena always enjoyed social contact but recently Joan says that she has started to lose her "sparkle" and appears more apathetic. She has also started waking early and seems to be more irritable in mood. She was always a very active lady and in her youth won numerous ballroom dancing awards. Until recently she went for a daily walk with Joan, which was her main form of exercise, but has now lost interest and refuses to go, saying "it's boring" or that the weather is too inclement. Xena is currently taking Razadyne 24 mg orally per day.

Literature Review

Dementia is a term used to describe a group of disorders that have common symptoms (Cahill, O'Shea, & Pierce, 2012). Globally, 35.6 million people have dementia (Alzheimer's Disease International, 2009) and this is expected to reach 81.1 million by 2040 (World Health Organization, 2012). Western Europe has the highest prevalence of dementia in the world (Ferri et al.,

2005, Prince & Jackson, 2009), calculated to be 7 million in 2013 (ALCOVE, 2013) and projected to increase to 13.4 million by 2050 (Prince & Jackson, 2009). Dementia affects people in different ways (Cahill et al., 2012). Common early problems include impaired memory, learning, judgment, communication, depression, and reduced physical activity due to impaired motor function (Eggermont & Scherder, 2006; Rolland, Abellan van Kan, & Vellas, 2008). Problems with balance and walking speed further compound these issues (O'Keefe et al., 1996; Pettersson, Engardt, & Wahlund, 2002). Declining physical function impacts on what a person can do and increases feelings of hopelessness that can in turn increase caregiver burden. With medication having limited effect, the development of new interventions that delay disability and reduce the care needs of people with dementia is critical (McLaren, LaMantia, & Callahan, 2013; Vreugdenhil, Cannell, Davies, & Razay, 2012). There is substantial evidence to suggest that physical activity can improve the quality of life (QOL) for people with dementia.

A number of systematic reviews have examined the effects of physical activity programs on people with dementia (Balsamo et al., 2013; Blankevoort et al., 2010; Crocker et al., 2013; Forbes et al., 2008; Heyn, Abreu, & Ottenbacher, 2004; McLaren et al., 2013; Potter, Ellard, Rees, & Thorogood, 2011; Rolland et al., 2008; Suttanon, Hill, Said, & Dodd, 2010; Teri et al., 2003). These studies conclude that different types and intensities of exercises are possible for people with dementia. However, there is uncertainty as to the optimal intensity, frequency, type, and duration of the exercise interventions required (Crocker et al., 2013; Kemoun et al., 2010). Potter et al. (2011) propose that regular exercise for older people with dementia can include a wide range of exercise modalities including aerobic strengthening, flexibility, and balance elements. Likewise, Blankevoort et al. (2010) found that physical activity programs that incorporate a combination of endurance, such as strength and balance, lead to larger improvements in gait speed, functional mobility, and balance compared to progressive resistance training alone. These findings would suggest that to achieve beneficial effects, different combinations of exercises are needed. Beneficial effects identified in the literature include improvements in mobility, flexibility, balance, and gait speed (Blankevoort et al., 2010; Crocker et al., 2013; Potter et al., 2011; Rolland et al., 2008; Suttanon et al., 2010). Physical activity has also been found to improve functioning in activities of daily living (ADLs; Blankevoort et al., 2010; Crocker et al., 2013; Suttanon et al., 2010). Chang, Chen, Shen, and Chiou (2011) found that people with dementia who had participated in a physical activity program had significant improvements in their ability to engage in self-care activities such as personal hygiene and self-grooming, but not in feeding, toileting, and dressing. Currently, Xena requires minimal assistance with her ADLs, but in order to maintain this level of independence, increasing her physical activity would help maintain and enhance her mobility, strength, and balance.

Many people with dementia may also suffer from depression, and physical activity has been found to reduce the symptoms of depression (Williams & Tappen, 2008) and cognitive decline (Balsamo et al., 2013; McLaren et al., 2013; Rolland et al., 2008). However, research exploring the impact of physical activity on depression is limited, and further work is recommended (Crocker et al., 2013; Forbes et al., 2008; Potter et al., 2011). It is important that Xena is assessed, because if she is depressed, treating her depression will improve her mood and may also improve her cognitive functioning. In addition, engaging in a physical activity program may reduce her symptoms, encourage social interaction, and enhance her overall quality of life. It is known that Xena was a keen ballroom dancer in the past. Therefore, developing a physical activity program that incorporates ballroom dancing may make engaging in physical activity more appealing to Xena.

The majority of the studies included in the aforementioned systematic reviews involved people with dementia living in residential settings. The needs and ability of people living in the community may differ from those in residential care and therefore need to be considered separately (Rolland et al., 2008; Suttanon et al., 2010). Vreugdenhil et al. (2012) conducted a randomized control trial (RTC) to examine the effectiveness of a community-based exercise program to improve functional ability in people with Alzheimer's disease (AD). The exercise program involved 10 exercises focusing on balance and strength, plus 30 minutes of brisk walking; participants were encouraged to do these daily. They found that participants in the intervention group showed significant improvements in cognitive and physical function and performance of ADLs. Trends toward improvement in depression and caregiver burden were also evident, but these were not significant.

It is also important to assess individual motivations, preferences, and capabilities of the person with dementia regarding physical activity programs, taking into consideration any existing comorbidities. If an exercise is too difficult for someone, he or she may get frustrated and refuse to participate (Logsdon, McCurry, & Teri, 2005). Blankevoort et al. (2010) discovered that people with higher MMSE scores (mild dementia) had higher participation rates in the physical activity program but also higher dropout rates. This has implications for Xena, who has mild cognitive impairment; therefore, strategies that motivate her to engage in physical activity need to be considered.

Galik, Resnick, and Pretzer-Aboff (2009) conducted focus groups with seven nursing assistants to explore the factors they considered important in motivating cognitively impaired older adults to participate in restorative care such as physical activity. Knowing the person with dementia was identified as a key motivator to promote participation in physical activity, which could be achieved by conducting the person's life history/life story. It is essential at all times to know the person with dementia, build authentic relationships, and be aware of the person's values about care (McCormack, 2003). The overall aim is to maintain personhood in the face of failing mental powers (Kitwood, 1997). Therefore, the focus should be on the person first and the dementia second. Flexibility was also identified by nursing assistants as important for motivating and engaging people with dementia in exercise programs as it allowed them to engage at their own pace (Galik, Resnick, & Pretzer-Aboff, 2009). Other strategies used to motivate and engage people with dementia to participate in physical activity programs involve the inclusion of social interaction and casual conversations throughout the exercise (Blankevoort et al., 2010; Rolland et al., 2008; Williams & Tappen, 2008). Introducing music or dancing and individualizing the activity were also highlighted as important in promoting participation (Kemoun et al., 2010; Logsdon, McCurry, & Teri, 2005). This is particularly pertinent to Xena because of her love of dancing.

The nurse must also be cognizant of potential barriers to exercise participation for people with dementia, including anxiety, agitation, fear of injury, and the side effects of medications, which may cause drowsiness and limit their ability to engage (Galik, Resnick, & Pretzer-Aboff, 2009). In addition, the presence of pain may also inhibit engagement in exercise. Plooij, Scherder, and Eggermont (2012) reviewed the impact of physical inactivity in dementia and its relationship to pain. They concluded that, on the basis of the few studies available, pain may cause physical inactivity in the person with dementia. It is important, therefore, that a pain assessment is conducted with Xena to detect whether this may be a factor that has led to her reluctance to engage in physical activity.

The burden of caring for Xena is clearly impacting on Joan as she is on her first holiday in 2 years. A useful strategy, therefore, would be to actively encourage and include Joan as a participant in the physical activity program, as this strategy has been found to enhance the health of the caregiver as they exercise beside the person with dementia (Vreugdenhil et al., 2012). Furthermore, caregivers reported that they enjoyed the social aspect of walking in the community and enjoyed doing something positive with the person rather than the usual routine of personal care tasks. Participating in exercise may also help reduce Joan's sense of care burden, quality of sleep, and overall QOL (Hirano et al., 2011). When developing an activity program, the nurse should therefore encourage Joan to actively participate in the planned exercise program.

Xena's well-being and QOL could be improved by the development of an individualized physical activity program that incorporates her love of dance, thereby enhancing her motivation and subsequent compliance with the program. Engaging in physical activity has the potential to help her maintain her current independence in performing her ADLs, improve her cognition, and enhance her physical well-being in terms of balance, strength, and flexibility. Working in partnership with Xena and Joan, the nurse can devise a physical activity program that meets their needs, preferences, and capabilities, and such a program will enhance the likelihood that the program will be implemented, ultimately improving both Xena's and Joan's QOL.

Role and Cultural Considerations

Most nurses are not provided with an adequate amount of education on the importance of physical activity for people with dementia or how to design an appropriate physical activity program. More education is needed, therefore, at both generalist and advanced practice levels. Assessment tools, such as the interview-administered physical activity questionnaire Assessment of Physical Activity in Frail Older People (APAFOP), which has been tested for use with older people who are cognitively impaired (Hauer et al., 2011), may be useful in supporting and guiding nurses to assess and subsequently develop a physical activity program for people with dementia. However, not all older adults with dementia may be willing to engage in physical activity. Therefore, taking the time to get to know the person and ascertaining his or her likes, dislikes, cultural norms, and values in regard to physical activity is crucial.

Strategies and Solutions

- Depression is common in people with dementia, so assess for depression.
- Assess Xena's capacity for physical activity, and devise a physical activity program tailored to her needs, mindful of any comorbidities and potential side effects from medications.
- Encourage Joan to also actively participate in the physical activity program.
- Encourage Xena to have a good diet to maintain nutritional and hydration status.

Clinical Reasoning Questions

1. What is your plan for follow-up care of Xena?
2. Are any referrals needed in this case? If so, to whom?
3. What if Xena were more inclined to lose her balance or is depressed?
4. Are there any standardized guidelines that you could use to assess or treat Xena?

References

ALCOVE. (2013). *Alcove synthesis report* [Alzheimer Cooperative Valuation in Europe. The European Joint Action on Dementia]. Retrieved from http://www.kbs-frb.be/uploadedFiles/2012-KBS-FRB/05)_Pictures,_documents_and_external_sites/12)_Report/ALCOVE%20SYNTHESIS%20REPORT.pdf

Alzheimer's Disease International. (2009). *World Alzheimer report*. Retrieved from http://www.alz.co.uk/research/files/WorldAlzheimerReport.pdf

Balsamo, S., Willardson, J. M., de Santana, F. S., Prestes, J., Balsamo, D. C., Nascimento, D. C., & Nobrega, O. T. (2013). Effectiveness of exercise on cognitive impairment and Alzheimer's disease. *International Journal of General Medicine, 6*, 387–391.

Blankevoort, C. G., van Heuvelen, M. J. G., Boersma, F., Luning, H., de Jong, J., & Scherder, E. J. A. (2010). Review of effects of physical activity on strength, balance, mobility and ADL performance in elderly subjects with dementia. *Dementia and Geriatric Cognitive Disorders, 30*(5), 392–402.

Cahill, S., O'Shea, E., & Pierce, M. (2012). *Creating excellence in dementia care: A research review for Ireland's National Dementia Strategy*. Dublin, Ireland: DSIDC's Living with Dementia Research Program, School of Social Work and Social Policy, Trinity College Dublin, & Irish Center for Social Gerontology, National University of Ireland Galway.

Chang, S. H., Chen, C. Y., Shen, S. H., & Chiou, J. H. (2011). The effectiveness of an exercise program for elders with dementia in a Taiwanese day-care center. *International Journal of Nursing Practice, 17*(3), 213–220.

Crocker, T., Forster, A., Young, J., Brown, L., Ozer, S., Smith, J., & Greenwood, D. C. (2013). Physical rehabilitation for older people in long-term care (Review). *The Cochrane Library, 2*, 1–190.

Eggermont, L. H. P., & Scherder, E. J. A. (2006). Physical activity and behavior in dementia: A review of literature and implications for psychosocial intervention in primary care. *Dementia, 5*(3), 411–428.

Ferri, C. P., Prince, M., Brayne, C., Brodaty, H., Fratiglioni, L., Ganguli, M., . . . Alzheimer's Disease International. (2005). Global prevalence of dementia: A Delphi consensus study. *Lancet, 366*(9503), 2112–2117.

Forbes, D., Forbes, S., Morgan, D. G., Markle-Reid, M., Wood, J., & Culum, I. (2008). Physical activity programs for persons with dementia. *The Cochrane Library, 3*, 1–75.

Galik, E. M., Resnick, B., & Pretzer-Aboff, I. (2009). "Knowing what makes them tick": Motivating cognitively impaired older adults to participate in restorative care. *International Journal of Nursing Practice, 15,* 48–55.

Hauer, K., Lord, S., Lindemann, U., Lamb, S., Aminian, K., & Schwenk, M. (2011). Assessment of physical activity in older people with and without cognitive impairment. *Journal of Aging and Physical Activity, 19,* 347–372.

Heyn, P., Abreu, B. C., & Ottenbacher, K. J. (2004). The effects of exercise training on elderly persons with cognitive impairment and dementia: A meta-analysis. *Archives of Physical Medicine and Rehabilitation, 85*(10), 1694–1704.

Hirano, A., Suzuki, Y., Kuzuya, M., Onishi, J., Ban, N., & Umegaki, H. (2011). Influence of regular exercise on subjective sense of burden and physical symptoms in community-dwelling caregivers of dementia patients: A randomized control trial. *Archives of Geronotology and Geriatrics, 53,* e158–e163.

Kemoun, G., Thibaud, M., Roumagne, N., Carette, P., Albinet, C., Toussaint, L., & Dugué, B. (2010). Effects of a physical training programme on cognitive function and walking efficiency in elderly persons with dementia. *Dementia and Geriatric Cognitive Disorders, 29(*2), 109–114.

Kitwood, T. (1997). *Dementia reconsidered: The person comes first.* Buckingham, England: Open University Press.

Logsdon, R. G., McCurry, S. M., & Teri, L. (2005). A home health care approach to exercise for persons with Alzheimer's disease. *Care Management Journals, 6*(2), 90–97.

McCormack, B. (2003). Researching nursing practice: Does person-centeredness matter? *Nursing Philosophy, 4,* 179–188.

McLaren, A. N., LaMantia, M. A., & Callahan, C. M. (2013). Systematic review of non-pharmacologic interventions to delay functional decline in community-dwelling patients with dementia. *Aging and Mental Health, 17*(6), 655–666.

O'Keefe, S. T., Kazeem, H., Philpott, R. M., Playfer, J. R., Gosney, M., & Lye, M. (1996). Gait disturbance in Alzheimer's disease: A clinical study. *Age and Aging, 25*(4), 313–316.

Pettersson, A. F., Engardt, M., & Wahlund, L. O. (2002). Activity level and balance in subjects with mild Alzheimer's disease. *Dementia and Griatric Cognitive Disorders, 13*(4), 213–216.

Plooij, B., Scherder, E. J. A., & Eggermont, L. H. P. (2012). Physical inactivity in aging and dementia: A review of its relationship to pain. *Journal of Clinical Nursing, 21*(21–22), 3002–3008.

Potter, R., Ellard, D., Rees, K., & Thorogood, M. (2011). A systematic review of the effects of physical activity on physical functioning, quality of life and depression in older people with dementia. *International Journal of Geriatric Psychiatry, 26*(10), 1000–1011.

Prince, M., & Jackson, J. (2009). *World Alzheimer report 2009*. London, England: Alzheimer's Disease International. Retrieved from www.alz.co.uk/research/files/WorldAlzheimerReport.pdf

Rolland, Y., Abellan van Kan, G., & Vellas, B. (2008). Physical activity and Alzheimer's disease: From prevention to therapeutic perspectives. *Journal of the American Medical Directors Association, 9*(6), 390–405.

Suttanon, P., Hill, K., Said, C., & Dodd, K. (2010). Can balance exercise programmes improve balance and related physical performance measures in people with dementia? A systematic review. *European Review of Aging and Physical Activity, 7*(1), 13–25.

Teri, L., Gibbons, L. E., McCurry, S. M., Logsdon, R. G., Buchner, D. M., Barlow, W. E., . . . Larson, E. B. (2003). Exercise plus behavioral management in patients with Alzheimer disease: A randomized controlled trial. *The Journal of the American Medical Association, 290*(15), 2015–2022.

Vreugdenhil, A., Cannell, J., Davies, A., & Razay, G. (2012). A community-based exercise program to improve functional ability in people with Alzheimer's disease: A randomized controlled trial. *Scandinavian Journal of Caring Sciences, 26*(1), 12–19.

Williams, C. L., & Tappen, R. M. (2008). Exercise training for depressed older adults with Alzheimer's disease. *Aging and Mental Health, 12*(1), 72–80.

World Health Organization. (2012). *Dementia: A public health priority*. Retrieved from http://apps.who.int/iris/bitstream/10665/75263/1/9789241564458_eng.pdf?ua=1

25 KNOWING ME

Adeline Cooney and Eamon O'Shea

Subjective

"Yohann and I have been together a long time. When the children got older we thought, 'Now's our time.' We liked puttering around together. We went out for a meal or a drink. Nothing fancy, but it was nice. We enjoyed each other's company. This disease robbed us of that. It broke my heart leaving him here (long-term care) but I couldn't manage any more. They're good here but they don't know him. How could they? He is really talented. He was the best carpenter for miles around—he could make anything. He didn't just put up shelves or fit kitchens. He liked to design things. The trickier the job, the better he liked it. When he retired, he started woodcarving for fun. He was really good at it. You should see the things he's carved—owls, dogs, trees. He loves nature, he loves being outside. He was always finding things to do outside, the garden, walking the dog. That's why he started carving, I suppose. It brought together the two things he loves most—wood and nature. He always said, 'I hate having nothing in my hands; I need to be doing something.' That's why it's so hard seeing him wandering around doing nothing. The nurses are really good. They try talking to him, but he either ignores them or shouts at them—I think they're leaving him alone so he doesn't disturb the others. I understand that, but it's sad because Yohann loves chatting. Maybe if they knew more about him, it would be easier for them to talk with him. I wish they could see him the way I see him. He is such a nice man."

Objective

Mr. Yohann Young, 84 years old, was admitted to the long-term care unit 1 month ago. Yohann has a clinical diagnosis of dementia. The major component of client evaluation is a comprehensive client history, including at least one informant other than the patient. Yohann's wife, Mary (80 years of age), reported that his memory gradually worsened. Initially, she put it down to absent-mindedness, but over time she recognized, "There was more to it." Yohann visited his general practitioner, who applied the Mini Mental State Examination (MMSE) (Folstein, Folstein, & McHugh, 1975). The MMSE, a screening test for cognitive impairment, assesses a broad range of cognitive functions: orientation, recall, attention, calculation, language, and constructional praxis (Shadlen & Larson, 2014). A score of 25 or higher (out of 30) indicates normal cognition. Scores below this may indicate severe (9 points or fewer), moderate (10 to 20 points), or mild (21 to 24 points) cognitive impairment (Crum, Anthony, Bassett, & Folstein, 1993). Yohann's scores have gradually deteriorated over time. His current score at 10 points indicates moderate cognitive impairment. Mary described Yohann's typical day. He wanders all day and most of the night, and on several occasions he has wandered away from home and got lost (example of deficits in visual spatial perception). He sleeps very little, and consequently she gets very little rest. He requires help with washing, dressing, and eating (example of problems with ideomotor praxis [i.e., the performance of learned motor movements]). She worries that he is not getting enough to eat. He is incontinent and wears an incontinence pad. Lately, he has become increasingly frustrated and sometimes aggressive. On one occasion he struck her, but this is out of character. Yohann still knows her and responds to her, but sadly, he does not always recognize their son or daughter. She still knows what he is saying or wants, but it is getting harder to understand him because he, increasingly, has difficulty finding words. This seems to be what frustrates him most. On questioning, Yohann knew his own identity, but was unsure of where he was and did not know the current date or month (example of recent memory deficits). His attention span is short, he is easily distracted, and he has difficulty focusing on questions and instructions (examples of attention and concentration deficits). Yohann tends to ramble and has difficulty naming objects presented to him (example of language deficits). He became visibly agitated with the questions and frequently replies, "I know the answer, but I'm not telling you." Yohann's clinical history suggests a diagnosis of dementia, or major neurocognitive disorder. The *DSM-5* describes this as a weakening or mental deterioration in one or more of the following: learning and memories, speech, function, attention, motor or perception, and cognition. These issues interfere with independence, and do not occur in isolated events, nor are they a product of another disorder.

A diagnosis of dementia requires absence of features of delirium and exclusion of nonorganic psychiatric disorders such as major depression or schizophrenia (American Psychiatric Association 2013). Yohann has no prior history of depression. Physical examination was normal. A routine blood screen was carried out including FBC, ESR, LFT, TSH, U&E, serum B_{12}, folate, ferritin, serum magnesium, phosphorus, and calcium. Shadlen and Larson (2014) note that the American Academy of Neurology recommend screening for B_{12} deficiency and hypothyroidism because of the high prevalence of hypothyroidism in older people and the potential benefits of treatment. However, the benefit of routine blood test screening is questionable (Shadlen & Larson, 2014). All were in normal range. A midstream specimen of urine was collected to rule out urinary tract infection, but nothing abnormal was detected.

Yohann needs assistance with activities of daily living (ADL). On observation, he needs help with cutting his food, but can eat simple foods (e.g., sandwiches) with cueing. He does, however, need full assistance with bathing, grooming, and dressing. He can do some tasks such as washing his face when cued. He is doubly incontinent. However, he is fully mobile and can walk independently. He scores 45 on the Barthel Index (Collin, Wade, Davies, & Horne, 1988). A normal score on the Barthel Index (BI) is 100, calculated across 10 basic aspects of self-care and physical dependency, with a lower score indicating increasing disability. A BI greater than 60 corresponds with assisted independence, and a BI of less than 40 corresponds with severe dependency (Granger, Dewis, Peters, Sherwood, & Barrett, 1979).

Yohann has not settled well into the unit. He is very agitated and on occasion verbally aggressive. He wanders constantly, rarely sitting down unless he is napping. On observation, he has a favorite place to stand, near a window where he can look out at the garden. He tries to get out the door, but because staff fear that he will fall, he is allowed outside only when supervised. If anybody tries to move him from the window or door, he becomes increasingly agitated and verbally aggressive. Staff have tried to integrate him into the social activities of the unit. However, he does not enjoy being in groups and is very disruptive if included. He lights up when he sees Mary and is content to sit with her while she chats. In contrast, he does not interact as well with staff. Mary sometimes brings gardening magazines or books with pictures of gardens, and he is interested in looking at the pictures with her. Staff have tried giving Yohann magazines to look at, but he shows no interest. Dementia Care Mapping (DCM, Bradford Dementia Group, 1997) was used to structure this observation of Yohann's behavior. The goal of DCM is to support the development of a person-centered care plan that enhances the dementia patient's quality of life (QOL). Kitwood (1997, p. 4) describes DCM as "a serious attempt to take the standpoint of the person with dementia, using a combination of empathy and observational skill." (See Kuhn, Ortigara, & Kasayka, 2000, for an overview of how DCM is implemented.)

Literature Review

An estimated 44.35 million people worldwide have dementia, a number that is expected to increase to 75.62 million in 2030 and 135.46 million in 2050 (Alzheimer's Disease International, 2013). Dementia is a clinical syndrome that includes a group of disorders (Alzheimer's disease, vascular dementia, dementia with Lewy bodies, and frontotemporal dementia are the most common) that have common symptoms but different causes (Batsch & Mittelman, 2012). Dementia is characterized by global cognitive impairment (affecting memory, understanding, language, judgment, decision making, and learning capability) of sufficient severity to affect functional abilities, in many cases accompanied by behavioral and psychiatric disturbances (National Collaborating Center for Mental Health [NICE-SICE], 2007). As the disease progresses, the person with dementia becomes increasingly reliant on caregivers. Around half of all people with dementia need personal care (Prince, Prina, & Guerchet, 2013), and most people with dementia move into long-term care at some stage in their illness. Prince et al. (2013, p. 6) comment that in high-income countries, long-term care "is mainly about" providing care for people with dementia and estimates that 80% of older people living in nursing homes have dementia. It is estimated that approximately 30% to 40% of those living in long-term care have moderate to severe cognitive impairment (Alzheimer's Association, 2013; Galik, 2010; Macdonald et al., 2002).

Neuropsychiatric, or behavioral and psychological symptoms of dementia—for example, agitation, aggression, delusions, and wandering—are observed in around 60% to 90% of people with dementia (Peters et al., 2006). One of the suggested causes of behavioral disturbances associated with dementia is expression of unmet physical or psychological needs (Kovach, Noonan, Schlidt, & Wells, 2005). For example, Yohann's constant attempts to get through the door may be his way of expressing a desire to be outside in the garden. Yohann is also verbally aggressive. Cohen-Mansfield, Libin, and Marks (2007) indicate the main causes of verbal agitation are physical pain, lack of social contacts, boredom or inactivity, hallucinations, and depression. Any or all of these causes could apply in Yohann's case. Interpreting unmet needs is difficult and these needs are sometimes dismissed or the behavior is treated more as a "problem for caregivers than as symptoms of unmet needs" (Kovach et al., 2005, p. 135). Consequently, the behavior may be treated rather than the need causing the behavior. Holistic assessment is critical to identifying and addressing unmet needs and should include a focus on "knowing" the person. Key to planning appropriate care to meet Yohann's needs is having an understanding of his life history and what is important to him. The remainder of this chapter explores biographical approaches in the context of managing behavior and psychological needs through knowing the person.

Biographical approaches draw on people's life histories to understand present needs and ambitions (Phillips, Ajdrouch, & Hillcoat-Nalletamby, 2010). Biographical approaches assume that who we are today is shaped by our past and unique life history (Phillips et al., 2010). Phillips et al. (2010, p. 40) explain that "only by understanding the meaning that an individual has placed on his or her social world and life history are we able to appreciate more fully their current lives, their wishes and fears and their future aspirations." The understanding of the person's biography is considered central to a needs-led approach to care (Keady & Jones, 2010). Biographical approaches include life story and reminiscence.

Life story work (LSW) involves compiling a life story and giving people opportunities to talk about their life experiences (Clarke, Hanson, & Ross, 2003; McKeown, Clarke, & Repper, 2006). The format used for documenting the life story varies and may take the form of a story book, a biography, a memory box, an album, a collage, or a pen portrait. Life story books, however, are probably the most commonly used format. Life story books are individual and creative and may contain narrative, photographs, timelines, postcards, pictures, or other memorabilia (McKeown et al., 2006; Reichman, Leonard, Mintz, Kazier, & Lisner-Kerbel, 2004). The content is typically structured around significant events in the person's life, for example, childhood, family, interests, and achievements (Gibson, 2011). The emphasis is on positive and pleasant events, and it is generally recommended that sensitive or traumatic events are best avoided (Clarke et al., 2003; Reichman et al., 2004; Thompson, 2010). The focus and format should match the person's interests and need; for example, Yohann enjoys looking at pictures of plants or gardens, so including these in a book would be meaningful to him. An alternative might be putting together a memory box with seed catalogues, seed packets, a trowel, and other bits and pieces so he has the pleasure of touching and holding the things included.

LSW is a dynamic and ongoing process rather than a task to complete (McKeown et al., 2006). It is important to understand that the benefits of LSW are not achieved through completing the book but through using the book to interact with Yohann, for example, looking at the pictures together or using the "stories" to generate conversation. The nature of dementia makes it impossible for Yohann to engage with the book on his own, which explains why giving him magazines to look at on his own does not work. Interacting with Yohann through his life story enables staff to learn about his life and interests, to understand his needs, and to interpret his current behavior in the context of his past behavior, for example, his looking out of the window and wanting to go outside. Consequently, LSW can help with finding strategies to manage behaviors that challenge. LSW also gives Mary a new way of interacting with her husband and confidence that staff know him as an individual and are seeing him as the "nice man" she knows. Studies have shown that LSW has the potential to improve care for the person through enabling staff to see the person behind the dementia (Heliker & Nguyen, 2010; McKeown, Clarke, Ingelton, Ryuan, & Repper, 2010). McKeown et al. (2010) explored the effect of using LSW on person-centered care with older people with dementia and their family carers. A multiple case study design was employed to explore the experience of all involved—staff, residents, and family. The cases were four people with dementia from four different health care settings—two assessment wards for people with dementia, an intermediate care ward, and a day center. The process of LSW was the unit of observation with key stakeholders interviewed on one or two occasions. A total of 21 interviews were conducted with nurses, support workers, care workers, and family carers. This was supported by documentary analysis of care plans, notes of meetings, and research diaries. The main researcher spent over 100 hours in the field. It was found that using LSW enhanced person-centered care for people with dementia. Three main themes were identified: "From patient to person"; "Can you hear me?" and "Pride and enjoyment." McKeown et al. (2010) found that using LSW helped staff to see, understand, and appreciate the person with dementia beyond the patient. It also enabled them to interpret current behavior in the context of the person's past experiences. Family carers valued the opportunity of LSW to allow their relative to be seen and heard. LSW also helped to preserve the person's self or personhood, for family as well as staff in the sense that it enabled sharing and connection with the person. The theme "Can you hear me?" described how LSW gave the person with dementia an opportunity for his or her voice to be heard through engaging with the life story book or through talking with the staff who had worked with them in developing the life story book in a different way. All staff reported enjoying the process, and the people with dementia demonstrated pride in their life story. McKeown et al. (2010) conclude that LSW has the potential to enhance person-centered care for people with dementia and their families because it enables staff to make links between past and present and promotes understanding of the person's preferences and current behavior. This suggests that LSW supports person-centered care planning. For example, an intervention based on taking Yohann for walks would meet both his need to be outside and contribute (in combination with other interventions around sleep hygiene) to changing his sleeping pattern. Others agree that LSW provides the context and framework for person-centered care (McKeown et al., 2010; Thompson, 2010). Increasingly, the importance of collecting life history data is recognized in clinical care guidelines, which recommend that the care plan for the person with dementia should be based on an assessment of his or her life history (Cass, Robbins, & Richardson, 2009; NICE-SCIE, 2007).

Reminiscence is another way to connect and engage with people with dementia. Reminiscence focuses on supporting people to think or talk about their past (Cotellli, Manenti, & Zanetti, 2012; Woods, Spector, Jones, Orrell, & Davis, 2005), using triggers (for example, photographs, music, dance, role-play) to help them unlock their preserved memories (i.e., drawing on the long-term memory) enabling them to engage with others (Gibson, 2011; O'Shea et al., 2011; Woods et al., 2005). Although focused on the past, reminiscence allows the person to communicate and interact with the listener in the present and looks to the future, bringing "new understanding, fresh perspectives, and courage for facing the future" (Gibson, 2011, p. 9). There are two broad types of reminiscence: *Simple or general reminiscence* is the planned use of open questions, usually with the aid of prompts or triggers (such as photographs, music, or artifacts), to stimulate recall of topics of interest to the person (Gibson, 2011; Woods et al., 2005). Simple reminiscence is least likely to stimulate painful memories (Gibson, 2011) and typically focuses on prompting positive memories that enhance positive feelings (Westerhof, Bohlemeijer, & Webster, 2010). Gibson (2011) points out that painful or sad memories should not, however, be excluded or ignored. This is somewhat at odds with the perspective of Westerhof et al. (2010), who argue the focus should always be on the "positive," and liken this type of reminiscence to "social reminiscence." In contrast, Gibson (2011, p. 31) argues that reminiscence is not about "nostalgic trips down memory lane," but takes a holistic view of life's ups and downs. She explains that the "modern reminiscence movement is primarily concerned with using recollection of past experience as a tool for coping in the present and anticipating the future" (Gibson, 2011, pp. 31, 32). In contrast, *specialized* or *specific reminiscence* is planned, structured, and encourages life review. The term "life review" is used in different ways across the literature. One form of life review, which we will term for clarity the "psychotherapeutic" interpretation of life review, is targeted at people who are struggling to find meaning or cope with adversities in their life. The goal of this type of life review is to help the person to achieve ego-integrity and involves the person, with the support of a trained professional, looking back at and evaluating his or her whole life, solving unresolved difficulties or conflicts, and searching for meaning (Gibson, 2011; Westerhof et al., 2010; Woods et al., 2005). The other, perhaps looser, interpretation involves a version of life review that focuses on promoting psychological well-being by confirming personal identity or enhancing self-esteem. NICE-SCIE (2007) indicate that life review's focus on enhancing adjustment and mood is appropriate for early stage dementia. This is analogous to what we have termed "psychotherapeutic" life review. In the later stages of dementia (i.e., Yohann's stage), reminiscence with a focus on well-being and QOL is more appropriate (NICE-SCIE, 2007).

Reminiscence can be planned (a formal interaction) or spontaneous (informal happening in the moment); it can be one-to-one or a group activity. In our experience, one-to-one interaction tends to work best for people with moderate to severe dementia. However, this must be judged on the basis of the individual's needs. There is no right way to implement reminiscence. Gibson (2011, p. 32) describes reminiscence work as a "loose collection of ideas" with the approach, activities, and practices varying in the context of the aims of the specific intervention and the person's individual preferences. Researchers have found that reminiscence has many positive outcomes, including promoting communication and sociability, reducing isolation, generating and maintaining personal relationships (Gibson, 2011; Schweitzer & Bruce, 2008), increasing self-esteem, continuity and preserving self-identity (Gibson, 2011; Schweitzer & Bruce, 2008), and improving cognition, preserving intact memories and skills, and promoting a sense of achievement and mastery (Gibson, 2011; Schweitzer & Bruce, 2008). However, the existing trials-based reminiscence therapy for people with dementia, which has been summarized in the form of a Cochrane review (Woods et al., 2005), is not entirely convincing. Only five randomized controlled trials were included in this review, of which only four had extractable data, comprising a maximum of 144 participants. The studies, therefore, were small in scale and also incorporated diverse forms of reminiscence, resulting in far from robust conclusions on overall effectiveness. The trials taken together only identified significant improvements in cognition and mood 4 to 6 weeks after treatment, and reduced stress in carers who participated with the person with dementia in a reminiscence group. It is unsurprising that the authors of the review recommended more and better designed trials of reminiscence therapy for dementia before a decision on overall effectiveness could be reached. This dearth of evidence is reflected in the NICE-SCIE (2007) guidelines on the management and treatment of dementia in the United Kingdom, which found insufficient evidence to recommend that reminiscence should be routinely offered to people with dementia, although its potential impact on the mood of the person with dementia was highlighted. Similarly, in the United States, O'Neil et al. (2011), in a systematic evidence review of nonpharmacological interventions for behavioral symptoms of dementia prepared for the Department of Veterans Affairs, concluded that the limited body of evidence on reminiscence therapy does not support its use for the treatment of behavioral symptoms of dementia.

Evidence of a more positive nature in relation to reminiscence is now emerging in Ireland from the delivery of a structured Dementia Education Program Incorporating Reminiscence to Staff (DARES) in long-term settings, who subsequently integrated reminiscence into the care of people with dementia, both formally and informally, over an 18-week period (O'Shea et al., 2011, 2014). The DARES trial was an attempt to provide new information on the effectiveness of reminiscence as a psychosocial intervention based on a robust trial methodology. The study yields some interesting and complex results that may help inform future research in this area. The results show that reminiscence had a positive effect on the QOL–AD care recipient measure of QOL. On an intention-to-treat basis, the difference between intervention and control just fails to reach the clinical significance of four points, whereas that difference is exceeded by one point when the data are analyzed on a per protocol basis. The DARES results are strongest, therefore, when analyzed on a per protocol basis, highlighting the presence of side effects and the importance of adherence to the program and completion of the intervention. The fact that there was a difference between intention to treat and per protocol is perhaps not that surprising given the pragmatic nature of the trial and the reality of trying to carry out the intervention in a busy, complex, and evolving long-term care sector, particularly in relation to care structures and processes, staff duties, and staff–management relationships. The DARES embedded grounded theory study (Cooney et al., 2014) provides insights into how residents and staff responded to reminiscence and shares the theory of "seeing me (through my memories)." This theory explains that through reminiscing and engaging with the person with dementia, staff begin to see the person (their personhood) through the mirror of his or her memories.

Role and Cultural Considerations

Changing practice, however, requires cultural change at the institutional, community, and policy levels. Most nurses are not provided with an adequate amount of education on caring for people with dementia. The care process within long-term care facilities is important in allowing residents to live well with dementia. There is no doubt that the medical and functional needs of residents dominate the care landscape within long-term care settings. Although to some extent this is understandable, psychosocial approaches are also needed to complement biomedical models of service delivery. In particular, psychosocial interventions can assist nurses to develop meaningful communication with patients, using all of the senses, through reminiscence, music, and various therapeutic and time-intensive activities. Furthermore, Beerens, Zwakhalen, Verbeek, Ruwaard, and Hamers (2013), who conducted a systematic review of the factors associated with QOL of people with dementia in long-term care facilities, concluded that psychosocial interventions may lower the level of agitation because lack of stimulation and activities in and of themselves may cause agitation. They argue that nursing staff should encourage activities that stimulate people with dementia.

Given the importance of connectivity for personhood within dementia, new ways of reaching into and out of long-term care settings should be encouraged through various forms of social interventions. Very few facilities have connectivity programs that link residents within long-term care facilities to the communities that surround them, both within and outside the long-term care setting. Education and training for nurses and care staff caring for people with dementia will be necessary to support the culture change involved in moving to a biopsychosocial framework of care provision that puts personhood at the core of the relationship between the carer and the person with dementia.

Strategies for Changing Practice

Policy makers tend to associate dementia with risk, resulting in a bias toward institutional care, where people with the disease can be cared for in a secure environment. It is as if people with dementia are deficient, pitiful, and need protection from society rather than being a living part of that society. Moving from a purely biological focus to a biopsychosocial world would allow greater discussion of the meaning of attachment, place, identity, and relationships, thereby challenging families and communities to develop and maintain a communal approach to care that prioritized connectivity and mutual support systems both for people living with dementia in the community and in long-term care. It would reinforce the need for, and benefit of, dementia-friendly communities at all levels of care provision. Replacing capabilities with risk would allow the potential of people with dementia to be realized during all stages of the disease, particularly in the early stages of the illness. For the most part, people with dementia should live in their own homes, where images of self and identity are easier to preserve in the face of ongoing cognitive decline. Even when people with the disease have to enter long-term care, the emphasis should be on homelike, small-scale provision, where biography and personality are central to the care process and autonomy is preserved as much as possible.

People with dementia are citizens with inalienable human and civil rights that must be protected whether they live at home or in long-term care. They continue to have roles and relationships within families, communities, and long-term care settings that serve to enhance overall well-being and preserve the integrity of the human spirit—their own and that of those around them. People with dementia are better off when treated with respect and dignity, but so too is society. The power of now should never be underestimated in the care of people with dementia. Making people with dementia happy by seeking to penetrate usable memory and latent connections should be central to the care process. Through a focus on direct engagement and inclusion, people with dementia will become more visible in society, leading to greater awareness of the disease and an acceptance of the need for a public response in the form of improved services and person-centered support systems at all levels of care.

Clinical Reasoning Questions

1. How can health care staff, at all levels and all care settings, engage with the person with dementia to learn about his or her individual life story, values, and aspirations?
2. How can the biopsychosocial model play a more prominent role in the care of people with dementia across all care settings?

3. What should education and training programs on dementia and dementia care look like for staff caring for people with dementia? When considering this question, identify your own learning needs and plan of action for implementing learning into your day-to-day practice.
4. How can more network connections be made between long-term care settings and the communities within which they are located to maximize connectivity opportunities for people with dementia?

References

Alzheimer's Association. (2013). 2013 Alzheimer's disease facts and figures. *Alzheimer's & Dementia, 9*(2), 131–168. Retrieved from http://www.alz.org/downloads/facts_figures_2013.pdf

Alzheimer's Disease International. (2013). *Policy brief for heads of government: The global impact of dementia 2013–2050.* London, England: Alzheimer's Disease International. Retrieved from http://www.alz.co.uk/research/GlobalImpactDementia2013.pdf

American Psychiatric Association. (2013). *Diagnostic and statistical manual of mental disorders* (5th ed.). Washington, DC: Author.

Batsch, N. L., & Mittelman, M. S. (2012). *World Alzheimer's report 2012: Overcoming the stigma of dementia.* London, England: Alzheimer's Disease International. Retrieved from http://www.alz.org/documents_custom/world_report_2012_final.pdf

Beerens, H. C., Zwakhalen, S. M. G., Verbeek, H., Ruwaard, D., & Hamers, J. P. H. (2013). Factors associated with quality of life of people with dementia in long-term care facilities: A systematic review. *International Journal of Nursing Studies, 50*(9), 1259–1270.

Bradford Dementia Group. (1997). *Evaluating dementia care: The DCM method* (7th ed.). Bradford, England: University of Bradford.

Cass, E., Robbins, D., & Richardson, A. (2009). *Dignity in care SCIE: Adults' services SCIE Guide 15.* London, England: Social Care Institute for Excellence. Retrieved from http://www.scie.org.uk/publications/guides/guide15/files/guide15.pdf

Clarke, A., Hanson, E., & Ross, H. (2003). Seeing the person behind the patient: Enhancing the care of older people using a biographical approach. *Journal of Clinical Nursing, 12*(5), 697–706.

Cohen-Mansfield, J., Libin, A., & Marks, M. S. (2007). Nonpharmacological treatment of agitation: A controlled trial of systematic individualized intervention. *The Journals of Gerontology. Series A: Biological Sciences and Medical Sciences, 62*(8), 908–916.

Collin, C., Wade, D. T., Davies, S., & Horne, V. (1988). The Barthel ADL Index: A reliability study. *International Disability Studies, 10*(2), 61–63.

Cooney, A., Hunter, A., Murphy, K., Casey, D., Smyth, S., Devane, D., . . . O'Shea, E. (2014). "Seeing me through my memories": A grounded theory study on using reminiscence with people with dementia living in long-term care. *Journal of Clinical Nursing, 23*(23–24), 3564–3574.

Cotellli, M., Manenti, R., & Zanetti, O. (2012). Reminiscence therapy in dementia: A review. *Maturitas*, 72, 203–205.

Crum, R. M., Anthony, J. C., Bassett, S. S., & Folstein, M. F. (1993). Population-based norms for the Mini-Mental State Examination by age and educational level. *Journal of the American Medical Association, 269*, 2386–2391.

Folstein, M. F., Folstein, S. E., & McHugh, P. R. (1975). "Mini-mental state": A practical method for grading the cognitive state of patients for the clinician. *Journal of Psychiatric Research, 12*(3), 189–198.

Galik E. (2010). Function-focused care for LTC residents with moderate-to-severe dementia: A social ecological approach. *Annals of Long-Term Care, 18*(6). Retrieved from http://www.annalsoflongtermcare.com/content/function-focused-care-ltc-residents-with-moderate-severe-dementia-a-social-ecological-approa

Gibson, F. (2011). *Reminiscence and life story work: A practical guide* (4th ed.). London, England: Jessica Kingsley.

Granger, C. V., Dewis, L. S., Peters, N. C., Sherwood, C. C., & Barrett, J. E. (1979). Stroke rehabilitation: Analysis of repeated Barthel index measures. *Archives of Physical Medicine & Rehabilitation, 60*(1), 14–17.

Heliker, D., & Nguyen, H. T. (2010). Story sharing enhancing nurse aide-resident relationships in long term care. *Research in Gerontological Nursing, 3*, 240–252.

Keady, J., & Jones, L. (2010). Investigating the causes of behaviours that challenge in people with dementia. *Nursing Older People, 22*(9), 25–29.

Kitwood, T. (1997). *Dementia reconsidered: The person comes first*. Buckingham, England: Open University Press.

Kovach, C. R., Noonan, P. E., Schlidt, A. M., & Wells, T. (2005). A model of consequences of need-driven dementia-compromised behavior. *Journal of Nursing Scholarship, 37*(2), 134–140.

Kuhn, D., Ortigara, A., & Kasayka, R. (2000). Dementia care mapping: An innovative tool to measure person centered care. *Alzheimer Care Quarterly, 1*(3), 7–15.

Macdonald, A., Carpenter, G. I., Box, O., & Roberts A. (2002). Dementia and use of psychotropic medication in non-"Elderly Mentally Infirm" nursing homes in South East England. *Age and Ageing*, 31, 58–64.

McKeown, J., Clarke, A., Ingelton, C., Ryuan, T., & Repper, J. (2010). The use of life story work with people with dementia to enhance person-centered care. *International Journal of Older People Nursing, 5*(2), 148–158.

McKeown, J., Clarke, A., & Repper, J. (2006). Life story work in health and social care: Systematic literature review. *Journal of Advanced Nursing, 55*(2), 237–247.

Murphy, K., O'Shea, E., & Cooney, A. (2007). Quality of life for older people living in long-stay settings in Ireland. *Journal of Clinical Nursing, 16*(11), 2167–2177.

National Collaborating Center for Mental Health. (2007). *Dementia: A NICE-SCIE guideline on supporting people with dementia and their carers in health and social care*. London, England: British Psychological Society and the Royal College of Psychiatrists. Retrieved from http://www.nice.org.uk/nicemedia/live/10998/30320/30320.pdf

O'Neil, M., Freeman, M., Christensen, V., Telerant, A., Addleman, A., & Kansagara, D. (2011). *Non-pharmacological interventions for behavioral symptoms of dementia: A systematic review of the evidence* (VA-ESP Project #05-225). Retrieved from http://www.ncbi.nlm.nih.gov/books/NBK54971/pdf/TOC.pdf

O'Shea, E., Devane, D., Cooney, A., Casey, D., Jordan, F., Hunter, A., . . . Murphy, K. (2014). The impact of reminiscence on the quality of life of residents with dementia in long-stay care. *International Journal of Geriatric Psychiatry*. Retrieved from http://onlinelibrary.wiley.com/doi/10.1002/gps.4099/pdf

O'Shea, E., Devane, D., Murphy, K., Cooney, A., Casey, D., Jordan, F., . . . Murphy, K. (2011). Effectiveness of a structured education reminiscence-based programme for staff on the quality of life of residents with dementia in long-stay units: A study protocol for a cluster randomised trial. *Trials, 12*(1), 4. Retrieved from http://www.trialsjournal.com/content/pdf/1745-6215-12-41.pdf

Peters, K. R., Rockwood, K., Black, S. E., Bouchard, R., Gauthier, S., Hogan, D., ... Feldman, H. H. (2006). Characterizing neuropsychiatric symptoms in subjects referred to dementia clinics. *Neurology, 66*(4), 523–528.

Phillips, J., Ajdrouch, J., & Hillcoat-Nalletamby, S. (2010). *Key concepts in social gerontology.* London, England: Sage.

Prince, M., Prina, M., & Guerchet, M. (2013). *World Alzheimer report 2013: Journal of caring—An analysis of long-term care for dementia.* London, England: Alzheimer's Disease International. Retrieved from http://www.alz.co.uk/research/WorldAlzheimerReport2013.pdf

Reichman, S., Leonard, C., Mintz, T., Kazier, C., & Lisner-Kerbel, H. (2004). Compiling life history resources for older adults in institutions: Development of a guide. *Journal of Gerontological Nurisng, 30*(2), 20–28.

Schweitzer, P., & Bruce, E. (2008). *Remembering yesterday, caring today.* London, England: Jessica Kingsley.

Shadlen, M. F., & Larson, E. B. (2014). Evaluation of cognitive impairment and dementia. *UpToDate.* Retrieved from http://www.uptodate.com/contents/evaluation-of-cognitive-impairment-and-dementia?topicKey=NEURO%2F5083&elapsedTimeMs=0&source=see_link&view=print&displayedView=full

Thompson, R. (2010). Realising the potential: Developing life story work in practice. *Foundation of Nursing Studies Dissemination Series, 5*(5), 1–4.

Westerhof, G. J., Bohlemeijer, E., & Webster, J. D. (2010). Reminiscence and mental health: A review of recent progress in theory, research and interventions. *Aging & Society, 30,* 697–721.

Woods, B., Spector, A., Jones, C., Orrell, M., & Davis, S. (2005). Reminiscence therapy for dementia. *Cochrane Database of Systematic Reviews, 2,* CD001120. Retrieved from http://onlinelibrary.wiley.com/doi/10.1002/14651858.CD001120.pub2/pdf

26

QUALITY OF LIFE FOR PERSONS WITH DEMENTIA LIVING IN THE COMMUNITY

JOHN KEADY AND SIMON BURROW

Subjective

"Who is who and what is happening?"

Objective

Mr. Zack Zagger is a 78-year-old married man from Stockport in Greater Manchester (UK) who was recently diagnosed with Alzheimer's disease following attendance at a local memory assessment treatment and support service. Following the clinical advice of Watts et al. (2010), Zack received a battery of neuropsychological testing to reach a diagnosis of Alzheimer's disease, which included the Cambridge Cognitive Examination-Revised (CAMCOG-R; Roth, Huppert, Mountjoy, & Tym, 1988) as a general cognitive screening instrument, the Wechsler Test of Adult Reading (WTAR; Wechsler, 2001) to indicate premorbid ability level, the Wechsler Memory Scale—third edition (WMS-III; Wechsler, 1997) to explore verbal and visual memory (both recall and recognition) and working memory, and the Delis-Kaplan Executive Function System (D-KEFS; Delis, Kaplan, & Kramer, 2001) to assess executive functioning. In line with best practice guidelines in the United Kingdom (Department of Health, 2009), Zack also received an MRI (magnetic resonance imaging) brain scan that revealed no evidence of significant vascular changes, but there were some changes to the temporal and parietal lobes that were consistent with Alzheimer's disease. Zack also achieved a score of 17/30 on the Mini Mental State Examination (MMSE; Folstein, Folstein, & McHugh, 1975) to indicate that he was in the moderate stages of the condition. The Bristol Activities of Daily Living Scale (Bucks, Ashworth, Wilcock, & Siegfried, 1996) also revealed that Zack required some help with his personal hygiene needs. Zack was prescribed the acetylcholinesterase inhibitor donepezil hydrochloride [Aricept] 10 mg once a day for the treatment of his Alzheimer's disease.

Zack spends most of his day in the family living room with the television on and the volume on high, although he is no longer able to follow the storylines in the programs and constantly asks Stella, his wife, to tell him who is who and what is happening. Stella finds these constant requests irritating and has stopped answering these requests. Zack previously worked as a high school teacher in Stockport for most of his adult life; as such, he is a well-known figure in the local community. Stella has had real difficulty in accepting and coming to terms with the diagnosis of Alzheimer's disease and thinks that this diagnosis may be "the last straw," as she nursed her father through the same condition many years ago and "knows what the future holds." Stella is therefore fearful for their future and for her own health needs, and says "she cannot face that again [the dementia]."

Zack leaves the family home only once a week when his wife takes him shopping to the local supermarket, a routine they have had all their married lives. However, for the past 2 or 3 weeks, Zack has begun to threaten to leave his home in order "to be with his children [Jane and Mark]," even though his children are now in their early 50s, both with families, and live in other cities in the United Kingdom (Edinburgh and Birmingham). Zack has become verbally aggressive toward Stella, saying that she is keeping their children from him and is threatening to report her to "the authorities." Zack often calls Stella by his mother's name [Joan] and is unable to recall the names of his children or where they are living. His concept of time is also wayward and Zack will often get up in the middle of the night to attempt to shave and get ready for the working day ahead.

Over the years Stella has built a trusting, productive, and friendly relationship with the supporting services and has recently shared her feelings about her husband's condition, indicating that she wants some help in managing her life; she says she still loves her husband, but is close to being overwhelmed by the situation. On a recent visit, the community support worker was present when Jane (Zack and Stella's daughter) was telling her mother to put her father "in a home," as she does not want her mother to be burdened for years to come. Mark (Zack and Stella's son) does not agree and wants his father to stay at home and has offered to help his mother "in whatever way she wants." Zack does not talk about his diagnosis of Alzheimer's disease and carries on as if nothing has changed in his life.

For the past 3 years, Zack has been receiving treatment by the district nursing service for his chronic obstructive pulmonary disease and osteoarthritis in both his knees. For his chronic obstructive pulmonary disease, intervention by the district nurses has centered on Zack's symptom management by teaching pursed lip and diaphragmatic breathing techniques through the use of visual prompts and reinforcement to Stella about when and how to use this approach for her husband. The district nurse has also attempted to improve the quality of Zack's life through pulmonary rehabilitation in the home, including the regulated use of oxygen, the prescription of long-acting inhaled bronchodilators (beta 2-agonists and anticholinergics to control Zack's symptoms and improve exercise capacity), and ensuring that Zack is no longer smoking. In the last week, Zack has said that he wants to start smoking again and does not understand why he stopped. For his osteoarthritis, the district nurses have been encouraging self-management techniques such as proper joint use, joint protection, exercise, medication scheduling, and weight control. Zack takes the over-the-counter pain relievers and aspirin, which Stella purchases for him. Owing to Zack's lack of mobility, he has the first signs of a pressure area sore on his sacral area.

Zack receives a monthly visit from the memory clinic nurse who checks on Zack's prescription of Aricept and repeats the MMSE (Folstein et al., 1975) and Bristol Activities of Daily Living Scale (Bucks et al., 1996) to compare present performance against the memory clinic baseline. The memory clinic nurse also spends time with the family carer and has introduced some stress-management treatment to help Stella cope with the demands that she faces. Stella often repeats that she needs to have some time for herself and that simply finding that time would help her cope better at home and in living with her husband.

Literature Review

Quality of life (QOL) is a complex and complicated construct. At one level it is concerned with a range of essential everyday issues that impact upon an individual, such as employment, income, housing and living conditions, family, health, work–life balance, and the perceived quality of society and public services (Bowling & Windsor, 2001). At another level, however, QOL is subjectively determined, imbued with personal meanings and values, and addresses the individual and his or her construction of life satisfaction and well-being (World Health Organization Quality of Life Assessment Group, 1995). By further distilling these broad domains, The World Health Organization (1997) defined QOL as "individuals' perception of their position in life in the context of the culture and value systems in which they live and in relation to their goals, expectations, standards and concerns" (p. 1).

Through the years, policy makers, economists, human geographers, health researchers, and social scientists have all attempted to measure these parameters and meanings through the application and evaluation of various QOL instruments. To take but one health-related example, derived from a European health and QOL initiative, the EQ-5D instrument (Ramos-Goñi et al., 2013) is divided into five sections—mobility; self-care; usual activities; pain/discomfort; and anxiety/depression—that are self-rated by the person him- or herself between the "worst imaginable health state" and the "best imaginable health state." This instrument continues to provide a cornerstone for many clinical and population studies (Ramos-Goñi et al., 2013), although it is the user control of domain applicability to the person's own health state that is crucial here in that there is a built-in acceptance that QOL is as it is experienced by the person and not what it is imagined to be by others.

In dementia studies, the literature has developed in recent years from a focus on the QOL experiences reported by family carers of people with dementia (Charlesworth et al., 2008; National Institute for Health and Clinical Excellence/

Social Care Institute for Excellence, 2007) to the construction of QOL reported by people with dementia themselves; however, there remains no reliable measure to document this latter experience (Alzheimer's Society, 2010a). On the other hand, there are indicators provided by people with dementia about what they consider to be a good QOL. For example, in the report *My Name Is Not Dementia* (Alzheimer's Society, 2010b), in which 44 people with dementia participated in a study via interviews, discussions, or postal survey, 10 key QOL indicators were identified: relationships and somebody to talk to, environment, physical health, sense of humor, independence, ability to communicate, sense of personal identity, ability or opportunity to engage in activities, ability to practice faith or religion, and experience of stigma. It is fair to say that it is unusual to find stigma mentioned in the general QOL literature, but for people with dementia and their carers it would appear that a life free from stigma would provide the foundations for a good QOL and underpin personal autonomy. As seen in the case study, Jane's demand to see her father placed "in a home," and her communicated wish to her mother that she oversee this transition, effectively positions Zack as "the other" in the relationship and negates Zack's choices and personal decision making.

Interestingly, in their top three QOL indicators, the Alzheimer's Society (2010b) study revealed that both carers and people with dementia placed "relationships" at the top of their list (p. 32); it was their only point of convergence. However, relationships can become easily fractured when living at home with a person with dementia, especially when carers begin to experience "role captivity" in their everyday lives (Aneshensel, Pearlin, Mullan, Zarit, & Whitlatch, 1995) and networks shrink so that time is spent indoors (Duggan, Blackman, Martyr, & van Schaik, 2008). Such a threat to QOL was evident in the case study, especially with Stella's vocalized need to find her own space and Zack's need to interact more with the outside world—his only time outside the confines of his own home being on escorted, weekly visits to the supermarket.

Role and Cultural Considerations

Previously, there has been little attention paid to understanding the ways in which the outdoor and built environment impacts and intersects with the lives of people with dementia and their care partners. In attempting to understand more about these issues, Keady et al. (2012) undertook a realist review of the literature on neighborhoods and dementia. They found 18 studies that matched their inclusion criteria, and they were able to group these findings under three themes: (1) outdoor spaces (defined as "life outside the front door and/or the practicalities of getting out and about in the neighborhood"); (2) built environment (defined as "the existence of dementia-friendly environments and/or how the environment can enable, or disable, people with dementia"); and (3) everyday technologies (defined as "how people with dementia interact/access technology outside the home and/or use technology to prepare to leave the home to engage with the outside world"). Interestingly, the review concludes that there had been no research that explores how people with dementia might define their own neighborhood or that explores everyday neighborhood practices for those living with the condition.

In many ways, these inherent tensions have been recognized at a macro level. For example, a recent World Health Organization (2012) report squarely positions dementia as a public health priority and places the rights of people with dementia at the forefront, such as the right to live in the community, the right to take part in activities, and the right to be involved in communal life (p. 47). The challenge is to find ways to help accommodate Zack within his own community and connect, should he wish to, to his long-held role of educator and skilled person of standing in the community.

Strategies and Solutions

It is inevitable that there will be multiple and complex impediments to achieving these ambitions for Zack, Stella, and their adult children, who will each have his or her own "take" on what is needed to have a good QOL. To help focus practice, it might be useful to consider these issues within the framework of Bartlett and O'Connor's (2010) multidimensional model for contextualizing dementia. This focuses attention on the complex interplay between a person's subjective and interpersonal experiences and the wider sociocultural context the person inhabits. For example, the work of Kitwood (1997) on the ill effects of "malignant social psychology" and Sabat's (2003) on the "malignant positioning" of people with dementia both illustrate how social identity, personhood, and well-being can be diminished by the values, actions, and inactions of "healthy others." These approaches, combined with the relationship-centered work of Nolan, Brown, Davies, Nolan, & Keady (2006), promote a more complete understanding of barriers to and enablers of well-being at the interpersonal and relational levels in which people are living.

However, Bartlett and O'Connor (2010) also urge us to focus on the influence that wider sociocultural factors exert on personhood and citizenship and, by extension, to QOL. Public discourse on dementia and the social location people inhabit are crucial determinants here. In this respect, ethnicity, gender, sexual orientation, and socioeconomic advantage or disadvantage may further shape a people's experiences within their situated contexts and exert their influence on QOL and well-being. By way of example, the relationship between social and economic disadvantage and poor health is clearly established (Marmot, 2010). It is difficult to imagine how an older person with dementia, living alone without family support, with limited economic means and in a socially deprived neighborhood, will not be confronted with significant barriers to life quality that may not be similarly experienced by persons living with dementia in a contrasting social context. Although this deviates a little from the provided case study in this chapter, driving improvements in health and care and creating dementia-friendly communities are worthy ambitions; note, however, that these need to be viewed alongside deep-rooted societal challenges to address inequalities and social justice.

Clinical Reasoning Questions

1. What type of relationship-based assessment or work would help Zack, Stella, and their family to achieve a good QOL?
2. What is the role of the community in helping to support QOL?
3. Do we need separate measures of QOL: one for carers and one for people with dementia? Or should we be looking at combined measures?
4. How can we start to assess QOL when the capacity of the person with dementia may be compromised?
5. What constitutes "the community" for people living with dementia?

References

Alzheimer's Society. (2010a). *My name is not dementia: Literature review*. London, England: Author.

Alzheimer's Society. (2010b). *My name is not dementia: People with dementia discuss quality of life indicators*. London, England: Author.

Aneshensel, C. S., Pearlin, L. I., Mullan, J. T., Zarit, S. H., & Whitlatch, C. J. (1995). *Profiles in caregiving: The unexpected career*. San Diego, CA: Academic Press.

Bartlett, R., & O'Connor, D. (2010). *Broadening the dementia debate: Toward social citizenship*. London, England: The Policy Press.

Bowling, A., & Windsor, J. (2001). Towards the good life: A population survey of dimensions of quality of life. *Journal of Happiness Studies, 2*, 55–81.

Bucks, R. S., Ashworth, D. L., Wilcock, G. K., & Siegfried, K. (1996). Assessment of activities of daily living in dementia: Development of the Bristol activities of daily living scale. *Age and Aging, 25*, 113–120.

Charlesworth, G., Shepstone, L., Wilson, E., Thalanany, M., Mugford, M., & Poland, F. (2008). Does befriending by trained lay workers improve psychological well-being and quality of life for carers of people with dementia, and at what cost? A randomised controlled trial. *Health Technology Assessment, 12*(4), iii, v–ix, 1–78.

Delis, D. C., Kaplan, E., & Kramer, J. H. (2001). *Delis-Kaplan executive function system (D-KEFS).* Oxford, England: Pearson.

Department of Health. (2009). *Living well with dementia, a national dementia strategy*. London, England: Author.

Duggan, S., Blackman, T., Martyr, A., & van Schaik, P. (2008). The impact of early dementia on outdoor life: A "shrinking world"? *Dementia, 7*, 191–204.

Folstein, M. F., Folstein, S., & McHugh, P. (1975). Mini mental state: A practical method for grading the cognitive state of patients for the clinician. *Journal of Psychiatric Research, 12*, 189–198.

Keady, J., Campbell, S., Barnes, H., Ward, R., Li, X., Swarbrick, C., . . . Elvish, R. (2012). Neighbourhoods and dementia in the health and social care context: A realist review of the literature and implications for UK policy development. *Reviews in Clinical Gerontology, 22*, 150–163.

Kitwood, T. (1997). *Dementia reconsidered: The person comes first*. Maidenhead, England: Open University Press.

Marmot, M. (2010). *Fair society healthy lives*. London, England: Institute of Health Equality. Retrieved from http://www.instituteofhealthequity.org/projects/fair-society-healthy-lives-the-marmot-review

National Institute for Health and Clinical Excellence/Social Care Institute for Excellence. (2007). *Dementia: Supporting people with dementia and their carers in health and social care. NICE clinical practice guideline 42*. London, England: Author.

Nolan, M. R., Brown, J., Davies, S., Nolan, J., & Keady, J. (2006). *The senses framework: Improving care for older people through a relationship-centered approach* (Getting Research into Practice [GRiP] Report No. 2). London, England: University of Sheffield.

Ramos-Goñi, J. M., Rivero-Arias, O., Errea, M., Stolk, E. A., Herdman, M., & Cabasés, J. M. (2013). Dealing with the health state "dead" when using discrete choice experiments to obtain values for EQ-5D-5L heath states. *The European Journal of Health Economics, 14*(1, Suppl.), 33–42.

Roth, M., Huppert, F. A., Mountjoy, C. Q., & Tym, E. (1988). *CAMDEX-R: The Cambridge examination for mental disorders in the elderly* (Rev. ed.). Cambridge, England: Cambridge University Press.

Sabat, S. R. (2003). Malignant positioning and the predicament of the person with Alzheimer's disease. In F. M. Moghaddam & R. Harré (Eds.), *The self and others: Positioning individuals and groups in personal, political, and cultural contexts* (pp. 85–98). Westport, CT: Greenwood Publishing Group.

Watts, S., Harkness, L., Domone, R., Shields, G., Moss, G., & Bilsborough, N. (2010). Memory services: Psychological distress, co-morbidity and the need for flexible working—The reality of late life mental health care. In J. Keady & S. Watts (Eds.), *Mental health and later life: Delivering an holistic model for practice* (pp. 104–124). London, England: Routledge.

Wechsler, D. (1997). *Wechsler memory scale—3rd UK edition (WMS-III UK).* Oxford, England: Pearson.

Wechsler, D. (2001). *Wechsler test of adult reading—UK edition (WTAR UK).* Oxford, England: Pearson.

World Health Organization Quality of Life Assessment Group. (1995). Position paper from the World Health Organization. *Social Science and Medicine, 41,* 1403–1409.

World Health Organization. (1997). *WHOQOL: Measuring quality of life.* Geneva, Switzerland: Author.

World Health Organization. (2012). *Dementia: A public health priority.* Geneva, Switzerland: Author.

27 MEDICATION USE AND OVERUSE

DIANA R. MAGER

Subjective

"I didn't do anything wrong. The doctor told me that he was doubling my blood pressure pill, so I took two. I didn't hear him say take one in the morning and one at night. How am I supposed to keep track of all this?"

Objective

Mrs. Adeline Ann Adams is an 83-year-old woman of Armenian descent living at home with her adult daughter. She was referred to home care services for medication education and management of her recently changed medication regimen. Despite independence with activities of daily living (ADL) and instrumental ADLs, along with her past history of medication adherence, a recent miscommunication regarding medication changes resulted in an adverse drug event (ADE). To prevent further ADEs, to monitor and assess her status, and to perform medication education in the home, a nurse practitioner was assigned for a short time to provide assessment and management of Mrs. Adams's health.

Upon the initial home visit, Mrs. Adams is alert and oriented to person/place/time and is dressed neatly and appropriately for the weather. Although pleasant and accommodating, she is slightly hard of hearing and asks the nurse to repeat herself throughout the exam. She is 61 in. (155 cm) tall and weighs 146 lbs. (66 kg) (BMI 27.58). Her vital signs are blood pressure: 166/84; pulse: 84 (apical/radial); respirations: 14/minute; temperature: 98.1°F; oxygen saturation:

97%. At 10 a.m., she has not yet taken her daily medications. Mrs. Adams's skin is warm, dry, and intact, slightly pale, and is without bruising, rashes, or wounds. Her lungs are clear with slightly diminished breath sounds bilaterally at the bases, and there is no sign of respiratory distress. Her cardiac exam is unremarkable, with normal S1 and S2 sounds, a regular pulse rate and rhythm, and no presence of S3 or S4 sounds. The exam reveals no jugular vein distention or carotid bruits. Her abdomen is soft, nondistended and nontender, with positive bowel sounds in all four quadrants. Her right ankle has a trace of nonpitting edema with no edema to the left lower extremity. Bilateral pedal pulses are present but weak, and feet are slightly cooler than lower extremities but are pink in color. A moderate amount of dry cerumen is found bilaterally upon ear examination. Her left eye has limited vision related to past damage from glaucoma. The oral examination reveals moist, pink mucous membranes and adequate dentition with no dentures present.

Mrs. Adams's past medical history includes hypertension, hypercholesterolemia, and glaucoma. She has had several surgical and laser procedures to both eyes to help control the glaucoma after numerous unsuccessful treatment regimens with eye drops alone. Her current oral medications include diltiazem (Cardizem) 240 mg twice a day; hydrochlorothiazide (HCTZ) 25 mg three times per week (Mondays/Wednesdays/Fridays); atenolol (Tenormin) 25 mg daily; atorvastatin (Lipitor) 20 mg daily; Nasonex, 2 sprays to each nostril daily; and Betagan, 1 drop to each eye twice daily.

During the history and physical examination, Mrs. Adams reports that over the past several weeks she has had elevations in blood pressure readings at the physician's office. During her last appointment, her blood pressure was 172/96, and her regimen at that time included Diltiazem 240 mg once daily. Owing to the continued elevation, her physician told her that he was going to "double her Diltiazem" by having her take one dose in the morning and one in the evening each day. Mrs. Adams did not hear him explain that she was to take the second dose in the evening; she only heard him say "double the dose." The morning after her visit to the physician, Mrs. Adams took two Diltiazem tablets at 8:30 a.m., thus doubling her dose as she thought she was supposed to do. Within 20 minutes of ingesting the tablets, she was dizzy, unsteady on her feet, and slightly nauseous. Her daughter immediately called the physician and reported the adverse event and resulting symptoms. The symptoms were managed at home with rest, increased fluid intake, and repeated blood pressure measurements with an electronic blood pressure cuff that Mrs. Adams owned. Her daughter was to call the physician back if the blood pressure dropped below 110/60, which, surprisingly, it did not. At that time, a referral was made to the Visiting Nurse Association to assist with medication management and to perform medication teaching.

Literature Review

Older adults consume up to 40% of all prescribed medications in the United States (Dierich, Mueller, & Westra, 2011). Trends suggest that the number of medications taken by older adults is increasing, and that in 2007 to 2008, 9 out of 10 older adults took at least one prescription drug daily (Gu, Dillon, & Burt, 2010). By 2010, approximately 39.7% of the noninstitutionalized population of Americans aged 65 and older consumed five or more prescription medications daily according to one government report (Centers for Disease Control [CDC], 2012, p. 282). More current statistics suggest that older adults take anywhere from 5 to 10 medications daily (Yetzer, Goetsch, & St. Paul, 2011), a phenomenon historically deemed "polypharmacy." Polypharmacy has more recently been defined as "the current use of more than one medication to treat a condition or number of conditions" (Dierich et al., 2011), and "the use of more medications than are clinically indicated" (Riker & Setter, 2013). Regardless of the definition, as the number of prescribed medications increases, so too does patient confusion over the regimen, potential for medication errors (Yetzer et al., 2011), and medication-related falls (Steinman, Lund, Miao, Boscardin, & Kaboli, 2011).

Many older adults suffer from a number of comorbidities requiring the prescription of multiple medications and creating a challenge for providers (Riker & Setter, 2013). Several factors can contribute to polypharmacy, including polyprescribers (having more than one provider prescribing medications), lack of communication between providers, and insufficient use of evidence-based practice when treating older adults (Riker & Setter, 2013). When present, polypharmacy may contribute to otherwise preventable hospitalizations (Dierich et al., 2011; Mager, 2013), drug–drug interactions (Mishra, Gioia, Childress, Barnet, & Webster, 2011; Riker & Setter), increased medication side effects, as well as other types of ADEs (Budnitz, Lovegrove, Shehab, & Richards, 2011; Chrischilles, VanGilder, Wright, Kelly, & Wallace, 2009; Yetzer et al., 2011).

ADEs have been defined as allergic reactions, undesirable pharmacologic and/or idiosyncratic effects, and unintentional overdoses, all of which contribute to otherwise preventable hospitalizations each year (Budnitz et al., 2011). In fact, the risk of ADEs increases 10% with each medication taken, approaching 100% with the use of 10 or more medications (Tinetti, 2005). A staggering reported 1.5 million ADEs occur annually in the United States (Institute of Medicine, 2006). Given the serious implications of ADEs, and the frequency of their occurrence, researchers are beginning to focus their work on ADEs and the effect on community-dwelling older adults, a population within a setting that is sometimes overlooked. In fact, a federal initiative called the Partnership for Patients has been instituted to try to decrease preventable hospitalizations related to ADEs (United States Department of Health and Human Services [USDHS], 2011).

Budnitz and colleagues (2011) studied emergency hospitalizations related to ADEs in older adults from 2007 to 2009 using a national databank of records. Among the 99,628 hospitalizations they studied, four medications, or classes of medications, contributed to ADEs leading to hospitalizations, including anticoagulants, oral antiplatelet drugs, and oral and injectable hypoglycemic agents. While results suggest that improved management of these medications is necessary for ADE reduction, other studies have also shown that any number of medications can cause ADEs and hospitalizations of older adults (Chrischilles et al., 2009; Mager, 2013).

In addition to ADEs and polypharmacy, another issue to consider when multiple drugs are ordered is medication adherence, or the extent to which patients follow the instructions given for prescribed treatments (Haynes, Ackloo, Sahota, McDonald, & Yao, 2008). Nonadherence has been linked to a number of problems including disease progression and complications, poor health outcomes, and increased numbers of hospitalizations and ADEs (Marck et al., 2010), making nonadherence a national concern (Berben, Dobbels, Kugler, Russell, & De Geest, 2011; Mishra et al., 2011).

A number of research studies have examined various interventions among community-dwelling older adults to measure medication adherence, including use of collateral and patient reports (Mager & Madigan, 2010), pill counts, electronic medication bottle monitoring, and any combination of these measures (Berben et al., 2011). Mager and Madigan surveyed older adults in their homes to determine medication adherence (n = 31) and found that 46% reported omitting a total of 45 medication doses, either purposefully or mistakenly, over the preceding 3 weeks. These and other findings suggest that adherence tends to decrease as the number of medications in a regimen increases (Mager & Madigan, 2010; Mansur, Weiss, Hoffman, Gruenewald, & Beloosesky, 2008). Similarly, Mishra and colleagues (2011) examined facilitators and barriers to adherence with multiple medications among low-income patients (n = 50). More than half of the sample experienced polypharmacy. This contributed to nonadherence due to both the complexity of the medication regimen and to financial constraints.

Although many factors contribute to nonadherence to one's regimen, medication cost is a frequently cited area of concern. As the number of prescriptions per person rises, so does the accompanying expense. The cost of prescription drug use in 2010 was $259 billion (CDC, 2012, p. 15), and the number of older adults who could not afford to purchase their prescriptions owing to cost rose from 2.8% in 1997 to 4.3% in 2011 (p. 235). When providers order medications for older adults, it is critical that they assess their socioeconomic status and their ability to secure the medications they need. Whenever possible, it may be more efficient to decrease the number of medications ordered and thus create a simpler regimen to follow that is more cost effective. It is important to remember that discontinuing medications can be challenging for the provider, and that some patients will not respond well to the changes, so clinicians must strategize to improve medication management and by analyzing whether medications are still beneficial to the patient (Riker & Setter, 2013).

As we saw in the case study of Mrs. Adams, a miscommunication between her and the provider caused her to experience an ADE. The taking of two doses of her blood pressure medication and the resulting symptomology could have easily caused her to be hospitalized. She was very fortunate that she did not fall, or suffer any other more serious effects of this mistake. It is critical to ensure that when medication changes are made, the patient is able to repeat the instructions to the provider so that miscommunications can be remedied before an ADE occurs.

Role and Cultural Considerations

Managing medication regimens with clients in their homes is a key component of many home care visits. In fact, Medicare home care guidelines state that medication teaching is considered a skilled and billable service (Center for Medicare and Medicaid Services, 2011, p. 2), validating the need for visits focused directly on medication management by a home care nurse. Patients can benefit dually by having an advanced practice registered nurse (APRN) with prescriptive authority perform the visit. APRNs have the ability to modify the medication regimen and teach about these changes all at the same time so as to avoid potential ADEs that can occur when patients do not fully understand the recommended changes.

It is important to consider cultural and socioeconomic needs when addressing medication regimens. Factors such as fasting, avoidance of certain types of treatments/products, and religious or cultural beliefs can all affect a patient's willingness or ability to take a given medication at a particular time of day. Additionally, the cost of and access to medications, along with the ability to physically obtain them, can also have an impact on adherence. When assessing a situation for medication use or misuse, it is necessary to consider all of these factors and to have a full understanding of the patient's ideas, values, and desires.

Assessment and Strategy

1. Lack of knowledge related to medication regimen
   - Provide education regarding current medication names, doses, and correct administration times; ask patient to repeat the regimen and assess for accuracy
   - Consider introduction of a medication box and evaluate the daughter's willingness and ability to prepour medications into the box for 1 week at a time
   - Provide education about signs and symptoms of low blood pressure to report to providers
   - Demonstrate how to rise slowly from lying to sitting, and sitting to standing, and educate the patient and family about prevention of orthostatic hypotension
   - Consider the use of a written medication list; educate the patient and family about the need to bring the list to the physician's office at every visit
2. Presence of bilateral dry cerumen in ears
   - Prescribe and teach the use of wax softener topically once a week
   - Perform ear irrigation after softening of cerumen occurs
   - Reassess patient's hearing after wax removal
   - Possibly refer to audiologist for hearing test and hearing aid as needed

Clinical Reasoning Questions

1. What is your plan for follow-up care for Mrs. Adams?
2. What referrals are needed in this case, if any?
3. How would your plan of care differ if Mrs. Adams lived alone?
4. What other factors could contribute to medication nonadherence for older adults?

References

Berben, L., Dobbels, F., Kugler, C., Russell, C. L., & De Geest, S. (2011). Interventions used by health care professionals to enhance medication adherence in transplant patients: A survey of current clinical practice. *Progress in Transplantation, 21*(4), 322–331.

Budnitz, D. S., Lovegrove, M. C., Shehab, N., & Richards, C. L. (2011). Emergency hospitalizations for adverse drug events in older Americans. *New England Journal of Medicine, 365*, 2002–2012.

Center for Disease Control. (2012). *Health, United States, 2012—With special feature on emergency care.* Retrieved from http://www.cdc.gov/nchs/data/hus/hus12.pdf#091

Center for Medicare and Medicaid Services. (2011). Home health services. In *Medicare benefit policy manual.* Retrieved from http://www.cms.gov

Chrischilles, E. A., VanGilder, R., Wright, K., Kelly, M., & Wallace, R. B. (2009). Inappropriate medication use as a risk factor for self-reported adverse drug effects in older adults. *Journal of the American Geriatrics Society, 57*(6), 1000–1006.

Dierich, M. T., Mueller, C., & Westra, B. L. (2011). Medication regimens in older home care patients. *Journal of Gerontological Nursing, 37*(12), 45–55.

Gu, Q., Dillon, C., & Burt, V. (2010). *Prescription drug use continues to increase: U.S. prescription drug data for 2007–2008* (Data Brief No. 42). Retrieved from http://www.cdc.gov/nchs/data/databriefs/db42.htm

Haynes, R. B., Ackloo, E., Sahota, N., McDonald, H., & Yao, X. (2008). Interventions for enhancing medication adherence. *Cochrane Database of Systematic Reviews, 4*(2), CD000011. doi:10.1002/14651858.CD000011.pub3

Institute of Medicine. (2006). *Report brief: Preventing medication errors.* Retrieved from http://iom.edu/~/media/Files/Report%20Files/2006/Preventing-Medication-Errors-Quality-Chasm-Series/medicationerrorsnew.pdf

Mager, D. (2013). Hospitalization of home care patients: Adverse drug events. *Home Health Care Management and Practice, 26*(1), 11–16. doi:10.1177/1084822313499772

Mager, D., & Madigan, E. (2010). Medication use among older adults in a home care setting. *Home Healthcare Nurse, 28*(1), 14–21.

Mansur, N., Weiss, A., Hoffman, A., Gruenewald, T., & Beloosesky, Y. (2008). Continuity and adherence to long-term drug treatment by geriatric patients after hospital discharge: A prospective cohort study. *Drugs & Aging, 25*(10), 861–870.

Marck, P. B., Lang, A., Macdonald, M., Griffin, M., Easty, A., & Corsini-Munt, S. (2010). Safety in home care: A research protocol for studying medication management. *Implementation Science, 5*(43), 1–9.

Mishra, S., Gioia, D., Childress, S., Barnet, B., & Webster, R. (2011). Adherence to medication regimens among low-income patients with multiple comorbid chronic conditions. *Health & Social Work, 36*(4), 249–258.

Riker, G. I., & Setter, S. M. (2013). Polypharmacy in older adults at home: What it is and what to do about it—Implications for home healthcare and hospice: Part 2. *Home Healthcare Nurse, 31*(2), 65–77.

Steinman, M. A., Lund, B. C., Miao, Y., Boscardin, W. J., & Kaboli, P. J. (2011). Geriatric conditions, medication use, and risk of adverse drug events in a predominantly male, older veteran population. *Journal of the American Geriatrics Society, 59*(4), 615–621.

Tinetti, M. (2005). Medication reduction strategy for older patients with multiple health conditions: Safe and effective medication decision-making. In *Fall risk assessment and interventions: A guide for clinicians* (pp. 1–6). New Haven: Connecticut Collaboration for Fall Prevention.

United States Department of Health and Human Services. (2011). *Partnership for patients: Better care, lower cost.* Retrieved from http://www.shea-online.org/Portals/0/Partnership%20for%20Patients%20Pledge%204.12.11.pdf

Yetzer, E. A., Goetsch, N., & St. Paul, M. (2011). Teaching adults SAFE medication management. *Rehabilitation Nursing, 36*(6), 255–260.

28 CONTINENCE CARE

TERESA MOORE AND MARCELLA KELLY

Subjective

"I'm fine really. Sure, for years I've had a bit of wetting. I was fine until I had my stroke and now I'm running to the toilet all the time."

Objective

Mrs. Beverly Bonnie Brown presents at the nurse-led continence clinic, having been referred by her public health nurse. She has had a long-term history of daytime wetting, but more recently experienced a need to use the toilet multiple times at night and during the day. Mrs. Brown is a 74-year-old retired hairdresser and a widow; she is a friendly, outgoing lady with two grown children, five grandchildren, and two great-grandchildren. Following the death of her husband some years earlier, Mrs. Brown sold her house and business and moved to a ground-floor apartment to be near her children and grandchildren. Mrs. Brown likes living alone, and her family both encourages and supports her to remain independent.

Prior to her husband's death she was actively involved with the local community, played golf, and enjoyed walking, reading, and gardening. She smoked cigarettes for most of her adult life, but gave them up in her forties following the death of her father at 70 from a CVA. Until recent years, her medical history was relatively uneventful—she had an emergency appendectomy in her teenage years, and at age 48 she had a cholecystectomy. Her obstetric history included the birth of two children via instrumental delivery over 50 years earlier.

Her first child was delivered via ventouse delivery due to delayed second stage of labor, and her second child was delivered via forceps delivery owing to shoulder dystocia and prolonged second stage of labor. Since the birth of her second child 47 years ago, Mrs. Brown has had intermittent urinary leakage that she has managed.

Since her late 50s, she has had a history of mild hypertension (BP ranging from 140/90 to 159/99 mmHg), which has been managed by a combination of medication, diet, and exercise. Two years ago, Mrs. Brown had a right-sided cerebrovascular accident (CVA), and although she rehabilitated well, her mobility and dexterity were reduced due to left-sided deficits. Her post-CVA medication includes 5 mg Lisinopril (Zestril) orally once a day, Simvastatin 10 mg orally daily, 500 mg aspirin, and Lasix, 40 mg orally daily.

After her CVA, Mrs. M's weight increased from 145 lbs. (66 kg) to 160 lbs. (72 kg). Her body mass index score of 30 suggests that for her height she is clinically obese (Todorovic, Russell, Stratton, Ward, & Elia, 2003). Concerned that the increase in weight was having a negative impact on her hypertension and on her mobility, the nurse practitioner referred Mrs. Brown to nutrition and physical therapy services. A combination of healthy eating and an exercise program enabled her to lose weight. With her new found confidence she started attending the local day center and other social events. While Mrs. Brown can wash, dress, and toilet independently, she does require support with bathing/showering and shopping. Her primary supports are her family, home help service provided by the public health community services, and private care, paid for by the family. Mrs. Brown goes to her family alternative weekends, and on the days she is not in the day center, Mrs. Brown has access to meals on wheels services.

Recently, Mrs. Brown stopped attending the center, and her family members were concerned as she was refusing to stay at the weekends. When contacted by day center staff, Mrs. Brown did not offer any explanation for the lack of attendance, but agreed to a home visit from the public health nursing services. Using a standardized protocol, the public health nurse completed a comprehensive assessment, the findings of which suggested that Mrs. Brown's reluctance to engage in social activities was due to a deterioration in her bladder control, as she was fearful of having a wetting accident in public or that her clothing might smell of urine. She also had a fear of falling, especially on the nights she stayed with her family. Symptoms of frequency, urgency, and urinary leakage resulted in Mrs. Brown becoming housebound. Although she missed going out, like many women, she was not willing to risk the potential embarrassment and stigma associated with incontinence (Elstad, Taubenberger, Botelho, & Tennstedt, 2010; Garcia, Crocker, Wyman, & Krissovich, 2005). As she lacked the motivation or interest to adhere to her diet and exercise plan, her weight had increased. Mrs. Brown consented to a referral to the nurse-led continence clinic and to sharing the findings from the assessment with the nurse continence advisor.

Literature Review

Stress urinary incontinence (SUI) is viewed as the most common type of incontinence, particularly in women (Getliffe & Dolman, 2007; Norton, 2001). SUI is associated with pregnancy and labor, in particular difficult labor that can cause pelvic floor trauma. It is also associated with postmenopausal deficiency of estrogen and the aging process, which affects the composition of the urethra and pelvic floor tissue, resulting in diminished elasticity and connectivity of these muscles (Charalambous & Trantafylidis, 2009). Poor pelvic floor muscle support can result in urinary leakage, particularly when there is an increase in intra-abdominal pressure caused by coughing, sneezing, or lifting (Charalambous & Trantafylidis, 2009; Melville, Delaney, Newton, & Katon, 2005). The aging process can also reduce the elasticity of the detrusor (bladder) muscle, which can result in incomplete bladder emptying and residual urine, which increases the risk of leakage and urinary tract infection (UTI) (Charalambous & Trantafylidis, 2009; Melville et al., 2005). Mrs. Brown's obstetrical history, age, and self-reported symptom of urinary leakage over a long number of years would indicate the likelihood of SUI.

Urgency urinary incontinence (UUI)/overactive bladder (OAB) is a set of conditions associated with a set of known symptoms including frequency, urgency, nocturia, and leakage. UUI/OAB is characterized by frequent and sudden urges to pass urine; the person may not be able to reach the toilet on time and as a result may be incontinent. In addition, the person may need to get up to pass urine many times during the night (Charalambous & Trantafylidis, 2009; Melville et al., 2005). Although the cause of UUI/OAB may be idiopathic (Charalambous & Trantafylidis, 2009; Melville et al., 2005) there are clear associations with neurological conditions such as cerebrovascular accident (Fritel, Lachal, Cassou, & Fauconnier, 2013; National Institute for Health Clinical Excellence [NICE], 2012). Neurological damage or trauma caused by a CVA may result in inappropriate or spontaneous voluntary contraction of the detrusor muscle during the filling phase, resulting in frequency and urgency. Coexisting conditions coupled with poststroke mobility or dexterity deficits can exacerbate incontinence (Fritel et al., 2013; NICE, 2012; Thomas et al., 2008). Temporary UUI/OAB symptoms are usually associated with local bladder irritation caused by infection or an increased intake of certain fluids such as alcohol or carbonated drinks or medication such as diuretics (Getliffe & Dolman, 2007; Norton, 2001). Mrs. Brown's medical history of CVA and self-reported symptoms of frequency, urgency, and incontinence would suggest UUI/ OAB.

Functional incontinence is not formally classified, but is recognized as a cause of incontinence in persons with impaired functional or cognitive ability (Getliffe & Dolman, 2007; Norton, 2001). The causative factors contributing to this type of incontinence are linked with functional and cognitive ability to manage bladder function, as opposed to bladder dysfunction (Getliffe & Dolman, 2007; Norton, 2001). Mrs. Brown's medical history of CVA with resultant hemiparesis of the left side is a potential contributory factor to functional incontinence.

As the cause of incontinence is multifactorial, the International Continence Society (Abrams et al., 2010) advocates effective management requiring a multidisciplinary approach. In the context of clinical governance, both assessment criterion and tools must be evidence based and linked with care pathways and clinical algorithms (Deneckere et al., 2012; Health Information and Quality Authority, 2012). Although evidence-based assessment criterion, care pathways, and algorithms have the potential to enhance the quality and safety of continence care, no algorithm or care pathway can be applied to every client, and therefore each client's care must be individualized (Abrams et al., 2010; NICE, 2012, 2013b).

Mrs. Brown was assessed using a standardized continence assessment protocol for poststroke clients (Health Service Executive [HSE], 2012). The assessment incorporated a comprehensive continence assessment and frequency volume monitoring using a bladder diary. A bladder diary serves as a diagnostic tool as well as providing objective data on symptoms and voiding patterns (Abrams et al., 2010). Mrs. Brown's bladder diary confirmed her fluid intake was less than 700 mL/24 hours, she passed urine more than 7 times/day, and she needed to go to the toilet 3 to 4 times at night. Despite constant use of disposable products, she experienced intermittent leakage/wetting accidents.

The data from Mrs. Brown's assessment was used to develop a plan of care and to provide visual feedback on improvements (Abrams et al., 2010; Getliffe & Dolman, 2007; Lucas et al., 2012). The assessment also confirmed that Mrs. Brown used fluid restriction and disposable pads as primary management strategies. The literature reveals that many women use fluid restriction as a coping strategy, in the belief that limiting intake lessens the risk of incontinence (Getliffe & Dolman, 2007; Wyman, Burgio, & Newman, 2009; Zimmern, Litman, Mueller, Norton, & Goode, 2010). While disposable products can be an effective intervention to prevent leakage, the type and absorbency of the product must align with the urinary output and needs of the client (Abrams et al., 2010; Getliffe & Dolman, 2007). Bladder training is also a frontline intervention for UI, which encompasses a suite of strategies aimed at reducing urinary frequency by delaying voiding as long as possible. Pelvic floor exercises also help manage urgency. The goal of the pelvic floor exercises is to improve pelvic floor muscle tone and strength so that Mrs. Brown can use these muscles to inhibit detrusor contractions (Eustice et al., 2009; NICE, 2012, 2013b; Santacreu, 2011; Thomas et al., 2008).

A urinalysis excluded abnormalities such as blood, glucose, protein, leucocytes, and nitrites. A physical inspection of the genital area indicated signs of mild excoriation, but no obvious evidence of vaginal prolapse. An ultrasound of Mrs. Brown's bladder revealed postvoid residual volume of less than 100 mL, which was deemed insignificant in the absence of recurrent UTIs (Lucas et al., 2012; NICE, 2013a, 2013b). There are a range of diagnostic investigations, such as voiding cystometry and videourodynamics, which can be used to verify symptoms; however, given Mrs. Brown's clear history of symptoms and in the absence of any abnormalities, the more invasive investigations were deemed unnecessary (Getliffe & Dolman, 2007; NICE, 2013b).

A further factor to consider in making a diagnosis of incontinence is the client's perception of how the symptoms are affecting his or her life. For example, if one considers the definition of urinary incontinence proffered as "the complaint of any involuntary leakage of urine" (Abrams et al., 2003, p. 38; Sand & Dmochowski, 2002, p. 3), arguably the word "any" suggests that any urine leakage irrespective of volume should be regarded as incontinence. This definition is important to consider as older women's individual perceptions of what constitutes urinary incontinence can vary, depending on age, culture, and social background (Charalambous & Trantafylidis, 2009; Lee, 2005). This gives rise to the rationale for conducting a holistic assessment of Mrs. Brown that incorporates her understanding of the symptoms and the impact of the symptoms on her quality of life (QOL). Charalambous and Trantafylidis (2009) highlight the impact urinary incontinence has on the QOL of women in particular and demonstrate, from a biopsychosocial perspective, the predominantly negative impact this condition can have on the individual's QOL irrespective of the category of urinary incontinence experienced.

The outcome of Mrs. Brown's assessment indicates the embarrassment and stigma linked with her symptoms of frequency, leakage, and odor had a negative impact on her QOL and caused her to withdraw from social interactions. The literature echoes the findings of Mrs. Brown's assessment (Charalambous & Trantafylidis, 2009; Melville et al., 2005). A further consideration as part of Mrs. Brown's holistic assessment included consideration of the impact this condition had on her physical well-being, particularly highlighting lifestyle factors.

The literature reveals again a potential trajectory linked with aging, reduced mobility, incontinence, and the propensity toward increased risk of falls (Fritel et al., 2013).

The literature also reveals an association between obesity and both urge and stress incontinence (Lucas et al., 2012). In the case of Mrs. Brown, obesity was viewed as a potential contributory factor to her incontinence and a risk to the effective management of her hypertension and mobility. Thus, the clinical picture revealed of Mrs. Brown is one of mixed urinary incontinence associated with the contributory factors of CVA, reduced functional mobility, obesity, and past obstetrical history.

Role and Cultural Considerations

Consideration of the impact urinary incontinence has from a psychosocial perspective should be a key aspect of Mrs. Brown's assessment and plan of care. The literature reveals the negative impact urinary incontinence can have on the individual associated with fear, embarrassment, diminished self-esteem, a sense of stigma, anxiety, depression, and shame (Avery, Braunack-Mayer, Stocks, Taylor, & Duggan, 2013; Heintz, DeMucha, Deguzman, & Softa, 2013; Siddiqui, Levin, Phadtare, Pietrobon, & Ammarell, 2013; Taylor, Weir, Cahill, & Rizk, 2013).

Siddiqui et al. (2013) alerts us to the impact on perceptions with regard to female urinary incontinence. Their systematic review highlights across different non-White racial/ethnic groups the sense of self-blame associated with incontinence symptoms, viewing this condition as a negative consequence of earlier life experiences and actions. The literature also identifies feelings of being unclean and of social stigma associated with symptoms of odor, fear of leakage, and of resultant withdrawal from social events in an attempt to conceal the condition (Avery et al., 2013; Heintz et al., 2013; Siddiqui et al., 2013; Taylor et al., 2013). Elstad et al. (2010) alerts us to the fear of being perceived of as unclean and indeed the impact this fear has with regard to "societal norms" of both body cleanliness and hygiene.

The sense of self-blame, shame, embarrassment, and lack of awareness as to what constitutes urinary incontinence would also appear to impact on treatment-seeking behaviors

(Elstad et al., 2010; Heintz et al., 2013; Siddiqui et al., 2013; Taylor et al., 2013). The literature review by Heintz et al. (2013) of stigma and microaggressions experienced by older women with urinary incontinence depicts the "silence" in both addressing and treating this condition. This silence they depict as the patients' role in not disclosing their condition and in health care providers not broaching the subject of urinary incontinence. The rationale provided in their review for lack of acknowledgment of this condition by health care providers would appear to be "inadequate education or expertise" in this area of practice (Heintz et al., 2013, p. 303). This finding is also echoed in Taylor et al. (2013, p. 97), revealing patients' reluctance to report their symptoms of urinary incontinence owing to a lack of awareness as to what constitutes incontinence and to "thinking that the condition could not be treated, feeling embarrassed, and thinking this is a normal part of ageing." Similarly, this study also revealed family physicians reporting their lack of being adequately trained and of their subsequent reluctance to both manage and treat this condition.

The literature suggests a need for more educational focus on the preparation of practitioners in both treating and managing this condition. This in turn, it is envisaged, would break the "silence" of this condition in that practitioners would feel equipped to address this condition with patients. Similarly, in breaking this silence, the patients' educational needs as to what constitutes "incontinence," the treatment options available, and, indeed, the reduced stigma of openly addressing their health needs associated with this condition can only serve to reduce the trauma of living with urinary incontinence.

Assessment and Strategies for Care

Establish a person-centered approach to care:

- Identify factors contributing to or exacerbating the symptoms that can be eliminated or managed (Abrams et al., 2010; Lucas et al., 2012; NICE, 2012, 2013b).
- Identify whether there is a need for referral to a specialist for evidence-based implementation of management options. Interventions may range from conservative management

to pharmacological or surgical options (Abrams et al., 2010; Lucas et al., 2012; NICE, 2012, 2013b).

Empowerment and decision making:

- Identify Mrs. M's knowledge deficits and address any myths in relation to cause, contributing factors, and type of urinary incontinence.
- Provide Mrs. Brown with information in a format and manner that would help her to understand the cause of her incontinence and enable her to make informed choices in relation to treatment options.

Behavioral interventions:

- Encourage Mrs. M to reduce the intake of tea and carbonated drinks and slowly increase her intake of water.
- Advise her to modify the intake of certain fluids instead of eliminating them to ensure long-term compliance (Getliffe & Dolman, 2007; Norton, 2001).
- Implement bladder training as a first-line treatment for women with UI or mixed urinary incontinence (International Urogynecological Association, 2011; NICE, 2013b).
- Teach pelvic floor exercises to help manage urgency.
- Consider a further home visit to identify environmental barriers to continence management and potential fall risks. Options that may be available to assist in incontinence management include a bedside commode, raised toilet seats, and grab rails in her bathroom.
- Encourage the use of clothing with elasticated waist bands, and replacing buttons with Velcro or easy-to-open zips.
- Consider fine motor exercises aimed at improving dexterity (Getliffe & Dolman, 2007; Supyk & Vickerman, 2004).

Clinical Reasoning Questions

1. What is the most likely diagnosis of the type of incontinence in this case and why?
2. What referrals are needed and why?

3. What is the key criterion when developing a plan of care for older people with urinary incontinence?
4. Are there standardized guidelines, protocols, or algorithms that clinicians should use to assess, plan, and evaluate care?
5. What is the plan for follow-up care?

References

Abrams, P., Andersson, K. E., Birder, L., Brubaker, L., Cardozo, L., Chapple, C., . . . The Members of the Committees. (2010). Fourth International Consultation on Incontinence Recommendations of the International Scientific Committee: Evaluation and treatment of urinary incontinence, pelvic organ prolapse, and fecal incontinence. *Neurourology and Urodynamics, 29,* 213–240.

Abrams, P., Cardozo, L., Fall, M., Griffiths, D., Rosier, P., Ulmsten, U. L. F., & Wein, A. (2003). The standardisation of terminology in lower urinary tract function: Report from the standardisation sub-committee of the International Continence Society. *Urology, 61,* 37–49.

Avery, J. C., Braunack-Mayer, A. J., Stocks, N. P., Taylor, A. W., & Duggan, P. (2013). Psychological perspectives in urinary incontinence: A metasynthesis. *OA Women's Health,* 1(1), 9.

Charalambous, S., & Trantafylidis, A. (2009). Review article: Impact of urinary incontinence on quality of life. *Pelviperineology, 28,* 51–53.

Deneckere, S., Euwema, M., Lodewijckx, C., Panella, M., Sermeus, W., & Vanhaecht, K. (2012). The European quality of care pathways (EQCP) study on the impact of care pathways on interprofessional teamwork in an acute hospital setting: Study protocol: For a cluster randomised controlled trial and evaluation of implementation processes. *Implement Science, 7*(47), 2–12.

Elstad, E. A., Taubenberger, S. P., Botelho, E. M., & Tennstedt, S. L. (2010). Beyond incontinence: The stigma of other urinary symptoms. *Journal of Advanced Nursing, 66*(11), 2460–2470.

Eustice, S., Roe, B., & Paterson, J. (2009). Prompted voiding for the management of urinary incontinence in adults. *Cochrane Database of Systematic Reviews, 2000*(2), CD002113.

Fritel, X., Lachal, L., Cassou, B., & Fauconnier, A. (2013). Mobility impairment is associated with urge but not stress urinary incontinence in community-dwelling older women: Results from the Ossebo study. *BJOG, 120,* 1566–1574.

Garcia, J. A, Crocker, J., Wyman, J. F., & Krissovich, M. (2005). Breaking the cycle of stigmatization: Managing the stigma of incontinence in social interactions. *Journal of Wound Ostomy Continence Nursing, 32*(1), 38–52.

Getliffe, K., & Dolman, M. (2007). *Promoting continence: A clinical research resource* (3rd ed.). London, England: Bailliere Tindall.

Health Information and Quality Authority. (2012). *National standards for safer better healthcare*. Dublin, Ireland: Author.

Health Service Executive. (2012). *Assessment and management of urinary incontinence in the stroke unit care pathway version: 1.2*. Dublin, Ireland: Author.

Heintz, P. A., DeMucha, C. M., Deguzman, M. M., & Softa, R. (2013). Stigma and micro aggressions experienced by older women with urinary incontinence: A literature review. *Urologic Nursing, 33*(6), 299–305.

International Urogynecological Association. (2011). *Bladder retraining: A guide for women*. Washington, DC: Author. Retrieved from http://c.ymcdn.com/sites/www.iuga.org/resource/resmgr/brochures/eng_btraining.pdf

Lee, J. J. (2005). The impact of urinary incontinence levels on the social lives of older Chinese in Hong Kong. *Hallym International Journal of Aging, 7*(1), 63–80.

Lucas, M. G., Bedretdinova, D., Bosch, J. L. H. R., Burkhard, F., Cruz, F., Nambiar, A. K, . . . Pickard R. S. (Eds.). (2012). *EUA guidelines on urinary incontinence*. Retrieved from http://www.uroweb.org/gls/pdf/16052013Urinary_Incontinence_LR.pdf

Melville, J. L., Delaney, K., Newton, K., & Katon, W. (2005). Incontinence severity and major depression in incontinent women. *Obstetrics and Gynecology, 106*(3), 585–592.

National Institute for Health and Care Excellence. (2013a). *Information document signposting to incontinence-specific quality-of-life scales: Urinary incontinence in women. NICE clinical guideline 171*. Retrieved from http://www.nice.org.uk/nicemedia/live/14271/65356/65356.pdf

National Institute for Health and Care Excellence. (2013b). *Urinary incontinence: The management of urinary incontinence in women. NICE clinical guideline 171*. Retrieved from http://guidance.nice.org.uk/CG171/NICEGuidance/pdf/

National Institute for Health Clinical Excellence. (2012). *Urinary incontinence in neurological disease: Management of lower urinary tract dysfunction in neurological disease. Clinical guideline 148*. Retrieved from http://www.nice.org.uk/guidance/cg148

Norton, C. (2001). *Nursing for continence* (2nd ed.). Buckinghamshire, England: Beaconsfield Publishers.

Santacreu, M. (2011). Evaluation of a behavioral treatment for female urinary incontinence. *Clinical Interventions in Aging, 6*, 133–139.

Sand, P., & Dmochowski, R. (2002). Analysis of the standardization of terminology of lower urinary tract dysfunction: Report from the standardisation sub-committee of the International Continence Society. *Neurology Urodynamics, 21*, 167–178.

Siddiqui, N. Y., Levin, P. J., Phadtare, A., Pietrobon, R., & Ammarell, N. (2013). Perceptions about female urinary incontinence: A systematic review. *International Urogynecology Journal*, 25(7), 863–871.

Supyk, J. A., & Vickerman, J. (2004). The hidden role of the occupational therapist in the management of incontinence. *International Journal of Therapy and Rehabilitation, 11*(11), 509–515.

Taylor, D. L., Weir, M., Cahill, J. J., & Rizk, D. E. E. (2013). The self-reported prevalence and knowledge of urinary incontinence and barriers to health care-seeking in a community sample of Canadian women. *American Journal of Medicine and Medical Sciences, 3*(5), 97–102.

Thomas, L. H., Cross, S., Barrett, J., French, B., Leathley, M., Sutton, C. J., & Watkins, C. (2008). Treatment of urinary incontinence after stroke in adults. *Cochrane Database of Systematic Reviews, 2008*(1), CD004462.

Todorovic, V., Russell, C., Stratton, R., Ward, J., & Elia, M. (Eds.). (2003). *The MUST explanatory booklet*. Redditch, England: British Association for Parenteral and Enteral Nutrition. Retrieved from http://www.bapen.org.uk/pdfs/must/must_explan.pdf

Wyman, J. F., Burgio, K. L., & Newman, D. K. (2009). Practical aspects of lifestyle modifications and behavioral interventions in the treatment of overactive bladder and urgency urinary incontinence. *International Journal of Clinical Practice, 63*(8), 1177–1191. Retrieved from http://www.ncbi.nlm.nih.gov/pmc/articles/PMC2734927

Zimmern, P., Litman, H. J., Mueller, E., Norton, P., & Goode, P. (2010). Effect of fluid management on fluid intake and urge incontinence in a trial for overactive bladder in women. *BJU International, 105*(12), 1680–1685. Retrieved from http://onlinelibrary.wiley.com/doi/10.1111/j.1464-410X.2009.09055x/pdf

29 PULMONARY REHABILITATION AND CHRONIC OBSTRUCTIVE PULMONARY DISEASE

DYMPNA CASEY AND KATHY MURPHY

Subjective

"There was a time when I could play hide-and-seek with all my grandchildren. Now I get so breathless that all I can do is sit and watch. It's so frustrating and so very scary. . . .

"My physician referred me to the consultant in the hospital a few years back because I was getting a lot of chest infections and he didn't have the equipment to accurately diagnose what was the matter. I had to wait three months for an appointment. In the hospital they carried out loads of tests and told me that I have something called COPD—not sure I understand it completely. It hadn't really affected me too much, but recently I'm getting a fit of coughing most mornings, and it takes me a good few minutes to clear it. I'm also beginning to lose my breath when I engage in even light physical activities, for example, playing with my grandchildren. It seems to me that the more I try to do the more breathless I become, and I'm so frightened when that happens. Maybe I should be doing less and forget about playing with the grandchildren, and then maybe I will begin to feel better."

Objective

Johnny is a 65-year-old man with chronic obstructive pulmonary disease (COPD) and hypertension attending his general practitioner. He reports that he now has a cough most days that generates a lot of mucus, particularly in the mornings, and over the past few weeks he has been feeling increasingly fatigued and getting more and more breathless on exertion. In particular, he recounts that it really upset him that he was not able to play hide-and-seek with his youngest granddaughter, Amelia, who is 5 years old, when she visited the previous weekend. Johnny's temperature is normal at 98°F. He appears breathless on exertion, and his oxygen saturation levels are 93%, reducing to 90% following exertion. His vital signs are BP 140/75, pulse 115, respirations 25/minute. Johnny quit smoking 10 years ago, but he used to smoke "about" 20 cigarettes a day, having commenced smoking at the age of 15. Johnny was reasonably active in his younger years, playing Gaelic football for his local community. On retirement, he commenced coaching the under-21 football team, but now he is no longer involved in any physical activity, stating that "it takes all my efforts to just breathe, never mind kick a football!" As his breathlessness has increased, he has become more and more sedentary. His waist circumference is 42 in. (107 cm) and his BMI is 41. His physical examination reveals hyperinflation of the chest, decreased breath sounds with a prolonged expiratory phase, scattered end expiratory wheezes, and crackles at the lung bases. There is no evidence of peripheral edema or digital clubbing. He is alert and oriented, and in no acute distress while resting. His skin is warm, dry, and intact; abdomen is soft and nontender; and bowel sounds are present in all four quadrants. His eyes are clear with normal sclera with pupils equal, round, reactive to light and accommodation (PERRLA). Johnny lives with his wife, Caroline, in the town of Saidbh. They have three children and six grandchildren, all of whom are healthy. Johnny's sister Christine (58 years) was also recently diagnosed with COPD. He is prescribed Exputex syrup 250 mg/5 mL three times daily, Symbicort turbohaler (budesonide/formoterol fumarate dehydrate) 400/12 mcg, 1 inhalation twice daily, 1 inhalation twice daily, and Micardis Plus (telmisartan 40 mg and hydrochlorothiazide) 40 mg/12.5 mg daily. His spirometery results reveal an FEV/FVC of 63% and an FEV1 68% predicted, indicating that he has moderate COPD.

Literature Review

COPD is a term used to describe progressive chronic lung diseases that cause obstruction in airflow that are not fully reversible, resulting in persistent breathlessness, productive coughing, fatigue, and recurrent chest infections (Global Initiative for Chronic Obstructive Lung Disease [GOLD], 2007, 2011). In the United States, more than 12 million people are diagnosed with COPD, and 120,000 people die each year (National Institute of Health [NIH], 2010). Worldwide, it is estimated that 210 million people are living with COPD (Franchi, 2009), and it is projected that by 2030 COPD will be the third most frequent cause of death (World Health Organization [WHO], 2008). There are numerous risk factors for COPD including genetics, sustaining recurrent respiratory infections, having a low socioeconomic status, exposure to air pollutants, poor nutrition, and asthma (Eisner et al., 2010; GOLD, 2011). However, smoking is recognized as a primary cause of COPD, and the more a person smokes during his or her lifetime, the more likely he or she is to develop this condition (Forey, Thornton, & Lee, 2011). Godtfredsen et al. (2008), in their narrative review of morbidity and mortality in COPD following smoking cessation, found that smoking cessation preserves lung function and improves survival in comparison with continued smoking. The fact that Johnny quit smoking 10 years ago is a positive step, and this will help modify the clinical course of his COPD. Traditionally, mortality rates from COPD were higher in men than in women (Shambou & O'Brien, 2009). However, Rycroft et al. (2012), in their epidemiological literature review on COPD, describe how in some countries, mortality rates in women have increased in comparison with those in men. For example, in the United States, since 2000, more women have died from COPD than men. The reasons for this disparity are varied and include increased susceptibility to the adverse effects of smoking, delayed diagnosis, and differences in smoking patterns (American Lung Association, 2013).

The symptoms of COPD make engagement in physical activity unpleasant, provoking anxiety that inevitably leads to further breathlessness, exacerbations of COPD symptoms, and panic. This is called the "anxiety–dyspnea–anxiety cycle" (Carrieri-Kohlman, Douglas, Gormley, & Stulbarg, 1993, p. 230), which results in increasing fatigue, more breathlessness, increased anxiety, and less activity. This inactivity leads to further muscle deconditioning, further reducing the capacity to engage in physical activity. In other words, it is a vicious circle (Bourbeau & Nault, 2007), which, as in the case of Johnny, ultimately leads to more inactivity (Troosters et al., 2013). In persons with COPD, physical inactivity is therefore a key predictor of mortality (Garcia-Aymerich, Lange, Benet, Schnohr, & Antó, 2006; Spruit et al., 2013; Waschki et al., 2011). Johnny needs to understand the symptoms of his COPD and the relationship between his sedentary lifestyle, his symptoms, and the progression of his condition. In particular, Johnny's fear of exercising will need to be allayed by explaining to him that the less activity he does, the worse he will feel. In contrast, the more physically active he is, the more improvement there will be in his COPD symptoms. Johnny may also benefit from learning relaxation techniques such as guided imagery/visualization and techniques to control his breathing. There is some evidence that breathing techniques such as pursed lip breathing, which slows down the breathing rate, can reduce exercise-induced dyspnea (Nield, Soo Hoo, Roper, & Santiago, 2007). It would therefore be beneficial to Johnny to be trained to use such strategies.

Pulmonary Rehabilitation Programs (PRP)

The Spruit et al. (2013) guidelines emphasize the importance of exercise in the management of COPD and endorse the central role of pulmonary rehabilitation (PR) as an interdisciplinary approach to the integrated care of persons with COPD. They define PRP as "comprehensive intervention based on a thorough patient assessment followed by patient tailored therapies that include, but are not limited to, exercise training, education, and behavior change, designed to improve the physical and psychological condition of people with chronic respiratory disease and to promote the long-term adherence to health-enhancing behaviors" (Spruit et al., 2013, p. e14).

Exercise training is recognized as the best method of increasing muscle function in persons with COPD (ATS/ERS, 2013). In PR, exercise training is a key component and is typically delivered in group settings, which use individually tailored exercise plans and are usually supervised, as supervised programs tend to yield the greatest benefit (Lacasse, Goldstein, Lasserson, & Martin, 2006). Most PRP's offer a range of exercise regimens, including strength and endurance training. Frequency, intensity, and specificity of the exercise sessions are the main determinants of the training effect, and the British Thoracic Society (2001) recommends twice weekly supervised exercise sessions with additional sessions undertaken by patients at home. The educational element of most PRPs is usually delivered during group teaching/discussion sessions and includes a variety of topics such as medications, O_2 therapy, energy conservation techniques, relaxation skills, breathing techniques, nutritional advice, what to do in emergencies, what to do when traveling with lung disease, and end-of-life issues (Hill, 2006).

Many studies reveal that PRPs lead to improvements in health-related quality of life (HRQL) for persons with COPD (Cambach, Wagenaar, Koelman, van Keimpema, & Kemper, 1999; Effing et al., 2007; Kruis et al., 2013; Lacasse et al., 2006). Cambach et al. (1999) undertook a meta-analysis of 18 studies, examining the outcome measures post-PRPs for exercise capacity and HRQL in patients with COPD. They found that there were significant improvements for maximal exercise capacity, endurance time and walking distance, and HRQL. In a Cochrane systematic review undertaken by Lacasse et al. (2006) examining PR in COPD, the findings of 23 RCTs were examined. This review concluded that PRPs statistically and clinically improved dyspnea and disease-specific quality of life (QOL) in persons with COPD. Likewise, Effing et al. (2007), in their Cochrane review on self-management education for adults with COPD, which focused predominantly on PRPs, found significant reductions in dyspnea and improvements in QOL. Kruis et al. (2013) also reported improved disease-specific QOL and exercise capacity in persons with COPD. They conducted a systematic review of 26 RCTs on integrated disease management (IDM) programs for COPD. Exercise training was a key component in the majority of the studies (n = 23) reviewed. Likewise, one of the largest PR trials to date, the PRINCE cluster randomized controlled trial, involving 32 primary care physicians and 350 participants, found that persons with moderate-to-severe COPD had a statistically significant improvement in QOL as measured by the total score of the Chronic Respiratory Questionnaire (CRQ) (Casey et al., 2013). The evidence therefore suggests that it is likely that Johnny will benefit from participating in a PRP.

The American College of Physicians (ACP) guidelines recommend that PRP be offered to all symptomatic patients with FEV1 less than 50% predicted and considered for individuals with FEV1 greater than 50% predicted (Qaseem et al., 2011). However, PRP is not recommended for patients who are immobile, have unstable angina, or who have recently suffered a myocardial infarction (National Institute for Health and Clinical Excellence [NICE], 2010). Therefore, Johnny would be considered a suitable candidate for a PRP, and the fact that he previously enjoyed sports and being active may be a motivating factor to participate. However, he is anxious about exercising.

Approximately 40% of persons with COPD have symptoms of anxiety or depression (Coventry, 2009). In some cases, depression rates of 50% have been identified in persons with COPD (Maurer et al., 2008), in comparison with a 6% to 8% rate in the general population (Wells, Golding, & Burnan, 1998). However, completing a PRP may reduce these symptoms. Güell et al. (2006) examined the impact of PR on psychosocial morbidity in a prospective trial involving 40 patients with COPD. They found that a 16-week PRP focused primarily on exercise leads to significant reductions in anxiety and depression compared with the control group. Coventry (2009), in a systematic review and meta-analysis of three RCTs of PRP, found a reduction in short-term anxiety and depression. Likewise, Bratås et al. (2010) reported a significant reduction in depression in COPD patients (n = 136) following a 4-week inpatient PRP. Similarly, Tselebis et al. (2013) found a statistically significant reduction in anxiety and depression in participants with COPD (n = 101) following a 3-month PRP, and these improvements were found irrespective of disease severity, gender, or education. Anxiety, depression, and lack of motivation may lead to exercise intolerance in persons with COPD (de Voogd, Sanderman, Postema, van Sonderen, & Wempe, 2011). It is important, therefore, that Johnny be assessed for depression and that he be given the opportunity to participate in a PRP.

Johnny's COPD symptoms and QOL could be improved by providing him with further education on the symptoms of COPD, and referring him to and encouraging him to participate in a PRP. Participating in a PRP has the potential to reduce his dyspnea and anxiety, prevent muscle decline, improve his exercise capacity, and allow him to play once more with his grandchildren.

Role and Cultural Considerations

In many European countries, spirometry testing is not undertaken routinely in the primary care setting (Jochmann et al., 2010; Lyngsø et al., 2010); therefore, patients like Johnny have to be referred to secondary settings to confirm diagnosis, and this takes time. The absence of early diagnosis makes the effective delivery of health care for people with COPD living in the community problematic. Early detection and appropriate treatment of COPD is crucial for alleviating patients' symptoms and reducing the economic burden of the disease. Nurses working in primary care, once they receive appropriate training, are optimally positioned to detect early stage COPD and undertake spirometery testing to confirm diagnosis and thereby implement early detection and treatment.

There is no agreed instrument for assessing depression in persons with COPD (Gilbody, House, & Sheldon, 2005). However, the Hamilton Depression Subscales (Stage, Middelboe, Stage, & Sorenson, 2006) have been identified as a useful tool for use with persons with COPD.

Accessibility to PRPs also differs from country to country, and in most countries, PRPs are based in secondary or tertiary care settings with few available in the community (Casey et al., 2013). In the review by Lacasse et al. (2006), only one program was delivered in the community (Cambach et al., 1997). In addition, recent trends are focusing on technology and the use of telemedicine and home monitoring systems in the management of COPD (ATS/ERS, 2013). The nurse would therefore need to identify the most appropriate PRP for Johnny. In so doing, transport and timing of program delivery would need to be discussed and agreed upon. In the event that a telehealth

PRP is available, Johnny's capacity to use and interact with the technology would also need to be considered.

Finally, it must be remembered that not all persons with COPD are willing to join a PRP. The nurse therefore needs to work closely with each person with COPD to identify his or her exercise preferences. In the event that a PRP is declined or is not an option, an appropriate exercise plan tailored to a person's needs and preferences must be devised.

Assessment and Plan

- Provide Johnny with information on COPD and the symptoms of COPD
- Assess Johnny for depression, and prescribe appropriate medications if required
- Encourage Johnny to engage in more physical activities
- Explain what a PRP is, and assess Johnny's motivation to participate in a PRP
- Identify an appropriate PRP for Johnny in terms of location, timing, and duration.
- Teach Johnny relaxation techniques and strategies to control his breathing such as pursed lip breathing

Critical Thinking Questions

1. What is your plan for follow-up care for Johnny?
2. Are any referrals needed in this case? If so, to whom?
3. What if Johnny is depressed?
4. Are there any standardized guidelines that you could use to assess or treat Johnny?

References

American Lung Association. (2013). *Taking her breath away: The rise of COPD in women* (Disparities in Lung Health Series). Chicago, IL: Author.

Bourbeau, J., & Nault, D. (2007). Self-management strategies in chronic obstructive pulmonary disease. *Clinics in Chest Medicine, 28*(3), 617–628.

Bratås, O., Espnes, G. A., Rannestad, T., & Walstad, R. (2010). Characteristics of patients with chronic obstructive pulmonary disease choosing rehabilitation. *Journal of Rehabilitation of Medicine, 42*, 362–367.

British Thoracic Society Standards. (2001). Standards of care subcommittee on pulmonary rehabilitation. *Thorax, 56*(11), 827–834.

Cambach, W., Chadwick-Straver, R. V. M., Wagenaar, R. C., van Keimpema, A. R. J., & Kemper, H. C. G. (1997). The effects of a community-based pulmonary rehabilitation programme on exercise tolerance and quality of life: A randomized controlled trial. *European Respiratory Journal, 10*, 104–113.

Cambach, W., Wagenaar, R. C., Koelman, T. W., van Keimpema, A. R. J., & Kemper, H. C. G. (1999). The long-term effects of pulmonary rehabilitation in patients with asthma and chronic obstructive pulmonary disease: A research synthesis. *Archives of Physical Medicine and Rehabilitation, 80*(1), 103–111.

Carrieri-Kohlman, V., Douglas, M. K., Gormley, J. M., & Stulbarg, M. S. (1993). Desensitization and guided mastery: Treatment approaches for the management of dyspnea. *Heart & Lung, 22*(3), 226–234.

Casey, D., Murphy, K., Devane, D., Cooney, A., McCarthy, B., Mee, L., . . . Murphy, A. W. (2013). The effectiveness of a structured education pulmonary rehabilitation programme for improving the health status of people with moderate and severe chronic obstructive pulmonary disease in primary care: The PRINCE cluster randomised trial. *Thorax, 68*, 922–928. doi:10.1136/thoraxjnl-2012-203103

Coventry, P. A. (2009). Does pulmonary rehabilitation reduce anxiety and depression in chronic obstructive pulmonary disease? *Current Opinion in Pulmonary Medicine, 15*, 143–149.

de Voogd, J. N., Sanderman, R., Postema, K., van Sonderen, E., & Wempe, J. B. (2011). Relationship between anxiety and dyspnea on exertion in patients with chronic obstructive pulmonary disease. *Anxiety Stress Coping, 24*, 439–449.

Effing, T., Monninkhof, E. M., van der Valk, P. P., van der Palen, J. J., van Herwaarden, C. L., Partidge, M. R., . . . Zielhuis, G. A. (2007). Self-management education for patients with chronic obstructive pulmonary disease. *Cochrane Database of Systematic Review, 2007*(4) [Art ID CD002990].

Eisner, M. D., Blanc, P. D., Yelin, E. H., Katz, P. P., Sanchez, G., Iribarren, C., & Omachi, T. A. (2010). Influence of anxiety on health outcomes in COPD. *Thorax, 65*, 229–234. doi:10.1136/thx.2009.126201

Forey, B. A., Thornton, A. J., & Lee, P. N. (2011). Systematic review with meta-analysis of the epidemiological evidence relating smoking to

COPD, chronic bronchitis and emphysema. *BMC Pulmonary Medicine, 11*, 36. doi:10.1186/1471-2466-11-36

Franchi, M. (2009). *EFA book on chronic obstructive pulmonary disease in Europe: Sharing and caring*. Brussels, Belgium: European Federation of Allergy and Airways Disease. Retrieved from http://www.efanet.org/wp-content/uploads/2012/07/EFACOPDBook.pdf

Garcia-Aymerich, J., Lange, P., Benet, M., Schnohr, P., & Antó, J. M. (2006). Regular physical activity reduces hospital admission and mortality in chronic obstructive pulmonary disease: A population based cohort study. *Thorax, 6*(61), 772–778.

Gilbody, S., House, A. O., & Sheldon, T. A. (2005). Review screening and case finding instruments for depression. *Cochrane Database of Systematic Review, 2005*(4) [Art ID CD002792].

Global Initiative for Chronic Obstructive Lung Disease. (2007). *Global strategy for the diagnosis, management and prevention of COPD*. Retrieved from http://www.goldcopd.org

Global Initiative for Chronic Obstructive Lung Disease. (2011). *Global strategy for the diagnosis, management, and prevention of chronic obstructive pulmonary disease* (updated 2010). Retrieved from http://www.csrd.org.cn/ppt/upload/201268164.pdf

Godtfredsen, N. S., Lam, T. H., Hansel, T. T., Leon, M. E., Gray, N., Dresler, C., . . . Vestbo, J. (2008, October). COPD-related morbidity and mortality after smoking cessation: Status of the evidence. *European Respiratory Journal, 32*(4), 844–853. doi:10.1183/09031936.00160007

Güell, R., Resqueti, V., Sangenis, M., Morante, F., Martorell, B., Casan, P., & Guyatt, G. H. (2006). Impact of pulmonary rehabilitation on psychosocial morbidity in patients with severe COPD. *Chest, 129*(4), 899–904.

Hill, N.S. (2006) Pulmonary rehabilitation. *Proceedings of the American Thoracic Society, 3*(1) 66–74.

Jochmann, A., Neubauer, F., Miedinger, D., Schafroth, S., Tamm, M., & Leuppi, J. D. (2010). General practitioner's adherence to the COPD GOLD guidelines: Baseline data of the Swiss COPD Cohort Study. *Swiss Medical Weekly*. Early online publication. Retrieved from http://www.smw.ch

Kruis, A. L., Smidt, N., Assendelft, W. J. J., Gussekloo, J., Boland, M. R. S., Rutten-van Mölken, M., & Chavannes, N. H. (2013). Integrated disease management interventions for patients with chronic obstructive pulmonary disease (Review). *The Cochrane Library 2013*(10). doi: 10.1002/14651858.CD009437.pub2

Lacasse, Y., Goldstein, R., Lasserson, T. J., & Martin, S. (2006). Pulmonary rehabilitation for chronic obstructive pulmonary disease. *Cochrane Database of Systematic Review, 2006*(4) 49. [Art ID CD003793]. doi:10.1002/14651858.CD003793

Lyngsø, A. M., Backer, V., Gottlieb, V., Nybo, B., Østergaard, M. S., & Frølich, A. (2010). Early detection of COPD in primary care—The Copenhagen COPD Screening Project. *BMC Public Health, 10*, 524. doi:10.1186/1471-2458-10-524

Maurer, J., Rebbapragada, V., Borson, S., Goldstein, R., Kunik, M. E., Yohannes, A. M., & Hanania, N. A. (2008). ACCP Workshop Panel on Anxiety and Depression in COPD: Anxiety and depression in COPD: Current understanding, unanswered questions, and research needs. *Chest, 13*(4 Suppl.), 43S–56S.

National Institute of Health. (2010). *Fact sheet: Chronic obstructive pulmonary disease (COPD)*. Retrieved from http://report.nih.gov/nihfactsheets/Pdfs/ChronicObstructivePulmonaryDisease(NHLBI).pdf

National Institute for Health and Clinical Excellence. (2010). *Chronic obstructive pulmonary disease: Management of chronic obstructive disease in adults in primary and secondary care*. London, England: National Collaborating Centre for Chronic Conditions NHS.

Nield, M. A., Soo Hoo, G. W., Roper, J. M., & Santiago, S. (2007). Efficacy of pursed-lips breathing: A breathing pattern retraining strategy for dyspnea reduction. *Journal of Cardiopulmonary Rehabilitation and Prevention, 27*, 237–244.

Qaseem, A., Wilt, T. J., Weinberger, S. E., Hanania, N. A., Criner, G., van der Molen, T., . . . Shekelle, P. (2011). Diagnosis and management of stable chronic obstructive pulmonary disease: A clinical practice guideline update from the American College of Physicians, American College of Chest Physicians, American Thoracic Society, and European Respiratory Society. *Annals of Internal Medicine, 155*, 179–191.

Rycroft, C. E., Heyes, A., Lanza, L., & Becker, K. (2012). Epidemiology of chronic obstructive pulmonary disease: A literature review. *International Journal of COPD, 7*, 457–494.

Shambou, A., & O' Brien, A. (2009). Fighting for breath. *WIN, 17*(4), 26–28.

Spruit, M., Singh, S. J., Garvey, C., ZuWallack, R., Nici, L., Rochester, C., . . . Wouters, E. F. M. (2013). An Official American Thoracic Society/European Respiratory Society Statement: Key concepts and advances in pulmonary rehabilitation. *American Journal of Respiratory and Critical Care, 188*(8), e13–e64.

Stage, K. B., Middelboe, T., Stage, T. B., & Sorenson, C. H. (2006). Depression in COPD—Management and quality of life considerations. *International Journal of COPD, 1*(3), 315–320.

Troosters, T., van der Molen, T., Polkey, M., Rabinovich, R. A., Vogiatzis, I., Weisman, I., & Kulich, K. (2013). Improving physical activity in COPD: Towards a new paradigm. *Respiratory Research, 14,* 115. Retrieved from http://respiratory-research.com/content/14/1/115

Tselebis, A., Bratis, D., Pachi, A., Moussas, G., Ilias, I., Harikiopoulou, M., . . . Tzanakis, N. (2013). A pulmonary rehabilitation program reduces levels of anxiety and depression in COPD patients. *Multidisciplinary Respiratory Medicine, 8,* 41. Retrieved from http://www.mrmjournal.com/content/8/1/41

Waschki, B., Kirsten, A., Holz, O., Müller, K. C., Meyer, T., Watz, H., & Magnussen, H. (2011). Physical activity is the strongest predictor of all cause mortality in patients with COPD: A prospective cohort study. *Chest, 140,* 331–342.

Wells, K. B., Golding, J., & Burnan, M. A. (1998). Psychiatric disorder in a sample of the general population with and without chronic medical conditions. *American Journal of Psychiatry, 145,* 976–979.

World Health Organization. (2008). *The global burden of disease: 2004 update*. Geneva, Switzerland: Author.

30 PROMOTING MENTAL HEALTH OF OLDER PEOPLE

JEAN M. O'CONNOR AND CHRISTINE CAUFFIELD

Subjective

The nurse reports that Mr. Daniel D. Davis has recently been behaving in a sexually inappropriate manner with females on the unit and fondling himself in public. He has frequent angry outbursts, and "cries at the drop of a hat." The nurse states that the staff has been excluding him from all social areas, including the dining room, in order to "protect the other residents."

Objective

Mr. Davis is an 84-year-old White male referred for psychiatric evaluation at the Veterans Administration from the nursing home where he resides. His vital signs are weight: 174 lbs. (79 kg); height: 70 in. (177 cm); BP: 128/76; pulse: 82 regular; respirations: 18. Mr. Davis originated in Philadelphia, Pennsylvania, the first born of three children. His parents were first generation British. He served 3 years in the army, where he saw active combat. He was discharged early from his service tour—honorably, although the reason for early discharge was unclear. After returning to Philadelphia, he completed a bachelor's degree in finance. He gained employment with a major oil company and rose to the rank of chief accountant. He was married for 48 years, and is father to two daughters, ages 53 and 58. The daughters live out of state, but maintain close telephone contact with their father. He was the primary caregiver for his wife, who had a prolonged period of illness (breast cancer) prior to her death 5 years ago. As his wife's illness progressed, he began to neglect maintenance and repairs of the Cape Cod home in which they resided. He began to look forward to his daily cocktail consumption, as his wife slept. The rural setting prevented regular visits from friends, and the aforementioned issues went largely unnoticed. His social circle disappeared over time as friends suffered similar circumstances to Mr. Davis. At the time of hospitalization for his CVA, his daughters were shocked to discover the house in significant disarray. Additionally, their father's unkempt appearance was a worrisome factor, as he had previously been impeccable with grooming and dress. The kitchen countertop was littered with over-the-counter medications, as well as numerous empty wine bottles. He was unable to accurately report his prescribed medication schedule.

His children report a loving relationship between parents and a happy childhood. They denied any history of domestic or family violence. Mr. Davis retired from his corporate position after 40 years at age 65. When his health began to fail 3 years ago, his daughters placed him in a nursing home. They have since moved back to the area in order to be closer to their father and are faithful visitors, as are other extended family members living locally.

Mr. Davis's father was reported to have "melancholia" per his daughter's report. She was not aware of the degree to which this interfered with his ability to function or whether he received treatment for this condition. He had episodes of depression following his service in Korea. He has had no psychiatric hospitalizations and denies suicidal ideation or attempts. Mr. Davis is a regular drinker—moderate to heavy in recent years. He has no history of illicit drug use or dependence. His medications include Trazodone 50 mg at bedtime for sleep, Lisinopril 20mg/12.5mg HCTZ, Metformin 500 mg bid, Aricept 10 mg daily.

Mr. Davis's past medical history includes hypertension, hyperglycemia, memory loss, depression, temporal lobe CVA in 2011 (last CT scan in 2012), and presbycusis (moderate), for which he has been prescribed bilateral hearing aids. His religion on record is Lutheran. He attends multidenominational services in the nursing home when available. On presentation, Mr. Davis is neat, clean, and appropriately dressed, walking slowly with the use of a cane. He appears his stated age. He is alert, and offers a friendly greeting. He remarks that he was not certain why he was being seen. He is aware of person, place, and time. His cognition is impaired—he is unable to report the date and is unsure of the president's name ("I know he's a very smart Black man"). His speech is clear, with slightly delayed responses and moderately increased volume. His activity level is appropriate for his age, and he is slightly unsteady on his feet. His affect and mood are depressed labile mood, anxious, and tearful/angry at times, with inappropriate sexual references toward interviewer ("I'd like to roll in the hay with you"). He denies feeling suicidal/homicidal and denies auditory or visual hallucinations. His concentration is fair; he appears distracted at times. His thought content shows preoccupation with sexual content, which is appropriate when directed to a subject. At times, it is relevant and organized. Mr. Davis's memory is poor for recent events, but his remote memory is somewhat clearer, and he minimizes and attempts to cover up his inability to remember information such as what was on the breakfast menu or when he last saw his daughters. His judgment is mildly to moderately impaired.

Literature Review

As life span continues to lengthen worldwide, the incidence of mental health-related conditions continues to grow (Administration on Aging, 2005). The Department of Economic and Social Affairs has projected that by 2030, the number of older adult Americans will double to 72.1 million people, or 1 in every 5 Americans. This projection applies around the globe.

In assessing overall well-being, mental health concerns are closely connected to physical health conditions (Healthy People, 2020; White House Conference on Aging, 2005). It is estimated that 20% of adults ages 55 and above will develop a mental health condition such as a mood disorder, generalized anxiety disorder, or cognitive impairment disorder (Administration on Aging, 2005; Goodwin, 1983). Alcohol abuse and prescription drug misuse are issues contributing to considerable morbidity in this population, yet are often overlooked in the assessment of the patient. Despite the significant incidence of these disorders in the population, less than 3% of those afflicted will receive appropriate intervention. The key issues regarding failing health, depression, dementia, substance use, and polypharmacy will be explored in this chapter.

There are numerous issues to further explore regarding Mr. Davis's potential mental health status. Obtaining a comprehensive assessment that includes biopsychosocial information is critical to enable the health care provider to make an accurate diagnosis. Cultural aspects of the client's life including gender, race, ethnicity, and spiritual/religious preferences are necessary components of the assessment, as these data can provide critical information for proper diagnosis and management as well.

In reviewing Mr. Davis's initial evaluation, an astute clinician will pay attention to historical information that requires further exploration. He is a Korean War veteran, with active combat experience. The history does not include whether Mr. Davis sustained head injury, loss of consciousness, or other compromising physical trauma that may have contributed to his dementing process. There was no mention that Mr. Davis was ever evaluated or treated for posttraumatic stress disorder, which has a long-lasting impact on soldiers. Although he received an honorable discharge after 3 years of service, the reason given for early release is listed as "unknown." Could there have been psychological reasons for early discharge?

A family history of depression (father) predisposes Mr. Davis to added risk for depression. His personal history indeed indicates that he has a history of depression. These risk factors place him in a high-risk position for suicide. This fact adds an eightfold risk for Mr. Davis to develop dementia.

Caregiver stress can be quite deleterious to one's health, and Mr. Davis was the sole caretaker for his wife's death. Did he seek professional help for grief/loss issues? Could a contributing factor to his current depression be unresolved grief and loss issues?

A review of medical records reveals that Mr. Davis's last CT scan was 3 years ago. It is imperative that treatment recommendations include a current imaging brain scan to determine whether there have been additional infarcts or other physiological changes in the brain. Inappropriate sexual behavior coupled with angry outbursts could be the result of damage to the frontal lobe region, which often manifests in frontal lobe disinhibition. A person's physical health and ability to function are affected by conditions such as depression and anxiety and ultimately adversely affect the outcome of the disease. Depression reduces body immune responses and may also affect a person's physical health (Bartels et al., 2002). For example, clients diagnosed with diabetes and co-occurring depression have a 38% higher all-cause mortality rate versus those clients diagnosed with diabetes who do not have clinical depression. Additionally, the risk of developing heart disease is doubled in people with depression. Men with clinical depression are more than twice as likely to develop coronary artery disease or suffer a heart attack.

Older adults with untreated depression are most at risk for suicide. The suicide rate of seniors is 21%, the highest of all age groups in the United States. Caucasian men over the age of 85 are at the highest risk of all age–gender–race groups. Alarmingly, 20% of elderly suicides over the age of 75 had visited their primary care physician in the 24 hours prior to the suicide. Seventy percent of older adult suicide victims had visited their primary care physician in the month prior to committing suicide. Contrary to popular belief regarding reasons for suicide, only a small percentage (2% to 4%) of suicide victims have been diagnosed with a terminal illness at the time of their death. It is estimated that elder suicide may be underreported by 40% or more. These sobering statistics reflect the need for health care professionals to include mood assessments as a routine component in every examination.

Mental health care for older people is often lacking. Barriers to utilizing mental health services include inadequate insurance, a dearth of trained geriatricians, lack of coordination of care with medical services, mental health stigmas, and denial of the presence of the disorder, as well as functional barriers including transportation to services (Bartels et al., 2002).

Depression is the most prevalent mental health condition facing older adults. Contrary to popular belief, depression is not considered to be a normal condition of aging (Evans & Mottram, 2000). There is no single definition of depression, as the spectrum of symptoms varies widely in presentation and severity. Patients may have mild depression with no obvious change in behavior or mood or may have major depressive disorder with severe symptoms of illness. Many older people deny the presence of depression, having grown up in an atmosphere that discouraged the expression of sadness or grief. Fear of stigmatization often prevents patients from addressing these concerns with a health care provider. Images of archaic psychiatric care often influence an elderly person's decision to seek help. Coupled with the number of physical ailments that often accompany aging, depression may be confused with physical disability, or conversely, a diagnosis could be improperly applied when the symptoms are just age related (stooped posture, slowed gait, etc.). This may interfere with identification and treatment of depression in the elderly (Mueller et al., 2004). The evidence is mounting to support the belief that late- and early-presentation depression are actually very different conditions.

Research has evidenced that depression is a disorder of the brain involving malfunction of critical neurotransmitters (American Psychiatric Association, 2013). Neurotransmitters are chemicals that affect mood, sleep regulation, appetite, cognition, and behavior. When they are imbalanced or disrupted, the effects often result in a diagnosis of clinical depression. Depression is a leading cause of disability worldwide and results in more years of lost productivity than any other disease (World Health Organization, 2001). Depression is implicated in a greater decline in function and overall health due to illnesses such as arthritis, asthmas, diabetes, and cardiovascular disease. It contributes to medical comorbidity and is a major cause of disability among older people (Alexopoulos & Kelly, 2009).

Researchers from the University of Rochester Medical Center identified key factors that predict which older adults are at risk for developing major depression. The factors identified were current low-level depressive symptoms, perception of poor social support system, and a past history of depression. Also recognized were the implications for the need for early detection and intervention for people in the high-risk group in order to prevent a major depressive episode.

There are several additional factors that influence the development of this disorder. These include isolation, unresolved grief and loss issues, polypharmacy, chronic comorbid illness, and cognitive impairment (Singh & Misra, 2009). In addition, substance use and dependence often mask an underlying depression, creating a co-occurring condition that is more difficult to treat.

Specific criteria have been identified in the *Diagnostic and Statistical Manual of Mental Disorders (DSM-5)* to accurately diagnose mental health disorders, including depression. According to this manual, the main feature of a major depressive episode is a period of at least 2 weeks during which there is either depressed mood or the loss of interest or pleasure in activities that previously provided a significant degree of entertainment. These symptoms may not be attributed to another medical condition.

Depression is frequently misdiagnosed as dementia and is termed *pseudodementia*. Many symptoms of depression can mimic dementia, including deficits in attention, concentration, responsiveness, and reported memory loss. Additional causes or contributors to depression include cerebrovascular disease. It is suggested that vascular disease might lead to depression through damage to specific brain circuits or less directly through inflammation. Other factors that exacerbate depression and vascular disease include overeating, sedentary lifestyle, diabetes, smoking, hypertension, arrhythmia, and nonadherence to medical recommendations.

Anhedonia presents as complete loss of interest in all activities that previously were a source of pleasure to the patient. Hobbies, sports, exercise, animals, and so on, are no longer important to the patient.

Insomnia, the most common sleep disturbance, may be classified as middle insomnia (i.e., waking up during the night and having difficulty returning to sleep) or terminal insomnia (i.e., waking too early and being unable to return to sleep). Initial insomnia (i.e., difficulty falling asleep) may also occur. Hypersomnia (i.e., excessive daytime or nighttime sleep episodes) may be reported as well. A symptom must either be newly present or must have clearly worsened compared with the person's pre-episode status. The episode must be accompanied by clinically significant distress or impairment in social, occupational, or other important areas of functioning.

Psychomotor reports may include agitation (e.g., the inability to sit still, pacing, hand-wringing; or pulling or rubbing of the skin, clothing, or other objects) or retardation (e.g., slowed speech, thinking, and body movements; increased pauses before answering; speech that is decreased in volume, inflection, amount, or variety of content, or muteness).

Decreased energy and fatigue are common complaints. Frequently, patients will suspect illness and undergo a variety of tests before depression is identified. Older adults often emphasize somatic complaints, including bodily aches and pains, gastrointestinal distress, and fatigue, rather than reporting feelings of sadness. Males often report increased irritability, anger, or frustration.

Depression, whether treated or untreated, is the psychiatric condition most closely associated with suicide (Gallo & Lebowitz, 1999). Statistics indicate that the elderly tend to be more successful at completing suicide than younger people. Suicide rates increase with age and are highest among males and females worldwide (World Health Organization, 2001). Males account for approximately 85% of suicides among people age 65 and older. The fastest growing rate for suicide occurs in males aged 80 to 84 years (Turvey et al., 2002). Caucasian men over the age of 85 are at the greatest risk of all age–gender–race groups. Suicide rates among older adults are highest in those who are single, separated, divorced, or widowed (Conwell, 2007). Most older suicide victims live with relatives or are in regular contact with family or friends. This group tends to make fewer attempts and uses highly lethal methods to ensure completion of suicide.

The presence of physical illness increases the risk of suicide for older adults. Conditions that have been closely associated with increased risk are chronic obstructive pulmonary disease, neurologic illness (in particular seizure disorders), cancer, bone fractures, visual impairment, and gastrointestinal disease (Juurlink, Herrmann, Szalai, Kopp, & Redelmeier, 2004; Quan, Arboleda-Flórez, Fick, Stuart, & Love, 2002; Turvey et al., 2002).

Approximately 75% of older adult suicide victims visited their primary care physician in the month prior to committing suicide. In fact, 25% to 50% of these individuals visited their physician within 24 hours of committing suicide (Conwell, 2007). Most older adults who successfully commit suicide had an Axis I psychiatric diagnosis. These statistics support the need for depression screening and evaluation as a routine part of all medical appointments. A tool with high validity and reliability that is specific for the older adult population is the Geriatric Depression Screening (Yesavage et al., 1983).

In reviewing the case study of Mr. Davis, there are many factors that position him for risk of suicide. He has a history of major depression, with a current diagnosis, as well. He has been isolated from his peers in his residence at the nursing home (Findlay, 2003). He maintains frequent contact with his daughters and is widowed. His age (84) and gender place him in the highest risk group for suicide.

Dementia is a condition characterized by the insidious onset and continuous progression of cognitive decline and dysfunction. Laboratory and radiological studies in these patients are invariably normal. Dramatic impairment in recent memory, decline in nonverbal abilities, and atrophy of the cerebrum with or without ventricular enlargement beyond all expectations based upon age assist in making the diagnosis. Taking a detailed history about the patients' life will often identify changes in mood, affect, judgment, memory, and concentration before orientation becomes a problem. Family members will often talk about changes in the personality of the patient long before disorientation becomes apparent.

A common mnemonic used by physicians who are sorting out differential diagnosis of dementia is listed below:

Drugs and alcohol
Emotional disorders, primarily depression
Metabolic and endocrine disorders
Eyes and ears (sensory loss)
Nutritional deficiency and normal-pressure hydrocephalus
Tumor and trauma
Infection
Arteriosclerotic complications

A misdiagnosis of dementia, particularly fatal Alzheimer's disease, can have a deleterious effect on both the patient and the family members (DeFina, Moser, Glenn, Lichtenstein, & Fellus, 2013). The current prevalence of dementia in older adults over the age of 80 is estimated at 10% to 30%. There is concern that the adoption of new diagnostic criteria will result in approximately 65% of older adults being diagnosed with Alzheimer's disease and up to 23% of nondemented older adults being diagnosed inaccurately with dementia (LeCouteur, Doust, Creasey, & Brayne, 2013). It is imperative that a complete neurologic examination with appropriate imaging studies, as well as a neuropsychological evaluation, be completed to ensure an accurate diagnosis is delivered.

Alcoholism is one of the eight leading causes of death for older adults. Alcoholism contributes to a myriad of comorbid health conditions, including osteomalacia, malnutrition, cirrhosis of the liver, dementia (including Korsakoff's syndrome), and falls, which may cause significant morbidity in an elderly patient.

Repeated intake of high doses of alcohol can affect nearly every organ system, most notably the gastrointestinal, cardiovascular, and central and peripheral nervous systems. Increased incidence of cancer of the stomach, esophagus, and other parts of the gastrointestinal tract has been observed, and hypertension and tachycardia are common side effects of alcohol abuse.

Alcohol, by nature, is a depressant, and seniors are at risk for exacerbating depression, which, as mentioned previously, has deleterious health consequences and contributes to high suicide risk during severe intoxication and in the context of a temporary alcohol-induced depressive and bipolar disorder.

The *DSM-5* (2013) lists 11 criteria of Alcohol Use Disorder, of which at least 2 must be manifested within a 12-month period to substantiate the diagnosis. The adapted criteria are:

1. One drinks more alcohol or drinks for a longer time period than previously planned
2. One cannot cut down alcohol use despite his or her wish to limit drinking

3. One spends exceeding amounts of time in order to get alcohol, use it, or recover from it
4. Intense pull or wish to use alcohol
5. Alcohol contributing to malfunctions at work, home, or school.
6. Persistent alcohol use despite having problems caused by its effects
7. Alcohol leading to abstinence from relationships, work, or hobbies.
8. Using alcohol in physically dangerous situations
9. Using alcohol in spite of its effect to aggravate psychological or physical problems.
10. Tolerance, as explained by:
    - Use of increased amounts of alcohol to reach intoxication
    - Weakening effects with use of the same amount of alcohol
11. Withdrawal, as explained by:
    - Withdrawal syndrome
    - Using controlled substances to avoid or diminish withdrawal

It is not uncommon for substance abusing older adults to have a co-occurring psychiatric disorder such as anxiety or depression. Often, these individuals have turned to alcohol or other substances to self-treat the presenting psychiatric symptoms.

It is estimated that 17% of older adults abuse alcohol and prescription medications. Approximately 87% of elderly patients receive regular care by a physician; however, 40% of those who are at risk for substance abuse-related problems neither divulge nor admit the actual degree of alcohol or drug consumption. This may prevent identification and potential treatment of this problem.

Substance abusers are often categorized as chronic or late onset. Chronic abusers have early onset usage, typically during the early teenage years, with progression of increased usage and increased tolerance. Their clinical histories often include a family history of substance abuse or failure to fulfill major role obligations at work, school, or home with continued usage despite the persistent or recurrent interpersonal problems.

Late-onset substance users typically do not have a problem with abuse until a triggering event later in life initiates the use of alcohol or other substances. Often the death of a spouse with increased isolation precipitates late-onset usage. Metabolic changes associated with aging, such as renal insufficiency and decreased liver function, often predispose an older adult to more rapid intoxication.

Treatment outcomes for substance-abusing older adults indicate that best practice should include a specialized, segregated unit, owing to the unique and often complex issues that seniors present with (Center for Substance Abuse Treatment, 1998). Medical detoxification is recommended to ensure the patient is medically cleared before beginning a structured treatment regimen that may include psychoeducational groups, individual and family therapy, and participation in the 12-step recovery model (Gfroerer, Penne, Pemberton, & Folsom, 2003).

Polypharmacy is a term used most commonly with reference to the elderly, describing the use of many drugs together, or the administration of excessive medication to patients. Medication misuse has not been well studied, but has been implicated as a cause of delirium and depression in older persons. It should be suspected in cases where a patient is:

- Using medicine prescribed to someone else
- Taking a medication with alcohol
- Taking a medication for a condition other than the one prescribed for
- Using a number of similar medications for one indication
- Taking less or more than prescribed
- Using medications that are incompatible
- Discontinuing prematurely, or taking longer than indicated (Beloosesky, Nenaydenko, Gross Nevo, Adunsky, & Weiss, 2013; Gallo & Lebowitz, 1999).

As the population of those over age 65 rises, so does the prevalence of polypharmacy. This is a phenomenon seen all over the world, with the highest rates occurring among nursing home residents. The relationship between polypharmacy and negative patient outcomes has been established, yet almost 50% of older persons take at least one medication that is unnecessary (Maher, Hanlon, & Hajjar, 2014).

Patients taking multiple unnecessary medications are at risk for a number of serious health consequences. This risk heightens with each additional medication. Health care costs increased from approximately 7.3% to 30% in studies in the United States and Sweden, respectively, when hospitalization was required because of inappropriate medication ingestion. Adverse drug events were responsible for approximately 4.3 million health care visits in 2005 (Burgeois, Shannon, Valim, & Mandl, 2010). Drug incompatibilities were reported in studies of the frail elderly at a rate of 15% to 40%, and functional capacity reduction leading to the patients' inability to perform ADLs was significantly affected. Cognitive impairment, including delirium and dementia, were strongly associated with polypharmacy. Falls resulting from medication effects are a major cause of morbidity and mortality. A study of older adults observed the fall risk to increase significantly with the number of medications prescribed. Patients are also at risk of developing physical conditions resultant to polypharmacy, including urinary incontinence and nutritional deficiencies, leading to a reduction in overall health status (Dwyer, Han, Woodwell, & Rechtsteiner, 2010; Patterson, Hughes, Kerse, Cardwell, & Bradley, 2012).

There are many medications that are contraindicated in the elderly because of age-related medical concerns. Older adults metabolize drugs less efficiently, and often exhibit a higher rate of side effects related to medication administration. In 2012, the American Geriatric Society updated the Beers Criteria for Potentially Inappropriate Medication Use in Older Adults. This document is a systematic, comprehensive, evidentiary review of drug-related issues and adverse drug events that have been reported in older adults (Campanelli, 2012). In creating this database, the evidence was rated for quality and strength of recommendation. A rationale is included that describes each drug-related risk. Medications prescribed to younger adults often have a different effect or consequence on an older person.

Some commonly prescribed medications in patients with mental disorders may be contraindicated in the older adult.

TABLE 30.1: Medications Contraindicated in Older Adults With Mental Disorders

Category of Drug	Rationale	Recommendation
Anticholinergics	Reduced renal clearance with age Tolerance risk Risk of confusion, toxicity	Avoid
Tertiary TCAs	Sedating May cause orthostatic hypotension	Avoid
Antipsychotics	Increased risk of CVA Increased mortality in patients with dementia	Avoid use for behavioral problems
Barbiturates	High incidence of dependence Increased sensitivity	Avoid
Benzodiazepines	Increased sensitivity/side effects Increased cognitive impairment	Avoid
Nonbenzo hypnotics	Similar to benzo	Avoid

CVA, cerebrovascular accident.

These criteria are recommended when prescribing medication to older adults with mental health disorders. Some of the medications to be used with caution in the elderly are listed in Table 30.1.

The challenge of treating mental health conditions is increasing as people are living longer. Several themes are seen in the literature and in practice (Abramson & Halpain, 2002). These themes include:

1. Care geared to maintaining function with a careful focus on quality of life (QOL)
2. A renewed interest in the integration of primary care and mental health; coordinating patient medications and improving collaborative communication between providers has the ability to greatly improve care
3. Increasing understanding of how culture influences care access and provision of care may lead to greater overall success in treatment outcomes (Douglas et al., 2011)

4. Preventing the potential consequences of mental health medications with careful patient monitoring
5. Meeting these challenges to ensure provision of a comprehensive, accessible health service for this population

Strategies and Solutions

- Older adults have a unique set of needs and health concerns, and acquiring all the necessary information from these patients can be challenging.
- Memory loss, either recent or remote memory, can limit the patients' ability to inform the interviewer.
- Elderly patients often enjoy reminiscing during an interview, making the interview difficult to direct.
- Information on family psychiatric history may be lacking, or patient may be reluctant to divulge.
- Patients may not be able to participate in a lengthy, detailed interview.

Recommendations for Assessment

- Attempt to develop a rapport with patient prior to assessment
- Schedule the assessment at a time when patient is rested and alert
- Collect collateral information regarding patient from willing family members or staff (if patient is residing in a facility)
- Review available records prior to assessment, including laboratory analysis, which may reveal clues to substance use (abnl INR, elevated MCV, elevated LFTs)
- Carefully note recent changes in weight, sleep patterns, mood, activity patterns
- Ask about specifics in terms of alcohol and drug use (prescribed and OTC)
- Pay particular attention to cognition, orientation, and memory (what are the names of grandchildren, birth dates, etc.)

Summary

Identifying and successfully managing the mental health needs of older people can be complex and challenging (American Geriatrics Society, 2013). Medication prescription must be monitored according to the patients' kidney and liver function as well as to his or her ability to tolerate the medication. Engaging the patient and family in the plan of care and allowing them to make decisions for care is critical to compliance as well as patient satisfaction and ensuring QOL (Taqui, Itrat, Qidwai, & Qadri, 2007).

Clinical Reasoning Questions

1. What is your plan for follow-up care of Mr. Davis?
2. Are any referrals needed in this case? If so, to whom?
3. What investigations should Mr. Davis have? Why?
4. Are there any standardized guidelines that could be used to assess or treat Mr. Davis?

References

Abramson, T. A., & Halpain, M. (2002, Spring). Providers of mental health services-now and in the future. *Generations, 26*(1), 107–110.

Administration on Aging. (2005). *A profile of older Americans* (pp. 1–15). Washington, DC: U.S. Department of Health and Human Services.

Alexopoulos, G., & Kelly, R. (2009). Research advances in geriatric depression. *Journal of the World Psychiatric Association, 8*(3), 140–149.

American Geriatrics Society. (2013). American Geriatrics Society identifies five things that healthcare providers and patients should question. *The Journal of American Geriatrics Society, 61*(4), 622–631.

American Psychiatric Association. (2013). *Diagnostic and statistical manual of mental disorders* (5th ed.). Arlington, VA: Author.

Bartels, S. J., Dums, A. R., Oxman, T. E., Schneider, L. S., Areán, P. A., Alexopoulos, G. S., & Jeste, D. V. (2002). Evidence-based practices in geriatric mental health care. *Psychiatric Services, 53*(11), 1419–1431.

Beloosesky, Y., Nenaydenko, O., Gross Nevo, R. F., Adunsky, A., & Weiss, A. (2013). Rates, variability, and associated factors of polypharmacy in nursing home patients. *Clinical Interventions in Aging, 8,* 1585–1590.

Burgeois, F., Shannon, M. W., Valim, C., & Mandl, K. D. (2010, September). Adverse drug events in the outpatient setting: An 11-year national analysis (U.S. national library of medicine). *National Institutes of Health, 19*(9), 901–910.

Campanelli, C. M. (2012). American Geriatrics Society updated Beers criteria for potentially inappropriate medication use in older adults. *Journal of the American Geriatrics Society, 60*(4), 616–631.

Center for Substance Abuse Treatment. (1998). *Treatment improvement protocol (TIP) #26: Substance abuse among older adults.* Rockville, MD: U.S. Department of Health and Human Services, Public Health Service, Substance Abuse and Mental Health Services Administration.

Conwell, Y. (2007, January). Suicide in older adults: Management and prevention. *Psychiatric Times*, 1–6.

DeFina, P. A., Moser, R. S., Glenn, M., Lichtenstein, J. D., & Fellus, J. (2013, July). Alzheimer's disease clinical and research update for health care practitioners. *Journal of Aging Research, 2013*, 1–9.

Douglas, M., Pierce, J. U., Rosenkoetter, M., Pacquiao, D., Callister, L. C., Hattar-Pollara, M., . . . Purnell, L. (2011). Standards of practice for culturally competent nursing care: 2011 update. *Journal of the Transcultural Nursing, 22*, 317–333.

Dwyer, L., Han, B., Woodwell, D. A., & Rechtsteiner, E. A. (2010, February). Polypharmacy in nursing home residents in the United States: Results of the 2004 national nursing home survey. *The American Journal of Geriatric Pharmacotherapy, 8*(1), 63–72.

Evans, M., & Mottram, P. (2000). Diagnosis of depression in elderly patients. *Advances in Psychiatric Treatment, 6*, 49–56.

Findlay, R. A. (2003). Interventions to reduce social isolation amongst older people: Where is the evidence? *Aging and Society, 233*, 647–658.

Gallo, J. J., & Lebowitz, B. D. (1999). The epidemiology of common late-life mental disorders in the community: Themes for the new century. *Psychiatric Services, 50*, 1158–1168.

Gfroerer, J., Penne, M., Pemberton, M., & Folsom, R. (2003). Substance abuse treatment need among older adults in 2020: The impact of the aging baby-boom cohort. *Drug and Alcohol Dependence, 69*(2), 127–135.

Goodwin, J. (1983, October). Common psychiatric disorders in elderly persons. *The Western Journal of Medicine, 139*, 502–506.

Healthy People 2020 (n.d.). Mental health and mental disorders. Retrieved from http://www.healthypeople.gov/2020/topics-objectives/topic/mental-health-and-mental-disorders

Juurlink, D., Herrmann, N., Szalai, J. P., Kopp, A., & Redelmeier, D. A. (2004, June 14). Medical illness and the risk of suicide in the elderly. *Archives of Internal Medicine, 164*(11), 1179–1184.

LeCouteur, D., Doust, J., Creasey, H., & Brayne, C. (2013). Political drive to screen for pre-dementia: Not evidence based and ignores the harm of diagnosis. *British Medical Journal, 347*, f5125.

Maher, R. L., Hanlon, J., & Hajjar, E. R. (2014, January). Clinical consequences of polypharmacy in elderly (U.S. National Library of Medicine). *National Institutes of Health, 13*(1), 57–65.

Mueller, T., Kohn, R., Leventhal, N., Leon, A. C., Solomon, D., Coryell, W., . . . Keller, M. B. (2004, February). The course of depression in elderly patients. *The American Journal of Geriatric Psychiatry, 12*(1), 22–29.

Patterson, S., Hughes, C., Kerse, N., Cardwell, C. R., & Bradley, M. C. (2012). Interventions to improve the appropriate use of polypharmacy for older people. *The Cochrane Database of System Reviews, 2012*(5). CD008165. doi: 10.1002/14651858.CD008165.pub2.

Quan, H., Arboleda-Flórez, J., Fick, G. H., Stuart, H. L., & Love, E. J. (2002, April). Association between physical illness and suicide among the elderly. *Social Psychiatry and Psychiatric Epidemiology, 37*(4), 190–197.

Singh, A., & Misra, N. (2009, January–June). Loneliness, depression and sociability in old age. *Industrial Psychiatry Journal, 18*(1), 51–55.

Taqui, A., Itrat, A., Qidwai, W., & Qadri, Z. (2007, October). Depression in the elderly: Does family system play a role? A cross-sectional study. *BMC Psychiatry, 7*, 1–12.

Turvey, C., Conwell, Y., Jones, M. P., Phillips, C., Simonsick, E., Pearson, J. L., & Wallace, R. (2002). Risk factors for late-life suicide: A prospective, community-based study. *American Journal of Geriatric Psychiatry, 10*, 398–406.

White House Conference on Aging. (2005, December). *The booming dynamics of aging: From awareness to action*. Report to the President and the Congress. Washington, DC: U.S. Department of Health and Human Services.

World Health Organization. (2001). *World health report 2001-mental health: New understanding, new hope*. Retrieved from http://www.who.int/whr/2001/en

Yesavage, J., Brink, T. L., Rose, T. L., Lum, O., Huang. V., Adey, M., & Leirer, V. O. (1983). Development and validation of a geriatric depression screening scale: A preliminary report. *Journal of Psychiatric Research, 17*, 37–49.

31 CARDIOVASCULAR HEALTH PROMOTION

KIMBERLY O. LACEY AND BERNADETTE MADARA

Subjective

"I'm so glad you're here. I'm not feeling well. I'm very tired and out of breath, and I can't stop coughing. I ran out of my blood pressure and water pills three days ago. Can you help me?"

Objective

Ms. Elaine E. Elliott is a 79-year-old widow who lives alone in an 84-unit condominium complex. She has had primary hypertension for 20 years and biventricular heart failure for 3 years. Since her husband died 11 months ago, she has had limited social interaction, although her neighbors check on her every few days. Her cat, Tabby, is a major source of companionship.

Three months ago, she was admitted to home care services after hospitalization for decompensated heart failure. Today, when the visiting nurse found Ms. Elliott in moderate respiratory distress, she called 911. The following report was given to the EMTs when they arrived: Vital signs: 170/98, 103, 32, 98.4°F. Bilateral crackles on auscultation. The patient complained of dyspnea, a frequent nonproductive cough, and bilateral 3+ pitting edema is present.

When Ms. Elliott arrived at the emergency room, the nurse practitioner noted the following: mild diaphoresis, cool extremities, jugular vein distention, bilateral expiratory wheeze, hepatic tenderness to palpation, and a diminished first heart sound. Lab work revealed a brain natriuretic peptide (BNP) of 480 pg/mL. The nurse practitioner ordered an indwelling catheter for 24 hours, 80 mg furosemide IV push STAT, then 20 mg furosemide by mouth daily, saline lock, vital signs every 2 hours times four, then every 4 hours, strict I/O, 2 gm Na diet, 1,500 mL fluid restriction, Lisinopril 20 mg by mouth daily, nasal oxygen at 2 L/min, discharge to rehabilitation facility when stable.

Thirty-six hours after admission, Ms. Elliott reported "feeling wonderful" and denied dyspnea. Her intake during the previous 24 hours was 1,300 mL, and her urine output was 3,860 mL. Her lung sounds were clear bilaterally, pedal edema reduced to 1+, BNP reduced to 98 pg/mL, vitals 136/74, 81, 22. The discharge planner discussed her pending transfer to Sunnyvale Rehabilitation Center that afternoon. Ms. Elliott voiced concern about going to a "nursing home where people wait to die" and stated, "I must go home. My cat needs me." Once the reason for rehabilitation was explained to her, and her neighbor promised to care for Tabby, Ms. Elliott expressed relief and said she was ready to give Sunnyvale a try.

During the admission process to Sunnyvale Rehabilitation Center, Ms. Elliott was assessed by the rehabilitation team composed of a registered nurse, a physical therapist, an occupational therapist, a dietitian, and a recreational therapist. Three physical and/or occupational therapy sessions a day were scheduled. The dietitian explained that she would be on a 2 gm Na low cholesterol diet. Ms. Elliott stated that, "Following the diet will be easy because I eat frozen meals and do not add any salt." She told the recreational therapist that she missed going to church, playing cards with her friends, and going to a restaurant once a week with her neighbors. She commented that, "Those days are really over now that I am on this diet, and the water pills sometimes make me leak urine, so I do not go out anymore anyway."

Literature Review

Approximately 5.1 million people in the United States have heart failure (HF), with an anticipated 25% increase between 2013 and 2030. The incidence of HF is approximately 10 cases/1,000 population in individuals age 65 and above, with a 20% lifetime risk for those 80 years of age and above.

HF is more common in men than in women, and in African Americans as compared with Caucasians and Hispanics. In 2009, HF was listed as a contributing factor in 1 in 9 deaths. Total costs (direct and indirect) associated with HF in the United States are estimated to be $32 billion annually (Go et al., 2013). Patients may have left-sided HF, right-sided HF, or both (American Heart Association [AHA], 2013). Depending on their HF symptoms and how they impact their activities of daily living and quality of life (QOL), they are classified according to the New York Heart Association Functional Classification for HFs (The Criteria Committee for the New York Heart Association, 1994).

Ms. Elliott has Class II HF (mild). People in Class II HF experience some fatigue, palpitations, or dyspnea with routine activity. Ms. Elliott decompensated from her usual state of health when she was unable to take furosemide and Lisinopril for 3 days. The emergency department nurse practitioner ordered a BNP level to help diagnose the cause of the dyspnea. Brain natriuretic peptide (BNP) is a natural diuretic released from the ventricles in response to increased preload. A prospective study of over 1,500 patients admitted to the emergency department with acute dyspnea demonstrated the usefulness of this blood test in arriving at a differential diagnosis of decompensated HF versus other causes of dyspnea. A BNP level below 50 pg/mL indicates no HF decompensation, while a level above 100 pg/mL is indicative of decompensation. BNP test results have been shown to be more accurate in diagnosing decompensated HF than physical exam or other lab values (Maisel et al., 2002).

HF is a clinical syndrome that may be caused by structural abnormalities such as mitral valve stenosis or a functional abnormality such as HTN. Both types of abnormalities prevent the ventricle(s) from filling with, and ejecting, blood in a normal pattern. Patients with HF present with dyspnea, fatigue, exercise intolerance, and fluid retention. This syndrome can negatively affect the patient's QOL and self-care ability. Patients cannot revert to a less serious class of HF, but with pharmacological and nonpharmacological interventions, their HF can be stabilized. When HF signs and symptoms worsen, it is termed decompensation. That is what happened when Ms. Elliott went without furosemide and Lisinopril for 3 days.

The nurse practitioner opted to send Ms. Elliott to a rehabilitation facility after her hospital stay in order to assure close monitoring, reconditioning, and education about HF. In 1995, the U.S. Department of Health and Human Services, Agency for Healthcare Policy and Research (AHCPR), and the NHLBI developed clinical practice guidelines for cardiac rehabilitation. These guidelines stressed a holistic, interdisciplinary cardiac health promotion approach including assessment, reduction of cardiac disease risk factors, and education. Approximately 25% of all patients over the age of 65 who are admitted to the hospital with HF will be readmitted for the same reason within 30 days of discharge (Krumholtz et al., 2009), 30% are readmitted within 60 to 90 days of discharge, and 50% are readmitted within 6 months of discharge (Desai & Stephenson, 2012). Use of a comprehensive education and discharge plan focused on disease management can reduce readmission rates and improve QOL survey scores (Krumholtz et al., 2009; Phillips et al., 2004). Research has demonstrated the vital role that cardiac rehabilitation plays in follow-up health care for women, elders, and those with HF (Wenger, 2008).

The importance of interdisciplinary patient-centered care for patients who have HF cannot be overemphasized. It is well known that HF negatively impacts QOL, and research suggests that poorer QOL is related to worse prognosis and survival in those diagnosed with CHF. Multidisciplinary programs have been associated with improved QOL and prognosis (Hoekstra et al., 2013; Hole, Grundtvig, Gullestad, Flonaes, & Westheim, 2010; Lupon et al., 2013). Using an integrated approach to management of patients with HF can lead to improvement in self-care, QOL, reduced mortality, and outcomes (Grady et al., 2000). The Institute of Medicine, based on the *Crossing the Quality Chasm* report, recommends patient-centered care that is evidence-based and promotes continuous improvement in quality of care and safety of patients (IOM, 2001). The report also recommends greater emphasis on teamwork and collaboration as strategies to improve the health care experience, avoid errors, and improve outcomes.

The American Geriatrics Society has called for improving the quality of transitional care for persons with complex care needs. It defines transitional care as "a defined set of actions designed to ensure coordination and continuity of health care as patients transfer between different locations or different levels of care within the same location" (Coleman, Boult, & American Geriatrics Society, 2003). It further states that "transitional care is based on a comprehensive plan of care and the availability of health care providers who are well-trained in chronic care and have current information about the patient's goals, preferences, and clinical status" and that such care "encompasses both the sending and receiving aspects of the transfers [and] is essential for persons with complex care needs" (Coleman et al., 2003). Coleman and colleagues (2006) demonstrated that care transitions reduced costs and were effective in reducing the likelihood of rehospitalization for 3 months post discharge.

Role and Cultural Considerations

In planning to discharge Ms. Elliott to cardiac rehabilitation it was important for the hospital team and the rehabilitation team to communicate regarding the precipitating factor(s) that led to the hospitalization as well as a summary of the care provided during the hospitalization. Identifying established goals for rehabilitation and ongoing management of HF was also important to discuss. Including Ms. Elliott in the discharge planning and establishment of goals was important so that patient preferences could be considered, thus alleviating some of the anxiety that she had regarding going to cardiac rehabilitation. Finally, at all steps along the way, the primary care physician and/or specialty physician(s) in the community was kept apprised of the status and treatment of Ms. Elliott. All too often, lack of communication between multiple providers leads to fragmented care, and that may result in preventable consequences experienced by patients as well as lower patient satisfaction. After a 4-day stay in the hospital, Ms. Elliott was discharged to Sunnyvale.

Ms. Elliott told the nurse at Sunnyvale that she did not understand why she needed to go to physical therapy so often. "Exercise can make you lose weight, and I am not heavy," she commented. The nurse explained that exercise has many benefits, including lowering her blood pressure and increasing her activity tolerance. "There is so much to learn about. How will I remember everything you have taught me?" Sunnyvale health care professionals use the teach-back method for patient education and the shared-decision model to guide their practice. The teach-back method of health care provider–patient communication has been shown to improve the effectiveness of information recall by patients (White, Garbez, Carroll, Brinker, & Howie-Esquivel, 2013). Guiding principles of the teach-back method include a caring demeanor including body language, eye contact, and tone of voice; use of plain language rather than medical jargon; posing open-ended questions (rather than "yes" or "no" questions) that prompt the patient to explain concepts in his or her own words; recognition that the responsibility for providing clear instructions is that of the health care provider; assessing the accuracy of patient responses and reteaching when necessary; supplementing verbal explanations with appropriate print material; and documenting the teaching sessions and patient responses (Xu, 2012).

Ms. Elliott benefitted from the teach-back method during her stay at Sunnyvale. When she was admitted to Sunnyvale, she believed that she was eating properly because she ate calorie-controlled frozen meals and did not realize the importance of adhering to her medication plan. After several diet teaching sessions, she was able to state the importance of fresh rather than frozen meals and the impact that salt had on fluid retention. She could also cite the reason for taking the prescribed diuretic and antihypertensive daily.

Using the shared-decision model, the staff at Sunnyvale helped Ms. Elliott develop a contingency plan for making sure that she did not run out of her medications or healthy meal choices. The shared-decision model stresses empowering patients to express their views and engage in critical thinking that leads to health care decisions geared toward their preferences (Elwyn et al., 2012; Hyde & Kautz, 2014). The dietitian at Sunnyvale listed a number of options for meal planning that would provide heart-healthy meal choices. After exploring the benefits and drawbacks for each choice, Ms. Elliott selected "Meals on Wheels" as the most viable option as she stressed that cooking for one was "no fun" and was the reason she used frozen meals. The registered nurse helped Ms. Elliott explore several ways of ensuring that she did not run out of medication such as purchasing the medications through a mail order pharmacy. When her neighbor visited her, she gave Ms. Elliott the name of a pharmacy that delivered medications to the condominium, and that was the option she selected.

After 3 weeks at Sunnyvale, she was discharged to home with a referral for home care. She was very happy to return home and see Tabby. Pet cats have been shown to reduce stress and lower the risk of fatal cardiovascular disease (Qureshi, Memon, Vasquez, & Suri, 2009), and are an important component of a high QOL for many elders, including Ms. Elliott.

The day after Ms. Elliott was discharged from Sunnyvale, a home care nurse from the Sun Valley Home Care Agency contacted her to schedule a home visit and admit her for home care services. In planning for the home visit, the nurse confirmed that Ms. Elliott had Medicare but no other insurance. After explaining the purpose of home care, the nurse asked a few questions about Ms. Elliott's status. The nurse determined that Ms. Elliott, despite her recent hospitalization, was no longer homebound and therefore ineligible for Medicare-covered home care services. Privately paying for service was not an affordable option for Ms. Elliott.

Patients who have HF are faced with a tremendous burden of self-managing their disease. They are required to safely manage multiple medications, adhere to complex medication regimens, adhere to dietary modifications, establish and maintain a healthy weight, remain active, and, in some cases, restrict fluid intake. These patients must recognize the symptoms of HF, which may sometimes be subtle; and changes in their heart rate, blood pressure, and respirations. Frequent follow-up with a health care provider may also be a challenge, depending on ability to drive or obtain transportation to medical appointments. The ability for patients to successfully manage their HF is influenced by the severity of the disease, the complexity of the plan of care, psychosocial support, and socioeconomic status. These factors also impact the ability to adhere to medications, to self-monitor, and follow-up appropriately (Reigel et al., 2009). HF patients are fragile; in some cases, gaining just 1 to 2 lbs. of fluid results in an acute exacerbation and hospitalization.

Prior to admission to the hospital, Ms. Elliott had missed medications, which led to an exacerbation of her HF.

Without any discharge follow-up, she was at risk for being re-hospitalized. Recognizing this, the nurse determined that Ms. Elliott was eligible for the Agency's care transitions program (Coleman et al., 2004; Parry, Coleman, Smith, Frank, & Kramer, 2003), a program that uses adult learning principles and focuses on education and support to promote self-management for patients with complex health conditions; this is provided free to eligible patients. The home care nurse notified the primary and specialty care providers and made the referral to the care transitions program.

According to Coleman et al. (2004), the term "care transitions" refers to "the movement patients make between health care practitioners and settings as their condition and care needs change during the course of a chronic or acute illness." Over a period of 4 weeks, patients and family members are provided with tools to help them reach or improve self-management, and a "transitions coach" from whom they will learn self-management skills that will ensure their needs are met during the transition from hospital to home. Typically, patients have one hospital visit, followed by one home visit and three follow-up phone calls. The interventions within the model focus on medication self-management, patient-centered personal health record, timely primary care/specialty care follow-up, and knowledge of red flags that indicate a worsening in their condition and how to respond.

The "teaching coach" (who is a nurse) at the care transitions program contacted Ms. Elliott that same day and explained the purpose of the program. Although a hospital visit was not made, the nurse believed Ms. Elliott would benefit from the program. The patient was receptive, and a home visit was scheduled for the next day. Before ending the call, the nurse discussed the importance of knowing medications and having a system for taking them in place. Ms. Elliott indicated that she did not have any further questions for today.

Assessment and Strategies

The nurse arrived to find Ms. Elliott sitting at her table with several bottles of medications. The goal for medication self-management is that the patient is "knowledgeable about medications and has a medication management system" (Coleman et al., 2004). Ms. Elliott informed the nurse prior to going into the hospital that she had been more forgetful and had missed 3 days of taking her medication. She also reported that she did not have a system in place, but just took her medication as scheduled. With the support of the nurse, Ms. Elliott decided that she would prefill her medications each week on Sunday morning. After reconciling the medications list with the medications in the home and confirming the medications with the physician, the nurse explained and demonstrated how to safely prepour the medications into a 7-day medication box. She also had Ms. Elliott write out a medication record and schedule along with side effects and purpose of the medications. Finally, they arranged for Ms. Elliott's daughter to double-check her medication boxes for accuracy the following week. Another goal for the program is to create a personal health record that the patient "understands and uses to facilitate communication and continuity of care plans across providers and settings" (Coleman et al., 2004). The nurse explained the purpose of the personal health record and reviewed the importance of keeping it updated and sharing it with her health care providers. Ms. Elliott was very pleased with the idea of the personal health record; she has had difficulty keeping track of "everything." The goal for follow-up is that the patient "schedules and completes follow-up visits with the primary care provider and/or specialist and is empowered to be an active participant in these interactions." During the home visit, the nurse explains the importance of follow-up visits with the primary care physician, especially in light of the recent hospitalization. She asks Mrs. Elliott to think of questions that she might want to ask at her appointment. They discuss the importance of asking questions and being sure to understand the responses from the health care provider. The final "pillar" of the intervention activities consists of "red flags" (Coleman et al., 2004), the goal of which is to ensure that the "patient is knowledgeable about indications that the condition is worsening and how to respond" (p. 1819). Although the patient has had some instruction in the past, it is important to reinstruct and assess the patient's knowledge and understanding of symptoms and drug reactions. The nurse has already reviewed the side effects of medications, and Ms. Elliott is now able to state them correctly. The nurse reminds the patient that there are also some uncommon side effects to medications and that Ms. Elliott should always consider this if she experiences something new or different. Finally, the nurse assesses Ms. Elliott's cardiorespiratory status to be stable: BP 128/72; apical heart rate 68 regular rate and rhythm; RR 18; lungs clear; no SOB/DOE or edema. The nurse reviews signs and symptoms and the need for prompt follow-up if changes in her status should occur. She instructs Ms. Elliott to monitor her weight daily and report gain of 2 lbs. or more to the physician. She also suggests that Ms. Elliott purchase a portable blood pressure machine so that she can monitor her blood pressure and pulse. The visit is finished and Ms. Elliott has no further questions. They determine a mutually agreeable time for the coaching calls.

Over the next 3 weeks, the nurse placed the follow-up calls as scheduled. During each phone call, Ms. Elliott was asked about her symptoms, medications, and any possible side effects. She is also given the opportunity to ask questions. The nurse reminded her to schedule follow-up appointments and to share her personal health record with her health care providers, and reinforced the importance of a low sodium diet, the need to watch for symptoms of worsening HF, and the consequent actions to take. During the first coaching phone call, Ms. Elliott reported that her weight was stable, she was taking her medications appropriately, and she was generally feeling well. She had gone out to lunch with friends and made a visit to the library and said that she had an appointment with her health care provider the next day. The nurse reminded her to take her personal health record with her and to record any new information. The following week, Ms. Elliott reported that her weight was up 2 lbs. but that she did not have shortness of breath. "Nothing else is different. I am taking my medication," she said. "I saw the doctor last week and everything was fine. He said I was doing great! I even remembered my personal health record." After further inquiry, the nurse learned that Ms. Elliott had attended a small party at a Chinese restaurant the day before. The nurse explained that Chinese food, although it does not taste salty, does in fact have a significant amount of salt in it. Ms. Elliott stated, "I did not know that; I am so glad that you told me! I will avoid Chinese food." The next week, when the nurse called Ms. Elliott for her last follow-up, everything was going well. Ms. Elliott had been correctly prepouring her medications, adhering to her medication regimen, and doing well overall. She reported that she was being careful to avoid foods high in salt and that she was walking at the mall with a friend a few times a week. She had also scheduled her next doctor's appointment and arranged for her daughter to accompany her. Through their conversation, the nurse learned that Ms. Elliott was feeling more confident in her abilities to manage her HF and now better understood not only how to manage her HF but also how to recognize early symptoms of worsening HF and the actions to take.

Clinical Reasoning Questions

1. What additional treatment plan topics would you plan to discuss with Ms. Elliott? How will you implement the teach-back method during these discussions?
2. What decisions may need to be made by Ms. Elliott concerning her treatment plan now that she is home?
3. What do you anticipate will be the most challenging self-management strategies for Ms. Elliott over the next 6 months?
4. Develop a short case study in which you apply the transitions care model to an elderly patient who has COPD.

References

Coleman, E. A., & Boult, C. & American Geriatrics Society. (2003). Improving the quality of transitional care for persons with complex care needs. *Journal of the American Geriatrics Society, 51*(4), 556–557.

Coleman, E. A., Parry, C., Chalmers, S., & Sung-joon, M. (2006, September 25). The care transitions intervention: Results of a randomized controlled trial. *Archives of Internal Medicine, 166*(17), 1822–1888.

Coleman, E. A., Smith, J. D., Frank, J. C., Min, S. J., Parry, C., & Kramer, M. (2004). Preparing patients and caregivers to participate in care delivered across settings: The care transitions intervention. *Journal of the American Geriatrics Society, 52*, 1817–1825.

The Criteria Committee of the New York Heart Association. (1994). Nomenclature and Criteria for Diagnosis of Diseases of the Heart and Great Vessels (9th ed., pp. 253–256). Boston, MA: Little, Brown & Co.

Desai, A. S., & Stevenson, L. W. (2012). Rehospitalization for heart failure: Predict or prevent. *Circulation, 126*, 501–506. doi:10.1161/circulationaha.112.125435

Elwyn, G., Frosch, D., Thompson, R., Joseph-Williams, N., Lloyd, A., Kinnersley, P., . . . Barry, M. (2012). Shared decision making: A model for clinical practice. *Journal of General Internal Medicine, 27*(10), 1361–1367. doi:10.1007/s11606-012-2077-6

Go, A. S., Mozaffarian, D., Roger, V. L., Benjamin, E. J., Berry, J. D., Borden, W. B. . . . . Turner, M. B. (2013). Heart disease and stroke statistic—2013 update: A report from the American Heart Association. *Circulation, 127*(1), e6–e245. doi:10.1161/CIR.0b013e31828124ad

Grady, K. L., Dracup, K., Kennedy, G., Moser, D. K., Piano, M., Stevenson, W., & Young, J. B. (2000). Team management of patients with heart failure: A statement for the healthcare professionals from the Cardiovascular Nursing Council of the American Heart Association. *Circulation, 102*, 2443–2456. doi:10.1161/01.CIR.102.19.2443

Hoekstra, T., Jaarsma, T., van Veldhuisen, D. J., Hillege, H. L., Sanderman, R., & Lesman-Leegte, I. (2013). Quality of life and survival in patients with heart failure. *European Journal of Heart Failure, 15*(1), 94–102. doi:10.1093/eurjhf/hfs14

Hole, T., Grundtvig, M., Gullestad, L., Flonaes, B., & Westheim, A. (2010). Improved quality of life in Norwegian heart failure patients after follow-up in outpatient heart failure clinics. *European Journal of Heart Failure, 12*, 1247–1252. doi:10.1093/eurjhf/hfq156

Hyde, Y. M., & Kautz, D. D. (2014). Enhancing health promotion during rehabilitation through information-giving, partnership-building, and teach-back. *Journal of Rehabilitation Nursing, 39*(4), 178–182. doi:10.1002/rnj.124

Institute of Medicine. (2001). *Crossing the quality chasm: A new health system for the 21st century.* Washington, DC: The National Academies Press.

Krumholtz, H. M., Merrill, A. R., Schone, E. M., Schreiner, G. C., Chen, J., Bradley, E. H., . . . Drye, E. E. (2009). Patterns of hospital performance in acute myocardial infarction and heart failure 30-day mortality and readmission. *Circulation: Cardiovascular Quality and Outcomes, 2*(5), 407–413. doi:10.1161/CIRCOUTCOMES.109.883256

Lupon, J., Gastelurrutia, P., de Antonio, M., Gonzalez, B., Cano, L., Cabanes, R., . . . Bayes-Genis, A. (2013). Quality of life monitoring in ambulatory heart failure patients: Temporal changes and prognostic value. *European Journal of Heart Failure, 15*(1), 103–109. doi:10.1093/eurjhf/hfs133

Maisel, A. S., Krishnaswamy, P., Nowak, R. M., McCord, J., Hollander, J. E., Duc, P., . . . McCullough, P. A. (2002). Rapid measurement of B-type natriuretic peptide in the emergency diagnosis of heart failure. *New England Journal of Medicine, 347*, 161–167.

Page, A. (Ed.). (2004). *Keeping patients safe: Transforming the work environment for nurses.* Washington, DC: The National Academies Press. Retrieved from http://www.nap.edu/catalog/10851.html

Parry, C., Coleman, E. A., Smith, J. D., Frank, J., & Kramer, A. M. (2003). The care transitions intervention: A patient-centered approach to ensuring effective transfers between sites of geriatric care. *Home Health Care Services Quarterly, 22*(3), 1–17. doi:10.1300/J027v22n03_01

Phillips, C. O., Wright, S. M., Kern, D. E., Singa, R. M., Shepperd, S., & Rubin, H. R. (2004). Comprehensive discharge planning with postdischarge support for older patients with congestive heart failure: A meta-analysis. *JAMA, 291*(11), 1358–1367. doi:10.1001/jama.291.11.1358

Qureshi, A. I., Memon, M. Z., Vazquez, G., & Suri, M. F. (2009, January). Cat ownership and the risk of fatal cardiovascular diseases. Results from the Second National Health and Nutrition Examination Study Mortality Follow-up Study. *Journal of Vascular Interventional Neurology, 2*(1), 132–135.

Reigel, B., Moser, B. K., Anker, S. D., Appel, L. J., Dunbar, S. B., Grady, K. L., . . . Whellan, D. J. (2009). State of the science. Promoting self-care in persons with heart failure: A scientific statement from the American Heart Association. *Circulation, 120*, 1141–1163. doi:10.1161/CIRCULATIONAHA.109.192628

Wenger, N. K. (2008). Current status of cardiac rehabilitation. *Journal of the American College of Cardiology, 51*(17), 1619–1631.

White, M., Garbez, R., Carroll, M., Brinker, E., & Howie-Esquivel, J. (2013, March–April). Is "teach-back" associated with knowledge retention and hospital readmission in hospitalized heart failure patients? *Journal of Cardiovascular Nursing, 28*(2), 137–146.

Xu, P. (2012, March). Using teach-back for patient education and self-management. *American Nurse Today, 7*(3). Retrieved from http://www.americannursetoday.com/Article.aspx?id=8848&fid=8812#

32 PROSTATE CANCER

MEREDITH WALLACE KAZER

Subjective

"My dad had prostate—died of the stuff. Now they think I might have it, too."

Objective

Mr. Frederick F. Fixer is a 69-year-old African American who lives at home with his wife, Donna. He has returned to the urology clinic today for his 6-month check-up and prostate-specific antigen (PSA) reading. Preceding this, Mr. Fixer had been seen every 6 months at the clinic for a gradually rising PSA level. When he first started at the clinic 4 years ago, his PSA was 4.4 ng/dL. Last month, it was 10.2 ng/dL.

Upon physical examination, Mr. Fixer is alert and oriented and ambulates independently. He is 69 in. (175 cm) tall, and weighs 185 lbs. (84 kg). His blood pressure is 128/82; his pulse is 84, and respirations are 16/minute. He is febrile with a temperature of 97.7°F. His oxygen saturation is 98%. His lungs are clear bilaterally with good symmetrical expansion, and there are no adventitious sounds noted. He has a regular heart rate; S1, S2 sounds are regular, with no adventitious sounds noted. His abdomen is soft, nontender, and his bowel sounds are present in all four quadrants. His skin is warm, dry, thin, and intact; his eye examination reveals clear sclera bilaterally and pupils equal, round, reactive to light and accommodation (PERRLA). His ear examination reveals normal tympanic membranes. His oral examination reveals normal moist, pink mucosa with adequate dentition. His neurological exam reveals 2+ deep tendon reflexes bilaterally and equal strength bilaterally. He has diminished sensation in his lower extremities upon microfilament testing. His current medications include Lisinopril 20 mg po daily, Crestor 10 mg po daily, and metformin 500 mg po twice daily.

In following up with the patient's chief complaint, Abigail, the nurse practitioner, questioned Mr. Fixer further on his concerns about prostate cancer. Mr. Fixer replied that his father had been diagnosed with the disease in his fifties after it spread to his bones. He died within a year of diagnosis, and Mr. Fixer is very fearful that the same thing will happen to him. He continues to question why he "just doesn't have the thing out, if they think it is cancer." He states that he would feel much better knowing it was gone. He does not know what the prostate does, but it does not seem to bother him, and he feels he would be better off without it.

Abigail assured Mr. Fixer that he was doing the right thing in coming to the urology clinic every 6 months. She explained that his father was probably diagnosed late, when the disease had already spread, which is why he passed away so quickly after diagnosis. She assured him that they examined him each month for the spread of the disease. Abigail explained that regular diagnostic testing was the best way to catch the disease at an early stage. She also explained that treatment has many adverse effects, including erectile dysfunction (ED) and may also result in urinary and bowel issues. However, at this point, his PSA had risen to the point that they should test him further and consider whether it was time to implement treatment. Mr. Fixer agreed that avoiding these adverse treatment effects was important and that he would continue to comply with visits and diagnostic testing at the clinic as directed.

Literature Review

Prostate cancer was the second most common cancer in adult American males in the year 2013 (American Cancer Society, 2014a), exceeded only by the incidence of skin cancer. It is also the second leading cause of death from cancer in men in the United States, surpassed only by lung cancer. In the United Kingdom, it is estimated that 36,000 men are newly diagnosed with prostate cancer each year (Lynch & Burgess,

2011). Prostate cancer is the sixth most common cancer in the world, with an estimated 238,590 new cases reported in 2013 (American Cancer Society, 2014a). Prior to the 1980s, prostate cancer was usually detected in the late stages, ensuing in impending death. However, the development and widespread use of the PSA has allowed clinicians to inexpensively and readily screen for prostate cancer, leading to a doubling of the incidence of prostate cancer between 1984 and 1994 (Parkin, Pisani, & Ferlay, 1999). This number has now stabilized in the United States. However, Casey et al. (2012) estimate that prostate cancer diagnoses will increase by 275% by 2025 in some European countries. Currently, about 1 out of every 6 men will be diagnosed with prostate cancer in his lifetime. Most prostate cancers are diagnosed in older men with an average age of diagnosis at 67 years (American Cancer Society, 2014a).

Given the prevalence of prostate cancer, especially among an increasingly aging population, it is imperative for nurse clinicians to cultivate a rich understanding of this disease and treatment options to ensure that patients do not experience unnecessary morbidity and mortality. Nurse clinicians assume a central role in recognizing men at high risk for the disease and diagnosing prostate cancer sufficiently early to ensure treatment effectiveness. African American men, such as Mr. Fixer, are at the highest risk for prostate cancer. In fact, nonmodifiable risk factors for developing prostate cancer include increased age, African American and Jamaican ethnicity, nationality, and family history of first-degree relatives with the disease. More recently, a genetic link to prostate cancer, including specific inherited mutations in the *BRCA1* or *BRCA2* genes, has undergone investigation in relation to the development of prostate cancer (American Cancer Society, 2014b).

In addition to these nonmodifiable risk factors, a number of lifestyle factors have been shown to play a role in the development of prostate cancer. Diets high in red meat and high-fat dairy products, obesity, and smoking are among the top high-risk health behaviors linked to prostate cancer. In addition, workplace exposure; history of prolonged inflammation of the prostate; sexually transmitted diseases, such as gonorrhea or Chlamydia; and men who had undergone an early age vasectomy younger than 35 may also be at increased risk for prostate

TABLE 32.1: Prostate Cancer Prevention Checklist for Men

Risk Factors	Risk Reduction	Early Detection
Over the age of 50 African American Diagnosis of patient's father, brother, or son before the age of 65 Diet high in red meat and high-fat dairy Overweight	Increase fruit, vegetable, and whole-grain diet Lower intake of red meat and high-fat processed meats Reach or maintain a healthy weight Be active Discuss pharmaceutical options to reduce cancer risk with doctor	Communicate with your doctor about the risks and benefits of prostate cancer testing Men of average risk should begin communication with their doctor at the age of 50. Men of high risk should begin communication at the age of 45 Men with at least one close relative with prostate cancer should discuss screening with their doctor at the age of 40 A prostate-specific antigen (PSA) blood test should be part of your screening. Doctors may also perform a digital rectal exam (DRE)

Adapted from the American Cancer Society (2014c).

cancer (American Cancer Society, 2014b). For full prostate cancer screening guidelines, see Table 32.1.

As in the case with Mr. Fixer, early stage prostate cancer often presents asymptomatically. In advanced prostate cancer, signs of disease specifically center on symptoms of bladder outlet obstruction and urethral obstruction with possible anuria, azotemia, uremia, anemia, and anorexia. In light of what is known about the rising incidence and risk factors for prostate cancer, the American Cancer Society recommends that all men over the age of 50 discuss screening for prostate cancer with their primary care provider (American Cancer Society, 2014c). Men at high risk, such as those who have had relatives who died from the disease, as well as African American men, should consider discussing screening with primary care providers at age 40 to 45. In addition, men who present with urinary symptoms should undergo a full physical examination and diagnostic assessment for the possibility of prostate cancer. This may include a digital rectal examination (DRE), magnetic resonance imaging (MRI), and possibly a transrectal ultrasound guided (TRUS) biopsy of the suspicious tissue, which is necessary for histological or cytological diagnosis of prostate cancer.

The prostate specific antigen (PSA) is a well-known serum marker for unusual prostate activity, as it detects both benign and malignant prostate disease. Caplan and Kratz (2002) first reported that a PSA cutoff value of 4.0 ng/mL provided the best specificity and sensitivity for prostate cancer. Since that time, more research has specified PSA values by age group. Lynch and Burgess reported age-specific PSA ranges as follows: Age 50–59, PSA 0.0–3.0; Age 60–69, PSA 0.0–4.0; Age 70–79, PSA 0.0–5.0. A more recent study by Casey et al. (2012) aimed at determining PSA cutoff values in different age groups in a sample of 660 healthy male patients without prostate cancer in Ireland. The results revealed a PSA velocity of 0.024 ng/mL/year with a near flat line of PSA values from age 20 to 50. After the age of 50, PSA median and 95th percentile for PSA values were reported as follows: 30–34 (0.73, 1.57), 35–39 (0.71, 1.65), 40–44 (0.73, 1.85), 45–49 (0.78, 2.17), 50–54 (0.88, 2.63), 55–59 (1.01, 3.25), 60–64 (1.20, 4.02), and 64–70 (1.43, 4.96). The authors concluded that PSA of the Irish men in the study was similar to that of other racial populations but not as high as Caucasians in the United States until the age of 65.

While drawing PSA levels is always recommended in men following a positive DRE, it is important to note that the availability of this inexpensive screening blood test has been thought to lead to overdiagnosis of the disease. This finding is increasingly controversial given that prostate tumors grow slowly, and detecting subclinical tumors often results in the initiation of treatment in the absence of clinically significant prostate cancer. Consequently, the U.S. Preventive Services Task Force (2008) recommended that men over the age of 75 years consider going without PSA screening.

If a diagnosis of prostate cancer is made, there are a variety of treatment options available to men in the early stages of the disease, such as Mr. Fixer, including active surveillance, surgery, and radiation. In later stage prostate cancer, hormonal therapy may also be an option. While the substantial treatment options for prostate cancer have reduced morbidity and mortality related to the disease, a great deal of confusion remains in selecting the most appropriate treatment for individual patients. While efforts have been made in the past to develop consensus around treatment decision making through the Prostate Outcomes Research Team (PORT) (Fleming, Wasson, Albertsen,

Barry, & Wennberg, 1993) and other similar groups, no universally accepted consensus treatment guidelines are available.

An active surveillance (AS) approach to the management of prostate cancer involves a system of watching for PSA and tumor progression, delaying treatment until necessary. Alonzo, Mure, and Soloway (2013) define AS "as a method to potentially delay or obviate the need for treatment in men with clinically insignificant PC or PC thought to be at low risk for progression" (p. 109). It is often a recommended management strategy for men over the age of 70, with less than a 10-year predicted survival, low-grade tumors, and no prostate cancer symptoms. The AS approach is not consistently popular with men and their families, as there is the perception that they are "doing nothing" to treat the disease. However, comparative research results reveal no significant differences in outcomes among those with low-risk PC who delay treatment within the AS approach (Alonzo et al., 2013). In addition, there are numerous benefits to AS, such as eliminating the risk of adverse treatment effects and opportunities to take advantage of continually developing state-of-the-art therapies as they develop in the future.

Two other treatments for men with localized prostate cancer, such as Mr. Fixer, include radical prostatectomy (RP) and radiation. RP is often recommended for men younger than 70 with organ-confined disease and a greater than 10-year survival. RP is a broad term that is used to describe several different procedures, including retropubic prostatectomy, perineal prostatectomy, laparoscopic prostatectomy, and robotic prostatectomy—all aimed at removing the prostate gland. This type of treatment may be delivered through external beam radiation in daily doses over a 7- to 8-week period, or through seed implantation. Internal radiation seed placement, also known as brachytherapy, refers to the placement of radioactive sources into the prostate. RP and radiation treatments for prostate cancer are considered curative. However, both treatments carry a high risk of ED and urinary symptoms (Mirza, Griebling, & Kazer, 2011). A final treatment option for men with localized prostate cancer is cryosurgery. The American Urological Association (AUA) reports that primary cryosurgery is appropriate for men with clinically organ-confined, nonmetastatic prostate cancer, regardless of grade, and salvage cryosurgery is reasonable in patients who have failed radiation therapy (AUA, 2007). This treatment works by freezing and destroying prostate tissue. Long-term results are still forthcoming on the effectiveness of this procedure for curing prostate cancer. However, as a minimally painful procedure that may be done as day surgery, cryosurgery is a promising alternative to traditional surgical and radiation procedures.

While not necessary for Mr. Fixer, treatment options for metastatic prostate cancer include androgen deprivation therapy (ADT) with luteinizing hormone releasing hormone (LHRH) agonists, also known as gonadotropin-releasing hormone (GnRH) antagonists (Turner & Drudge-Coates, 2014). These treatments are usually delivered intramuscularly every 1 to 4 months. Adverse effects include pain and swelling at injection site, hot flashes and loss of libido, impotence, gynecomastia, nocturia, and urinary frequency. Long-term effects may also include decreased bone mineral density and anemia.

Role and Cultural Considerations

The many treatment choices for localized prostate cancer and the lack of consensus regarding the efficacy of one treatment over the other leaves patients such as Mr. Fixer with a great amount of ambiguity and uncertainty. To assist in the decision-making process, nurses and advanced practice clinicians play a role in educating prostate cancer patients and their families regarding the disease, as well as the risks and the benefits of each treatment option. Nurses may use pictures and diagrams of the prostate gland and surrounding structures to help enhance understanding about the possible impact of the disease and treatment. Patient and family perception of the prostate cancer may be influenced by past history with cancer, fears about treatment, cultural and educational backgrounds, and literacy and language abilities (Wallace, Bailey, & Brion, 2009). As a result, anxiety and misunderstanding about the disease and treatment must be assessed and managed through the development of strong communication and education.

The risk of ED and urinary incontinence (UI) are elevated with most prostate cancer management approaches. Thus, it is critical that patients become knowledgeable about these risks prior to commencing treatment. Additionally, discussion about these adverse treatment effects should be reinitiated after treatment completion to determine the presence of continuing adverse treatment effects. Cultural norms and values must be considered in addressing sensitive topics, such as ED and UI, as patients may be embarrassed and ascribe the effect to another cause or to personal failure. In the case of Mr. Fixer, it is important to discuss the impact of these potential adverse effects on his relationship with his wife.

Research has supported the use of oral erectile agents (phosphodiesterase type 5 [PDE5] inhibitors) to manage ED following RP (Miles et al., 2007). In addition, intracorporeal injection therapy and vacuum erection devices are also available to assist men to achieve erections following prostate cancer treatment. Men are not always comfortable initiating the discussion of ED and thus should be assessed to determine its presence and impact on quality of life. UI is estimated to occur in 5% to 60% of men undergoing RP (Hunskaar et al., 2002), and slightly less among men undergoing radiotherapy. UI may begin immediately after treatment for prostate cancer and extend for several months after treatment. Patients should be assessed for the presence of UI and counseled to use a bladder diary to document the frequency of UI incidents. Oral anticholinergic medications and voiding schedules may be helpful in regaining urinary continence. Kegel exercises may also be taught to improve continence. In addition, nurses should direct patients and families to supportive educational and other support services such as the American Cancer Society and local hospital groups.

Solutions and Strategies

In order to treat Mr. Fixer, the nurse practitioner will implement the following plan:

1. Progressing prostate cancer
   - Schedule Mr. Fixer for follow-up PSA testing
   - Conduct digital rectal examination
   - Refer to urologist for ultrasound-guided biopsy of prostate gland

2. Prostate cancer treatment decision making
   - Provide teaching regarding prostate cancer treatments
   - Provide teaching regarding adverse effects
   - Encourage communication between the patient and his family
   - Refer to credible evidence-based resources and support networks
   - Encourage healthy lifestyle habits throughout decision-making process
3. Erectile dysfunction secondary to prostate cancer treatment
   - Encourage continued sexual health and activity, assuring patient of the safety and health benefits of a good sex life
   - Encourage good communication with partner
   - Consider prescription for oral erectile agent or other erectile devices as needed
4. Urinary incontinence secondary to prostate cancer treatment
   - Encourage patient to keep a bladder diary
   - Provide teaching regarding Kegel exercises
   - Consider prescription for anticholinergic, if appropriate

Clinical Reasoning Questions

1. What is your plan for follow-up care of Mr. Fixer?
2. Are any referrals needed in this case? If so, to whom?
3. What if Mr. Fixer became depressed upon diagnosis?
4. Are there any standardized guidelines that could be used to assess or treat Mr. Fixer?

References

Alonzo, D. G., Mure, A. L., & Soloway, M. S. (2013). Prostate cancer and the increasing role of active surveillance. *Postgraduate Medicine, 125*(5), 109–116.

American Cancer Society. (2014a). *What are the key statistics about prostate cancer*. Retrieved from http://www.cancer.org/cancer/prostatecancer/detailedguide/prostate-cancer-key-statistics

American Cancer Society. (2014b). *Prostate cancer risk factors*. Retrieved from http://www.cancer.org/cancer/prostatecancer/detailed guide/prostate-cancer-risk-factors

American Cancer Society. (2014c). *Prevention checklist for men*. Retrieved from http://www.cancer.org/acsgroups/content/@nho/documents/webcontent/acsq-009104.pdf

American Urological Association. (2007). *Best practice policy statement on cryosurgery for the treatment of localized prostate cancer*. Retrieved from http://www.auanet.org/education/guidelines/cryosurgery.cfm

Caplan, A., & Kratz, A. (2002). Prostate-specific antigen and early diagnosis of prostate cancer. *American Journal of Clinical Pathology, 117* (Suppl.) S104–S108.

Casey, R. G., Hegarty, P. K., Conroy, R., Rea, D., Butler, M. R., Grainger, R., . . . Thornhill, J. A. (2012). The distribution of PSA age-specific profiles in healthy Irish men between 20 and 70. *ISRN Oncology, 2012,* 832109.

Fleming, C., Wasson, J. H. Albertsen, P. C., Barry, M. J., & Wennberg, J. E. (1993). A decision analysis of alternative treatment strategies for clinically localized prostate cancer. Prostate Patient Outcomes Research Team. *JAMA, 269,* 2650–2658.

Hunskaar, S., Burgio, K., Diokno, A. C., Herzog, A. R., Hjalmas, K., Lapitan, M. C. (2002). Epidemiology and natural history of urinary incontinence. In P.C. Abrams, S. Khoury, & A. Wein (Eds.), *Incontinence: 2nd international consultation on incontinence* (pp. 165–200). Plymouth, UK: Health Publication.

Lynch, T., & Burgess, M. (2011). Prostate specific antigen test: An informed choice. *Primary Health Care, 21*(3), 16–21.

Miles, C. L., Candy, B., Jones, L., Williams, R., Tookman, A., King, M. (2007). Interventions for sexual dysfunction following treatments for cancer. *Cochrane Database of Systematic Reviews, 2007*(4), 005540.

Mirza, M., Griebling, T. L., & Kazer, M. W. (2011). Erectile dysfunction and urinary incontinence after prostate cancer treatment. *Seminars in Oncology Nursing, 27,* 278–289.

Parkin, D. M., Pisani, P., & Ferlay, J. (1999). Global cancer statistics. *CA: A Cancer Journal for Clinicians, 49*(1), 33–64.

Turner, B., & Drudge-Coates, L. (2014). Pharmacological treatment of patients with advanced prostate cancer. *Nursing Standard, 28*(23), 44–48.

U.S. Preventive Services Task Force. (2008). Screening for prostate cancer: U.S. Preventive Services Task Force recommendation statement. *Annals of Internal Medicine, 149*(3), 185–191.

Wallace, M., Bailey, D. E., & Brion, J. (2009). Prostate cancer update. *Nurse Practitioners Journal, 34*(10), 24–34.

33 PREVENTING TYPE 2 DIABETES

DYMPNA CASEY AND PAULINE MESKELL

Subjective

"I feel fine, really—okay, so I've gained a few pounds in the last year, and my skirt feels a bit tighter on the waist, but my blood pressure is under control, and that's the main thing really isn't it? It's just a nuisance having to come back every 6 months for my repeat prescription. . . .

"I have to go to the GP again next week to get a new prescription—I hate having to go every time. I feel good, but I'm not too happy with the way I look at the moment. I feel a bit frumpy—I knew I had gained a few pounds, but it didn't really bother me until I tried on my favorite skirt yesterday, and it's too tight on me and too uncomfortable to wear. I'm baffled really as I don't eat that much rubbish, just a few chocolate biscuits at night with my tea when I settle down to watch the TV, and of course the odd slice of apple pie that I have with Joan twice a week, but it's all homemade, with the apples direct from Joan's orchard. I have even started to cut down on sweet things since my last visit to the GP. I used to take cream with the apple pie, but now I have ice cream instead, so that has to be better for me. I also now make sure that I get the low fat drinks and yogurts. It's so hard to bother with cooking, especially when you live on your own, as cooking for one is such a chore—it's so much easier to get the readymade meals from the supermarket. No doubt the GP will be telling me that I have to lose weight again and that I must exercise. I have to admit I have become a bit lazy recently when it comes to exercise. It's difficult when you don't have that many friends as I love the social aspect of exercising. I so

loved being a member of the Ballina walking club—we had such fun during the walks, and on the nights away we had such chats and great singsongs. But when I went back after my ankle sprain, two of my best friends had left the club. Anne went to live with her sister in Dublin, and Jane went to live with her daughter in Sliabh Luchra. It wasn't the same for me anymore, the others all had their old friends, but I had no one, so I stopped going. I did try and start going for a walk after work in the evenings, but the weather was cold, and it was rather boring on my own without the company."

Objective

Georgiana G. Garth is a 61-year-old single lady who lives alone; she is attending her GP for a routine blood pressure checkup and repeat prescription for antihypertensive medications as she has been treated for hypertension for the past 10 years. She is currently on Exforge 5/160 mg (OD). She has a family history of hypertension, and her older brother (63) has type 2 diabetes mellitus (T2DM). Georgiana is a librarian in the local town, Ballina, having moved there 4 years ago from Caher (30 miles away) when the library there closed. She had worked in the Caher library for 20 years and was an active member of that community. When she moved to Ballina, she joined the local walking club, but a sprained ankle about 12 months ago curtailed her involvement, and she has never really gone back to the walking club since. She now leads a more sedentary lifestyle and has gained 14 lbs. (6 kg) in the past year. She reports that she does not feel any more fatigued than normal, and there is no evidence of polyuria or polydipsia. Mrs. Garth quit smoking 20 years ago and only takes the occasional glass of red wine when dining out with friends, which she reports is "about once a fortnight at most." At her last visit, her HbA1C (IFCC) was 31 mmol/mol (5.9%), and she was encouraged to lose weight and exercise at least 30 minutes/day. Mrs. Garth reports that she is making an effort and has reduced her intake of sweet things. She says that she tries to go for a walk in the evenings but the inclement weather has hindered her ability to do so. She reports that she "feels fine, no major health problems." Her current HbA1C is 42 mmol/mol (6.4%) (an increase of 11 mmol/mol/5%). Her waist circumference is 90 cms (35.4 in.), BMI 32 kg/m2, and blood pressure 130/80 mmHg. Her HDL cholesterol is low (30 mg/dL), and her triglyceride level is high (185 mg/dL). The LDL was mildly elevated (132 mg/dL), and total cholesterol was 199 mg/dL. Her fasting glucose was elevated at 115 mg/dL. Mrs. Garth scores 24 points on the FINDRISK (Lindstrom & Tuomilehto, 2003) questionnaire, which consists of eight questions used to screen and identify persons at risk of T2DM. This indicates that Georgiana is in a prediabetes stage and at a high risk of developing T2DM.

Literature Review

T2DM accounts for 85% to 95% of all diabetes in high-income countries (International Diabetes Federation [IDF], 2013). Meanwhile, it is predicted that global prevalence will increase from 171 million in 2000 to 366 million by 2030 (WHO, 2004) and the largest group affected will be the 60- to 79-year age group (Bailey, Barner, & Weems, 2012; Ryden et al., 2007; IDF, 2013). International Diabetes Federation (IDF) (2013). International trends in the management of T2DM now focus on identifying persons at high risk of diabetes (Ryden et al., 2007), often classified as "prediabetes." "Prediabetes is where blood sugar levels are higher than normal but not high enough to be classified or diagnosed as diabetes. Persons diagnosed as having prediabetes are at an increased risk of developing type two diabetes mellitus (T2DM). Furthermore, persons classified as having prediabetes are also at increased risk of cardiovascular disease (CVD; Pratley & Matflin, 2007; Ryden et al., 2007). Similar to T2DM, age is a risk factor for the presence of prediabetes (European Diabetes Working Party, 2004; Paulweber et al., 2010). In a review of 7,267 participants in the U.S. National Health and Nutrition survey, Cowie et al. (2009) report a crude total prediabetes prevalence rate of 36.8% in the 60 to 74 age group and 46.7% in those aged >75. Within the literature, two main approaches to the prevention of T2DM have been identified: pharmacological interventions and lifestyle modifications.

There have been several large pharmacological T2DM prevention trials, including the Troglitazone in Prevention of Diabetes study (TRIPOD) in the United States (Azen et al., 1998): the STOP-NIDDM trial (Chiasson et al. 2002) in Canada and Europe, and the Xendos study in Sweden (Torgerson, Hauptman, Boldrin, & Sjostrom, 2004). The troglitazone (TRIPOD) study evaluated the incidence of diabetes in women of Hispanic ethnicity (n = 93) with previous gestational diabetes and a history of positive glucose tolerance tests (PGC less than or equal to 625 mg/dL). Women were assigned to placebo or 400 mg/day troglitazone. After a median follow-up of 30 months, women randomized to troglitazone had a 55% reduction in the risk of diabetes. Likewise, Chiasson et al. (2002) found that participants who received the intervention drug (Acarbose) were at a reduced risk of developing T2DM. This double-blind placebo-controlled randomized trial across nine countries investigated the effect of acarbose with people with impaired glucose tolerance (IGT) on the incidence of diabetes, hypertension, and cardiovascular disease. Patients were randomly allocated to receive placebo (n = 715) or Acarbose 100 mg 3 times a day (n = 714) and were followed up for 3.3 years. Acarbose treatment resulted in a 25% relative risk reduction in the development of T2DM.

The Xendos study (Torgerson et al., 2004) was a double-blind, randomized prospective study that ran over 4 years. Participants were 30 to 60 years old with a BMI greater than 30.0 kg/m^2 (mean 37 kg/m^2). All enrolled subjects were non-diabetic with normal glucose tolerance tests (GTT) (79%), but some (21%) had IGT. Participants (n = 3305:55% females, 21% with IGT) were randomly assigned to 120 mg of orlistat 3 times a day or placebo. All patients had lifestyle interventions also, such as reducing dietary regime and exercise. After 4 years' treatment, the cumulative incidence of diabetes was 9.0% with placebo and 6.2% with orlistat, corresponding to a risk reduction of 37.3% (P = 0.0032). Over the entire study period, a significantly higher proportion of patients treated with orlistat compared with those treated with placebo achieved weight losses of greater than 5% and 10%.

Systematic reviews examining specific pharmaceutical products used in the prevention of T2DM have also confirmed their benefits (Abuissas, Jones, Marso, & O'Keefe, 2005; Lily & Godwin, 2009; Orchard et al., 2005). These reviews conclude that there is merit in using hypoglycemic agents in addition to lifestyle modifications and antiobesity agents to prevent T2DM. Lily and Godwin (2009) particularly focused on metformin and concluded that even without the lifestyle interventions, metformin decreased the rate of conversion to T2DM at both a higher (850 mg twice daily) and lower (250 mg twice daily) dosage. In particular, hypoglycemic agents are recommended for individuals who are at risk of diabetic complications and exacerbations from existing cardiovascular diseases (Abuissas et al., 2005), as is the case with Georgiana.

Metformin suppresses hepatic gluconeogenesis by activating AMP (activated protein kinase), a liver enzyme responsible for insulin activation and the metabolism of glucose and fats (Lily & Godwin, 2009). Metformin is the only medication recommended for use with patients with IGT or impaired fasting glucose (IFG) (i.e., patients at high risk of T2DM; Nathan et al., 2007). Following their double-blind RCT (metformin vs. placebo) and their 7- to 8-year open-label extension and analysis of adverse events and tolerability, The Diabetes Prevention Program Research Group (2012) concluded that metformin is effective and safe to use in the prevention of T2DM. Prescribing metformin for Georgiana should therefore be considered.

The literature reveals that lifestyle intervention programs targeted at persons at high risk of developing T2DM (prediabetes) are viable, cost effective, and may delay and prevent the development of T2DM (Roumen et al., 2009). Furthermore, many of these large lifestyle intervention programs are also associated with improvements in CVD risk factors (Pratley & Matfin, 2007). The major lifestyle intervention studies include the Finnish Diabetes Prevention Study (FDPS), the Da Quing study, and the American Diabetes Prevention Program (DPP). The 3-year FDPS trial examined whether an intensive diet and exercise lifestyle intervention could delay, or prevent, the onset of T2DM in 522 high-risk overweight adults with impaired IGT (Tuomilehto et al., 2001). They found a 58% reduction in T2DM over a median of 4 years in participants allocated to the intervention (n = 265) compared with those allocated to the control (n = 257). The Da Quing cluster randomized trial also found that a community-based diet and exercise intervention reduced the cumulative 6-year occurrence of T2DM in all intervention groups (41%–46%) compared with the control group (68%) (Li et al., 2008). Likewise, the U.S. DPP trial demonstrated that an intensive diet and exercise intervention reduced the onset of T2DM by 58% in participants with IGT ($n = 1,079$) over a mean follow-up of 2.8 years, compared with a control group ($n = 1,082$) who received brief lifestyle advice and a placebo (Knowler et al., 2002; Orchard et al., 2005). All of these studies demonstrate that a relatively small change in lifestyle (increasing fiber [an increase of 15 g/1,000 kcal or more], reducing total fat [less than 30% of energy consumed] and saturated fat [less than 10% of energy consumed], and engaging in moderate physical activity [30 mins/day or more] and weight reduction [5%]) can significantly reduce the onset of T2DM in adults with IGT.

Several systematic reviews and meta-analyses of trials, evaluating different lifestyle interventions for people at high risk of developing T2DM, have also been undertaken. A Cochrane review conducted by Nield et al. (2008) concluded that, although only two RCTs had examined dietary interventions and control groups, dietary interventions are effective at reducing the risk of developing T2DM. In relation to exercise, one systematic review concluded that increasing physical activity by even a modest amount can have an impact on the prevention of T2DM (Jeon, Lokken, Hu, & van Dam, 2007). Another systematic review of 30 systematic reviews on lifestyle intervention trials examining the elements associated with increased modifications in diet and/or exercise in persons at risk of T2DM was undertaken by Greaves et al. (2011). They concluded that the interventions achieved clinically meaningful weight loss and increased physical activity. They also report that the effectiveness of interventions is increased through targeting diet and exercise, use of clearly defined behavior change techniques, and use of clearly defined strategies for supporting the maintenance of behavior change, for example, motivational interviewing. Baker et al. (2011), in their systematic review of behavioral change strategies used in diabetes prevention programs, conclude that interventions targeted at several physical activity and dietary goals simultaneously are most successful in comparison with usual care or pharmacological interventions. Furthermore, Lindström et al. (2008) found that lifestyle intervention was most effective in those over 61. Georgiana should therefore be encouraged to join a lifestyle intervention program—for example, the "Let's Prevent Diabetes" structured education program, which is based on the FDPS trial (Troughton et al., 2008), or the America National Diabetes Prevention Programs (NDPP), which translates the U.S. DPP trial into community-based diabetes prevention programs. Georgiana therefore needs to modify her diet and physical activity levels. The nurse needs to work with her to review her diet—this may be done by asking Georgiana to keep a weekly food diary that they can then analyze and work through together. In addition, the nurse should identify Georgiana's preferred physical activity and what supports she may need to help motivate her to engage in it.

Systematic reviews of randomized controlled trials that examined lifestyle and pharmacological interventions to prevent T2DM have also been conducted (Burnet et al. 2005; Gillies et al., 2007; Hays, Galassetti, & Coker, 2008; Yuen, Sugeng, Weiland, & Jelinek, 2010). These reviews concluded that a dual approach to delaying or preventing the onset of T2DM appears to be effective. Burnet et al. (2005) argue that interventions to prevent the onset of diabetes are cost effective but that lifestyle changes should be supported as a first-line approach. This is supported by the International Diabetes Federation ([IDF], 2013), who also note that lifestyle intervention is the more successful intervention for older people (Alberti, Zimmet, & Shaw, 2007; Lindström et al., 2008). However, it is unclear whether lifestyle interventions or pharmacological interventions are most effective (Gillies et al., 2007; Yuen et al., 2010). Concerns are raised that both intervention strategies have problems relating to side effects and adherence (Yuen et al., 2010). Adherence to a treatment regimen that includes dietary restrictions and physical activity may be a problem for Georgiana. The nurse must therefore consider how best to support Georgiana to successfully achieve her goals.

Social support—which includes relationships with peers, family, friends, and colleagues, as well as other persons with diabetes and Internet contacts—is considered a key element of effective diabetes management (Lindstrom et al., 2010).

There is no single definition of the concept of social support, and no agreement as to how it should be measured. Typically, social support is the physical and emotional comfort given to us by family, friends, and significant others in our social network. The social support network consists of a system of social ties and usually consists of friends, family, and health care professionals. The social network has the potential to provide the social support and assistance the individual requires when needed (Schwarzer, Knoll, & Rieckmann, 2004). House (1981) described four main types of social support: appraisal support, informational support, instrumental support, and emotional support. Appraisal support (validatory support) is when others in the social network confirm the appropriateness of actions taken or of statements made by the person (Payne & Walker, 1998). Informational support involves the provision of relevant knowledge. Instrumental support involves the concrete/tangible direct form of explicit social support, including, for example, providing help with household tasks or driving someone to the clinic. These are supports that help the individual overcome a particular problem. Finally, there is emotional support, which is the verbal and nonverbal expressions of empathy, trust, and caring. The consensus from the literature is that social support is a key element of effective prediabetes self-management (Jacob & Serrano-Gil, 2010; van Dam et al., 2005).

Van Dam et al. (2005) undertook a systematic review involving six RCTs to examine the impact of social support interventions on care outcomes for persons with T2DM in primary or outpatient care. Although social support was measured differently across studies, they tentatively reached conclusions on a number of issues: that group consultations improved HbA1C and lifestyle outcomes; that web-based and telephone-based peer support improved perceived support; and that exercise and social support groups led to increased knowledge levels and psychosocial functioning. Studies have found that high levels of support from spouses and family are associated with higher rates of adherence to diabetic medical regimes (Garay-Sevialla et al., 1995; Glasgow & Toobert,

1988). Miller and Davis (2005) found that T2DM patients believed that social support was crucial to effective self-management; likewise, the DPS study (Kronsbein et al., 2011) found that social support received from sharing experiences of physical activity with others and the experiences of exercising together facilitated engagement in exercise. Furthermore, they suggest that regular counseling and support are an important element in promoting exercise in older adults. Greaves et al. (2011), in their systematic review of lifestyle intervention trials, also concluded that the effectiveness of interventions is increased through the use of social support. They found that interventions that included social support, typically provided by family members, resulted in an additional weight loss of 3.0 kg at up to 12 months. Furthermore, if lifestyle changes are to be maintained, then ongoing support is necessary (Funnell, 2010; Penn, 2009). Social support can therefore act as a catalyst for patients to successfully embrace the required lifestyle and management regimes (Miller & DiMatteo, 2013). Currently, Georgiana appears to have limited social support. It would therefore be important for the nurse to help establish new social support networks with her, which may make it more likely that she will adhere to a new diet and exercise regime. The nurse also needs to exploit Georgiana's enjoyment of the social aspects of exercising to help her adhere to any exercise program.

T2DM is a serious chronic condition that in Georgiana's case may be prevented or at least whose onset may be delayed. Georgiana may be perceived to be particularly vulnerable as she is an older lady who lives alone and appears to have few friends or social networks. However, for some individuals, these factors are not considered problematic as they may have lived very independent lives, predominantly preferring their own company to that of others. The nurse therefore needs to be cognizant of individual personal preferences and cultural norms when assessing Georgiana's situation and circumstance, and actively listen to Georgiana so that what is important to Georgiana is identified and effective strategies can be developed with her that have the greatest potential for success as she introduces lifestyle changes to reduce the likelihood of her developing T2DM.

Strategies and Solutions

- Listen to Georgiana, and identify how important it is for her to make lifestyle changes in light of her current physical examination.
- Work with Georgiana to help her to identify realistic diet and exercise goals. For example, in terms of weight loss a realistic goal may be to lose 1 lb. per week.
- Locate a "Let's Prevent Diabetes" program in an accessible venue, and encourage Georgiana to join the program, focusing on the social aspects of exercising that are important to Georgiana.
- Teach Georgiana how to recognize healthy and unhealthy foods, and assist her in understanding food labels so she can more easily select a healthy food option.
- Teach Georgiana to recognize the early signs/symptoms of diabetes.
- Consider commencing Georgiana on metformin, and monitor effectiveness and possible side effects.
- Plan to monitor Georgiana's HbA1C every 3 to 6 months.

Clinical Reasoning Questions

1. What is your plan for follow-up care of Georgiana?
2. Are any referrals needed in this case? If so, to whom?
3. What if Georgiana was also depressed?
4. Are there any standardized guidelines that you could use to assess or treat Georgiana?

References

Abuissas, H., Jones, P. G., Marso, S. P., & O'Keefe, J. H. (2005). Angiotensin-converting enzyme inhibitors or angiotensin receptor blockers for prevention of type 2 diabetes. A meta-analysis of randomized clinical trials. *Journal of the American College of Cardiology, 46*(5), 821–826.

Alberti, K. G., Zimmet, P., & Shaw, J. (2007). International diabetes federation: A consensus on type 2 diabetes prevention. *Diabetic Medicine, 24*, 451–463.

Azen, S. P., Peters, R. K., Berkowitz, K., Kjos, S., Xiang, A., & Buchanan, T. A. (1998). TRIPOD: A randomized placebo-controlled trial of troglitazone in women with prior gestational diabetes mellitus. *Control Clinical Trials, 19*, 217–231.

Bailey, G., Barner, J., & Weems, J. (2012). Assessing barriers to medication adherence in underserved patients with diabetes in Texas. *Diabetes Education, 38*, 271–279.

Baker, M. K., Simpson, K., Llyod, B., Bauman, A. E., & Singh, M. A. (2011). Behavioral strategies in diabetes prevention programs: A systematic review of randomized controlled trials. *Diabetes Research and Clinical Practice, 91*(1), 1–12.

Burnet, D., Elliot, L., Quinn, M., Plaut, A., Schwartz, P. E., & Chin, M. (2005) Preventing diabetes in the clinical setting. *Journal of General Internal Medicine, 21*, 84–93.

Chiasson, J-L., Josse, R., Gomis, R., Hanefeld, H., Karasik, A., Laakso, M., & STOP-NIDDM Trail Research Group. (2002). Acarbose for prevention of type 2 diabetes mellitus: The STOP-NIDDM randomized trial. *Lancet, 359*(9323), 2072–2077.

Cowie, C. C., Rust, K. F., Ford, E. S., Eberhardt, M. S., Byrd-Holt, D. D., Li, C., . . . Geiss, L. S. (2009). Full accounting of diabetes and pre-diabetes in the U.S. population in 1988–1994 and 2005–2006. *Diabetes Care, 32*(2), 287–294.

The Diabetes Prevention Program Research Group. (2012). Long-term safety, tolerability, and weight loss associated with metformin in the Diabetes Prevention Program Outcomes Study. *Diabetes Care, 35*(4), 731–737.

DiMatteo, M. R. (2004). Social support and patient adherence to medical treatment: A meta-analysis. *Health Psychology, 23*, 207–218.

Division of Diabetes Translation National Center for Chronic Disease Prevention and Health Promotion. (2013). *National diabetes prevention program.* Retrieved from http://www.cdc.gov/diabetes/prevention/about.htm

European Diabetes Working Party for Older People. (2004). Clinical guidelines for type 2 diabetes mellitus. Retrieved February 21, 2015, from http://www.eugms.org/search.html?tx_solr%5Bq%5D=European+Diabetes+Working+Party+for+Older+People+%282004%29rch&id=24&L=0

Funnell, M. M. (2010). Peer-based behavioural strategies to improve chronic disease self-management and clinical outcomes: Evidence, logistics, evaluation considerations and needs for future research. *Family Practice, 27*(Suppl 1), i17–22. doi:10.1093/fampra/cmp027

Garay-Sevialla, M., Nava, L., Malacara, J., Huerta, R., Jorge, L., Mena, A., & Fajardo, M. (1995). Adherence to treatment and social support in patients with non-insulin dependent diabetes mellitus. *Diabetes Complications, 9,* 81–86.

Gillies, C., Abrams, K., Lambert, P., Cooper, N., Sutton, A., & Khunti, K. (2007). Pharmacological and lifestyle interventions to prevent or delay type 2 diabetes in people with impaired glucose tolerance: Systematic review and meta-analysis. *British Medical Journal, 334*(758), 299–302.

Glasgow, R. E., & Toobert, D. (1988). Social environment and regimen adherence among type 2 diabetic patients. *Diabetes Care, 11,* 377–386.

Greaves, C. J., Sheppard, K., Abraham, C., Hardeman, W., Roden, M., Garth, P. H., . . . Schwartz, P. (2011). Systematic review of reviews of intervention components associated with increased effectiveness in dietary and physical activity interventions. *BMC Public Health, 11,* 119.

International Diabetes Federation. (2013). *IDF diabetes atlas* (6th ed.). Brussels, Belgium: Author. Retrieved from http://www.idf.org/diabetesatlas

Jacob, S., & Serrano-Gil, M. (2010). Engaging and empowering patients to manage their type 2 diabetes. Part II: Initiatives for success. *Advances in Therapy, 27,* 665–680.

Jeon, C. Y., Lokken, R. P., Hu, F. B., & van Dam, R. M. (2007). Physical activity of moderate intensity and risk of type 2 diabetes: A systematic review. *Diabetes Care, 30*(3), 744–752.

Knowler, W. C., Barrett-Connor, M., Fowler, S., Hanman, R., Lachin, J., & Walker, E. (2002). Reduction in the incidence of type 2 diabetes with lifestyle intervention or metformin. *New England Journal of Medicine, 346*(6), 393–403.

Kronsbein, P., Fischer, M. R., Tolks, D., Greaves, C., Puhl, S., Stych, K., . . . Schwarz, P.E.H. (2011). IMAGE: Development of a European curriculum for the training of prevention managers. *British Journal of Diabetes & Vascular Disease, 11,* 163–167.

Li, G., Zhang, P., Wang, J., Gregg, E., Yang, W., Gong, Q., . . . Bennett, P. (2008). The long-term effect of lifestyle interventions to prevent diabetes in the China Da Qing Diabetes Prevention Study: A 20-year follow-up study. *Lancet, 371*(9626), 1783–1789.

Lily, M., & Godwin, M. (2009). Treating prediabetes with metformin: Systematic review and meta-analysis. *Canadian Family Physician, 55*(4), 363–369.

Lindstrom, J., Neumann, A., Sheppard, K. E., Gilis-Januszewska, A., Greaves, C. J., Handke, U., . . . Yilmaz T. (2010). Take action to prevent diabetes—The IMAGE toolkit for the prevention of type 2 diabetes in Europe. *Hormone and Metabolic Research, 42*(Suppl. 1), S37–S55.

Lindström, J., Peltonen, M., Eriksson, J., Aunola, S., Hamalainen, H., Ilanne-Parikka, P., . . . Tuomilehto, J. (2008). Determinants for the effectiveness of lifestyle intervention in the Finnish Diabetes Prevention Study. *Diabetes Care, 31*(5), 857–862.

Lindstrom, J., & Tuomilehto, J. (2003). The diabetes risk score: A practical tool to predict type 2 diabetes risk. *Diabetes Care, 26*(3), 725–731.

Miller, C. K., & Davis, M. S. (2005). The influential role of social support in diabetes management. *Topics in Clinical Nutrition, 20*, 157–165.

Miller, T. A., & DiMatteo, M. R. (2013). Importance of family/social support and impact on adherence to diabetic therapy. *Diabetes, Metabolic Syndrome and Obesity: Targets and Therapy, 6*, 421–426.

Nathan, D. M., Davidson, M. B., DeFronzo, R. A., Heine, R., Henry, R., Pratley, R., . . . Zinman, B. (2007). Impaired fasting glucose and impaired glucose tolerance: Implications for care. *Diabetes Care, 30*, 753–759.

National Institute for Health and Clinical Excellence. (2003). *Guidance on the use of patient education models on diabetes: Technology appraisal guidance 60*. London, England: Author.

Nield, L., Summerbell, C.-D., Hooper, L., Whittaker, V., Moore, H. (2008). Dietary advice for the prevention of type 2 diabetes mellitus in adults. *Cochrane Database of Systematic Reviews, 2008*(3). Art. No.: CD005102.

Orchard, T., Temprosa, M., Goldberg, R., Haffner, S., Ratner, R., Marcovina, S., . . . Fowler, S. (2005). The effect of metformin and intensive lifestyle intervention on the metabolic syndrome: The diabetes prevention program randomized trial. *Annals of Internal Medicine, 142*(8), 611–619.

Paulweber, B., Valensi, P., Lindström, J., Lalic, N. M., Greaves, C. J., McKee, M., . . . Yilmaz, T., (2010). A European evidence-based guideline for the prevention of type 2 diabetes. *Hormone and Metabolic Research*, 42 (Suppl 1), S3–S36.

Payne, S., & Walker, J. (1998). *Psychology for nurses and the caring professions*. Philadelphia, PA: Open University Press.

Penn, L., White, M., Oldroyd, J., Walker, M., Alberti, K. G. M. M., & Mathers, J. C. (2009). Prevention of type 2 diabetes in adults with impaired glucose tolerance: The European Diabetes Prevention RCT in Newcastle upon Tyne, UK. *BMC Public Health, 9*, 342. Retrieved February 21, 2015, from http://www.biomedcentral.com/content/pdf/1471-2458-9-342.pdf

Pratley, R., & Matfin, G. (2007). Review: Pre-diabetes: Clinical relevance and therapeutic approach. *British Joural of Diabetes & Vascular Disease, 7*(3), 120–129.

Roumen, C., Blaak, E. E., Corpeliijn, E. (2012). Lifestyle intervention for prevention of diabetes: Determinants of success for future implementation. *Nutrition Reviews, 67*(3), 132–146.

Ryden, L., Standl, E., Bartnik, M., Van Den Berghe, G., Betteridge, J., de Boer, M. J., Cosentino, F., . . . Tuomilehto, J., Thrainsdottir, I. (2007). Guidelines on diabetes, pre-diabetes, and cardiovascular diseases: Executive summary: The Task Force on Diabetes and Cardiovascular Diseases of the European Society of Cardiology (ESC) and of the European Association for the Study of Diabetes. *European Heart Journal, 28*, 88–136

Schwarzer, R., Knoll, N., & Rieckmann, N. (2004). Social support. In A. Kaptein & J. Weinman (Eds.), *Health psychology* (pp. 158–182). Oxford, England: Blackwell.

Torgerson, J., Hauptman, J., Boldrin, M., & Sjostrom, L. (2004). XENical in the prevention of diabetes in obese subjects (XENDOS) study. A randomized study of orlistat as an adjunct to lifestyle changes for the prevention of type 2 diabetes in obese patients. *Diabetes Care, 27*(1), 155–161.

Troughton, J., Jarvis, J., Skinner, C., Robertson, N., Khunti, K., & Davies, M. (2008). Waiting for diabetes: Perceptions of people with prediabetes: A qualitative study. *Patient Education and Counseling, 72*(1), 88–93.

Tuomilehto, J., Lindstrom, J., Eriksson, J., Valle, T., Hamäläinen, H., Ilanne-Parikka, P., . . . Uusitupa, M. (2001). Prevention of type 2 diabetes mellitus by changes in lifestyle among subjects with impaired glucose tolerance. *The New England Journal of Medicine, 344*, 1343–1350.

van Dam, H. A., van der Horst, F. G., Knoops, L., Ryckman, R. M., Crebolder, H. F., & van den Borne, B. H. (2005). Social support in diabetes: A systematic review of controlled intervention studies. *Patient Education and Counseling, 59*(1), 1–12.

World Health Organization. (2004). *Diabetes action now: An initiative of the World Health Organization and the International Diabetes Federation.* Geneva, Switzerland: Author

Yuen, A., Sugeng, Y., Weiland, T., & Jelinek, G. A. (2010). Lifestyle and medication interventions for the prevention or delay of type 2 diabetes mellitus in prediabetes: A systematic review of randomized controlled trials. *Australian and New Zealand Journal of Public Health, 34*(2), 172–178.

34 A RESTFUL SLEEP

KATHLEEN LOVANIO

Subjective

"I'd be happier than a bird with a french fry, if I can only get a good night's sleep. I've tried everything but nothing helps."

Objective

Mrs. Harriet H. Henderson is a 70-year-old obese retired schoolteacher, who presented herself today at the clinic for her annual physical. She is alert, well groomed, and cooperative. Vital signs: afebrile, 97.8°F, BP 156/78, P 96 regular rhythm, RR 18 nonlabored, O_2 sat 96% on room air, knee pain 5/10 scale; BMI 34; pupils equal, round, reactive to light and accommodation (PERRLA), arcus senilis, lower lids slightly ectropic. Her vision and hearing are grossly intact, her oral mucosa are pink, and dentition is good. Carotid pulses are without bruits, her thyroid is supple, and her trachea is midline. She has no adenopathy, and her cranial nerves are intact. Mrs. Henderson's lungs are clear to auscultation (CTA), with no adventitious breath sounds. S1, S2, and no extra heart sounds, no murmurs. Her upper extremities reveal no obvious deformities, tenderness, or swelling, with the exception of a Heberden's node on her distal interphalangeal joint of the right index finger. She has full range of motion and equal hand-grip strength. Her lower extremities are warm and without edema. Her peripheral pulses are 2+ and symmetrical. She has superficial varicosities. Both knees are enlarged, and crepitus is noted with flexion and extension. Her gait is steady, but her "timed get up and go" test took 18 seconds (normal is 7 to 11 seconds). Mrs. Henderson is independent with all activities of daily living (ADL) and instrumental activities of daily living (IADL). Her Mini Mental State Exam score (MMSE) is 30/30, revealing no deficits, and her Geriatric Depression score (GDS) is 6, indicating depression and requiring further follow-up.

Ms. Henderson presented at the clinic with complaints of sleep problems that started about 8 months ago, shortly after her retirement. She stated that all her life she had been a very good sleeper, averaging 7 to 8 hours a night. But since she retired, it has been downhill. She reports difficulty falling asleep, sometimes taking longer than 2 hours to fall asleep. Staying asleep is also a problem: "It seems like after an hour or two, I'm wide awake looking at the clock and watching the time go by. I'm also running to the bathroom once or twice during the night and that doesn't help with my sleep problem at all." She reports that a good night is never more than 4 to 5 hours of sleep.

Because of her lack of sleep, she finds herself exhausted and napping more during the day. To help her fall asleep, she stated that a glass of wine before bed works like a charm to help her to fall asleep, but finds herself waking up to use the bathroom more and unable to get back to sleep right away, sometimes lying in bed awake for an hour or more. Some nights when she cannot fall back to sleep, she will get up and watch a movie in the living room and have a snack. For the last 6 months, she has been taking Tylenol PM in place of regular Tylenol that she normally takes for her knee osteoarthritis, and found that it does help her get a better night's sleep, but she wakes more tired and unrefreshed, which leads to more daytime napping, calling it a "losing battle."

When asked what she thought might be causing her sleep problems, she stated that she was very concerned that this might be the start of dementia. She remembers that her mother, who was diagnosed in her early seventies with dementia, experienced similar sleep disturbances throughout her illness. She added, "Lately, my memory is not as good as it used to be, and my memory problem is worse after a bad night. I've been having a hard time recalling things, and this month I missed a luncheon date with the girls. What do you think is happening to me—am I losing my mind? If it's not my mind, what can I take that will boost my energy level so I can have a social life again? I feel like I'm missing out on what should be a time of my life."

Ms. Henderson's diagnosis includes hypertension (HTN); hyperlipidemia; osteoarthritis (knees); and gastroesophageal reflux disease (GERD). Her current medications include hydrochlorothiazide, 25 mg daily; Diovan, 80 mg daily; Crestor, 40 mg daily; Nexium, 40 mg daily; OTC Tylenol for knee pain, PRN. She is allergic to penicillin and codeine.

Ms. Henderson has lived alone since the death of her mother 10 years ago and is financially secure. She was never married and proudly announces that she has no regrets, stating, "I love having my get-up-and-go lifestyle." She has three sisters, who live locally, and many nieces and nephews. She taught math at the local high school, where she was a well-respected and a highly regarded teacher. Along with her family, she has a large circle of friends and was very active in the community both before and after her retirement. However, lately, she no longer enjoys or has the energy to go to concerts, travel, shop, or even visit family and friends as she had in the past. She has a living will and has appointed her younger sister, who is a nurse, as her durable power of attorney. She is of Catholic faith and attends church regularly.

Literature Review

Problematic sleep has adverse effects on all individuals regardless of age, but older adults typically show an increase in disturbed sleep that can create a negative impact on their quality of life (QOL). Overall, older adults have a decrease in "sleep efficiency," relative percentage of time in bed spent asleep, and increased "sleep latency," defined as a delay in the onset of sleep. Older adults may also report an earlier bedtime, earlier morning awakenings, more awakenings during the night, nonrestorative sleep, and more daytime napping (Vaz Fragoso & Gill, 2007). Although the ability to sleep becomes more difficult, the need to sleep does not decrease with age.

Sleep complaints are common among older adults, and the incidence of sleep problems increases with age. However, aging alone does not lead to sleep disturbances, and they are strongly related to many issues in later life. Vaz Fragoso and Gill (2007) referenced sleep problems to a "multifactorial geriatric syndrome," with predisposing, precipitating, and perpetuating factors contributing to sleep complaints. Predisposing factors are changes in sleep physiology; precipitating factors or usual aging may include a reduction in health status, loss of physical function, and primary sleep disorders; and perpetuating factors are psychosocial in nature—for example, social isolation, inactivity, inadequate sleep hygiene, caregiving, and bereavement.

Changes in sleep with aging affect sleep architecture, sleep/wake cycle, and circadian rhythm. Sleep architecture refers to the basic structural organization of normal sleep and is made up of two phases—nonrapid eye movement (NREM) sleep and rapid eye movement (REM) sleep. NREM sleep is made up of four stages. Stage one is the lightest level of sleep, and one can be easily disturbed by a disruptive noise. Stage two requires more intense stimuli than in stage one to awaken. Stages three and four sleep are referred to as slow-wave sleep (SWS), with stage four having the highest arousal threshold. During the SWS sleep, the body repairs and regenerates tissues, builds bone and muscle, and appears to strengthen the immune system. With aging, less time is spent in stages three and four, and more time is spent awake or in the lighter stages of sleep. REM sleep follows NREM sleep and is characterized by complete atonia of muscles and bursts of rapid eye movements; it is the stage of sleep in which dreaming occurs. The loss of muscle tone and reflexes serves an important function because it prevents an individual from "acting out" his or her dreams. REM sleep is important for memory consolidation, learning, and daytime concentration. REM sleep occurs cyclically every 90 to 120 minutes throughout the night.

Circadian rhythms are 24-hour physiological rhythms important in determining sleep patterns. Changes in the sleep/wake cycle are likely due to changes in the core body temperature cycle, decreased light exposures, and environmental factors (Vaz Fragoso & Gill, 2007). Both endogenous pacemakers and exogenous zeitgebers help to maintain and control the sleep/waking cycle. Endogenous pacemakers are internal "biological clocks" that manage our rhythms. The main pacemaker is housed in the suprachiasmatic nucleus (SCN), located in the hypothalamus. This detects sunlight and alters our sleep/wake cycle when needed, putting the biological rhythm in time with the environment. This is the result of the SCN stimulating the pineal gland to produce more melatonin, which induces sleep. Exogenous zeitgebers are external cues or time-givers that help to keep these rhythms in tune with the changing external environment. As people age, the sleep/wake circadian rhythm may become less synchronized (Ancoli-Israel & Cooke, 2005), taking longer to have the same response to endogenous cues and becoming less effective, resulting in less reliable periods of sleep/wake across the 24-hour day.

Age is a risk factor of advanced phase sleep disorder (APSD). APSD is characterized by a stable sleep schedule that starts several hours earlier than the conventional time. Bedtime tends to occur between 6 p.m. and 9 p.m., and individuals tend to wake up between 2 a.m. and 5 a.m. The sleep rhythm is shifted so that 7 or 8 hours of sleep are still obtained, but the individual will wake up extremely early because he or she has gone to bed quite early. There is no strict definition of how advanced the sleep schedule is to be pathologic (Sack et al., 2007). Although it can be impairing, the disorder is not necessarily unhealthy. Most older adults do not seek help unless it starts to severely affect their social life.

Precipitating factors, or usual aging, have an enormous impact on sleep disturbances and QOL. Chronic disease has been associated with sleep disruption more than age-related changes. Results of the National Sleep Foundation's (NSF) 2003 poll showed that 43% of older adults reported having two to three chronic conditions, and 24% had four or more (NSF, 2003). Physiologic changes in chronic obstructive pulmonary disease (COPD) have been shown to lead to fragmented sleep (Scharf et al., 2011). To explore the relationship between sleep disturbance and QOL, Martin, Fiorentino, Jouldjian, Josephson, and Alessi (2010) found that poor sleep was associated with declining functional status, QOL, and greater depression. Another suggested that poor sleep quality can be an early sign of cognitive decline (Potvin et al., 2012). More recently, a study was conducted that found that too much or too little sleep is linked to chronic disease (Liu, Wheaton, Chapman, & Croft, 2013). The study found that people who sleep 6 hours or less on the average had a higher prevalence of coronary heart disease, stroke, diabetes, obesity, and mental distress compared with people who sleep 7 to 9 hours on average.

Many sleep-related disorders are most prevalent in the older population, with insomnia being the most common (Ancoli-Israel & Cooke, 2005; Colten & Altevogt, 2006). Insomnia is defined as a complaint of insufficient sleep and nonrestorative sleep despite the opportunity for adequate sleep. The complaint may consist of difficulty initiating sleep, nighttime awakening or difficulty maintaining sleep, waking too early, or nonrestorative or poor quality sleep. The National Sleep Foundation's America poll reported that 44% of older adults experience one or more of the nighttime symptoms of insomnia at least a few nights per week or more (NSF, 2003). In view of the many possible causes of insomnia, identifying the underlying problem causing the insomnia is key to successful treatment.

Sleep-disordered breathing (SDB), or sleep apnea, is characterized by partial cessation of breathing (hyponea) and/or complete cessation of breathing (apnea) lasting at least 10 seconds that repeats frequently throughout the night. Consequences of this disorder cause sleep fragmentation, which leads to excessive sleepiness during the day and oxygen desaturation nightly. Morning headaches, confusion, and decreased cognitive functioning are common (Shochat & Ancoli-Israel, 2006). SDB is also an independent risk factor for HTN and is strongly associated with obesity and several other cardiovascular disorders (Budhiraja, Budhiraja, & Quan, 2010; Wolk, Shamsuzzaman, & Somers, 2003).

Restless leg syndrome (RLS) is a common neurological movement disorder associated with a sleep complaint, and its prevalence increases with age. Older adults with RLS can suffer an irresistible urge to move their legs, which is worse during inactivity, resulting in discomfort, sleep disturbances, and fatigue. It has been estimated that 90% of individuals with RLS have periodic limb movements in sleep disorder (PLMS). PLMS is a disorder of unknown etiology characteristic of episodes of repetitive involuntary movements (primarily of the legs) lasting between 0.5 and 5 seconds and occurring about every 20 to 40 seconds. The kicks are often accompanied by arousals, but often too short to recall and associated with complaints of insomnia or excessive daytime sleepiness.

Psychosocial influences, such as bereavement, caregiving, and social isolation, are prevalent in older adults. These influences can lead to sleep complaints by augmenting the effect of predisposing or precipitating factors, but may also perpetuate a sleep complaint (Vaz Fragoso & Gill, 2007). The severe and emotional strain and profound changes of lifestyle that often accompany the loss of a loved one may lead to sleepless nights and subsequent sleep complaints. Caregivers frequently experience depression and physical and emotional exhaustion that may result in highly disrupted sleep/wake cycling, especially with day and late night caregiving responsibilities. Retirement, change in structured daily routines, and social isolation can result in poor sleep hygiene. In the NSF poll (2003), older adults who felt socially isolated were more likely to report insomnia and drowsiness.

Role and Cultural Considerations

Sleep disturbances are prevalent among older adults and often go undiagnosed and untreated by health care practitioners and underreported by older adults. Unfortunately, many of the consequences of sleep disturbances in older adults are thought to be typical of old age (Salzman, 2006). This important unmet need could be readily addressed during office visits and could potentially minimize adverse outcomes. Communication is key, and nurses and advanced practice nurses need to ask patients on a regular basis about their sleeping habits. It is also important to know about any self-treatments used for sleep problems. Older adults frequently choose treatments for their sleep problems that can potentially worsen their sleep symptoms (Gooneratne, 2011). The Pittsburgh Sleep Quality Index (PSQI) is an effective instrument for measuring the quality and patterns of sleep in the older adult (Division of Nursing, Hartford Institute for Geriatric Nursing, New York University, 2012). The PSQI can be used for both an initial assessment and ongoing comparative measurements. In addition to good patient–provider communication, critical to the success of managing the complexity of sleep problems in older adults is the communication between health care providers. The more complex the decision making, the more important the quality of communication. Successful management of sleep in older adults may result in significant improvement in QOL and daytime functioning.

As the aging population continues to grow, it will become increasingly important for nurses and advanced practice nurses to become aware of and sensitive to the needs and concerns of older adults. Unfortunately, many studies suggest that age bias is prevalent among health care providers today. Because of ageist attitudes, health concerns and symptoms in the older adult may be overlooked or dismissed as the normal aging process. Additionally, many older adults are conditioned to accept declines in health function and cognition as inevitable as they age. It is important for nurses and advanced practice nurses who care for older adults to be aware of their own attitudes and beliefs about aging and the effect of these attitudes on providing care for this population.

Solutions and Strategies

Insomnia—What is needed is a more detailed description of Ms. Henderson's insomnia. Many sleep-related disorders are most prevalent in the older population, with insomnia being the most common. Ms. Henderson's request for medications to help her sleep and additional medication to help her feel more alert will only target her symptoms, rather than the underlying problem. There are many possible causes for insomnia, including medical, psychiatric, drug and medication use, changes in circadian rhythms, and psychosocial issues (Bloom et al., 2009). Identifying the underlying problem causing the insomnia is key to successful treatment.

- Sleep diary—A sleep diary completed by the patient can be very helpful to understand the severity of his or her symptoms, and to guide further evaluation and treatment. Each morning, for 1 to 2 weeks, patients log:
  - Time they went to bed
  - Number of awakenings
  - Time of morning awakening

  - Time they got out of bed for the day
  - Any symptoms that occurred during the night
  - Any medications taken or other self-treatments used for sleep (alcohol and OTC sleep medications are often used and should be avoided)
  - If available, sleep log should be supplemented by information from a bed partner
  - Focused physical examination depends on evidence from the history
  - Reports of pain should be followed up by a careful examination of the affected areas
  - Reports of nocturia that disrupts sleep should be followed by evaluation for cardiac, renal, or diabetes mellitus, and prostatic disease
  - Medical problems that can contribute to sleep difficulties (paresthesia, cough, dyspnea from cardiac or pulmonary illness, gastroesophageal reflux disease [GERD])
  - Mental status testing should be considered, with a focus on memory and mood, particularly depression
- Sleep hygiene education
- Cognitive behavioral therapy (CBT) is first-line treatment for chronic insomnia
- Pharmacological intervention
  - Considered in individuals with transient sleep problems
  - Start on the smallest dose with the least risk of adverse events

Advanced Phase Sleep Disorder

- Refer patients with significant disturbance to the sleep laboratory for evaluation.
- APSD may respond to appropriately timed light therapy.

Sleep-Disordered Breathing—Diagnostic criteria for SDB are based on clinical signs and symptoms and findings identified by polysomnography (PSG). PSG or a sleep study is the "gold standard" to confirm the diagnosis and severity of SDB (Adult Obstructive Sleep Apnea Task Force of the American Academy of Sleep Medicine, 2009). A comprehensive PSG includes measurements to document SDB (oxygen saturation, rib cage and abdominal movement, nasal and oral airflow, and snoring sounds); data regarding sleep and stages of sleep (electroencephalography [EEG], electrical activity of the brain, electrooculography [EOG], recording of eye movements, and electromyogram [EMG], to evaluate and record the electrical activity produced by skeletal muscles); and electrocardiogram and leg electromyogram to document the presence of periodic leg movements.

- Refer to sleep laboratory for evaluation
- Continuous positive airway pressure (CPAP)

Restless Leg Syndrome/Periodic Limb Movements in Sleep—As stated earlier, it is estimated that 90% of individuals with RLS have PLMS disorder.

- Diagnosis based on patient's descriptions of symptoms
- Dopaminergic agent is the initial medication of choice
- PLMS disorder—diagnosis requires polysomnography when PLMS disorder is associated with sleep complaints not explained by another sleep disorder

Clinical Reasoning Questions

1. What additional information would be helpful to develop a plan of care?
2. What is your plan for follow-up care?
3. What health promotion interventions would you recommend?
4. What if this patient was living with dementia?
5. What if this patient lived in a long-term care setting?

References

Adult Obstructive Sleep Apnea Task Force of the American Academy of Sleep Medicine. (2009). Clinical guideline for the evaluation, management and long-term care of obstructive sleep apnea in adults. *Journal of Clinical Sleep Medicine*, *5*(3), 263–276

Ancoli-Israel, S., & Cooke, J. R. (2005). Prevalence and comorbidity of insomnia and effect on functioning in elderly populations. *Journal of the American Geriatric Society, 53*(7), S264–S271. doi:10.1111/j.1532-5415.2005.53392.x

Bloom, H. G., Ahmed, I., Alessi, C. A., Ancoli-Israel, S., Buysse, D., Kryger, M. H., . . . Zee, P. C. (2009). Evidence-based recommendations for the assessment and management of sleep disorders in older persons. *Journal of the American Geriatric Society, 57*(5), 761–789. doi:10.1111/j.1532-5415.2009.02220.x

Budhiraja, R., Budhiraja, P., & Quan, S. F. (2010). Sleep-disordered breathing and cardiovascular disorders. *Respiratory Care, 55*(10), 1322–1332.

Colten, H. R., & Altevogt, B. M. (2006). *Sleep disorders and sleep deprivation: An unmet public health problem.* Retrieved from http://www.ncbi.nlm.nih.gov/books/NBK19956/

Division of Nursing, Hartford Institute for Geriatric Nursing, New York University. (2012). The Pittsburg sleep quality index (PSQI). *Try this: Best practices in nursing care to older adults.* Retrieved from http://consultgerirn.org/uploads/File/trythis/try_this_6_1.pdf

Gooneratne, N. S., Tavaria, A., Patel, N., Madhusudan, L., Nadaraja, J. D., Onen, F., & Richards, K. C. (2011). Perceived effectiveness of diverse sleep treatments in older adults. *Journal of the American Geriatric Society, 59*(2), 297–303.

Liu, Y., Wheaton, A. G., Chapman, D. P., & Croft, J. B. (2013). Sleep duration and chronic diseases among US adults age 45 years and older: Evidence from the 2010 Behavioral Risk Factor Surveillance System. *Sleep, 36*(10), 1421–1427.

Martin, J. L., Fiorentino, L., Jouldjian, S., Josephson, K. R., & Alessi, C. A. (2010). Sleep quality in residents of assisted living facilities: Effect on quality of life, functional status, and depression. *Journal of the American Geriatric Society, 58*(5), 829–836. doi:10.1111/j.1532-5415.2010.02815.x

National Sleep Foundation. (2003). *Sleep in America poll.* Retrieved from http://www.sleepfoundation.org/sites/default/files/2003SleepPollExecSumm.pdf

Potvin, O., Lorrain, D., Forget, H., Dube, M., Grenier, S., Preville, M., & Hudon, C. (2012). Sleep quality and 1-year incident cognitive impairment in community-dwelling older adults. *Sleep, 35*(4), 491–499.

Sack, R. L., Auckley, D., Auger, R. R., Carskadon, M. A., Wright, K. P., Vitiello, M. V., . . . Zhdanova, I.V. (2007). Circadian rhythm sleep disorders, Part II: Advanced sleep phase disorder, delayed sleep phase disorder, free-running disorder, and irregular sleep-wake rhythm. An American Academy of Sleep Medicine review. *Sleep, 30*(11), 1484–1501.

Salzman, B. (2006). Myths and realities of aging. *Care Management Journals 7*(3): 141–150

Scharf, S. M., Maimon, N., Simon-Tuval, T., Bernhard-Scharf, B. J., Reuvenj, H., & Tarasiuk, A. (2011). Sleep quality predicts quality of life in chronic obstructive pulmonary disease. *International Journal of Chronic Obstructive Pulmonary Disease, 6*, 1–9.

Shochat, T., & Ancoli-Israel, S. (2006). Sleep and sleep disorders. In C. K. Cassel, R. M. Leipzig, H. J. Cohen, E. B. Larson, & D. E. Meier (Eds.), *Geriatric medicine: An evidence-based approach* (p. 1032). New York, NY: Springer.

Vaz Fragoso, C. A., & Gill, T. M. (2007). Sleep complaints in community-living older persons: A multifactorial geriatric syndrome. *Journal of the American Geriatric Society, 55*(11), 1853–1866. doi:10.1111/j.1532.5415.2007.011399.x

Wolk, R., Shamsuzzaman, A. S., & Somers, V. K. (2003). Obesity, sleep apnea, and hypertension. *Hypertension, 42,* 1067–1074. Retrieved from http://hyper.ahajournals.org/content/42/6/1067

35 DYING WELL

Alison E. Kris

Subjective

"I can't even walk to the mailbox to get the mail without running out of breath."

Objective

Approximately 3 weeks ago, Mrs. Irene I. Ireland visited her health care provider following an extended bout of what she thought was the flu. She states that she has had a cough for months that just will not subside. Mrs. Ireland also reports a 20 pack/year history of smoking, having quit approximately 2 years ago when she was initially diagnosed with COPD. Although she has never needed oxygen to manage her COPD in the past, she states that she now gets short of breath with even small tasks. She considers herself to be in otherwise good health, and she has mixed feelings about her recent 20-lb. (10-kg) weight loss. Although normally she would not be upset about losing weight so easily, she reports that she has not had very much of an appetite lately and the weight loss seems very much unexpected. Mrs. Ireland reports that she lost her husband approximately 1 year ago. She has three daughters, only one of whom lives nearby.

Following a concerning chest x-ray, she was sent for a follow-up MRI. After a fine needle biopsy revealed small cell lung cancer, she was initially admitted to San Rio University Medical Center. Additional workup determined the presence of extensive disease, and she was diagnosed with stage IV small cell lung cancer. It was determined that given the extent of the disease, comorbid conditions, and age, chemotherapy would not be an appropriate course of therapy. She was discharged to Cold Springs Subacute Nursing Facility for palliative care.

Upon assessment, Mrs. Ireland is extremely short of breath on exertion, and is most comfortable sitting upright at all times. Her oxygen saturation is 90% on room air. Her anxiety is 7/10 at rest, but she becomes increasingly anxious upon exertion. At 5 foot 5, 98 lbs. (44 kg), she is extremely thin. BP is 120/80, p100, respirations 30/minute with a nonproductive cough. She is afebrile with a temp of 98.0°F. Lung sounds are diminished at the bilateral bases, with wheezes upon expiration and a prolonged expiratory phase. Cardiac exam reveals a regular heart rate, S1, S2, and no adventitious sounds. Abdomen is soft, nontender, nondistended, positive BS in all four quadrants. She has a 10 × 10-cm area of nonblanchable erythema on her buttocks, as a result of continuous pressure associated with sitting upright for extended periods of time in an effort to alleviate some of her shortness of breath. Her lips are cracked and her mouth is dry, and she wears a partial upper denture. Her hearing is slightly diminished bilaterally, and she does not wear a hearing aid. Mrs. Ireland has had some problems with stress incontinence in the past, and self-limits fluid to avoid any potential episodes of incontinence. Prior to visiting her health care provider, she was not taking any prescribed medications. She took a multivitamin daily, and had been taking over-the-counter Guaifenesin to aid her cough. Her MRI revealed the presence of stage IV metastatic small cell lung cancer, with metastases to the liver and brain.

Although Mrs. Ireland had initially wanted to be discharged back to her home, she eventually decided that it might be best for her to be discharged to the nursing home as she was afraid to be alone. Following admission to the nursing home, Mrs. Ireland was started on oxygen, 2 liters, via nasal cannula, to aid with her shortness of breath. She was initially also prescribed an air mattress overlay; however, as she found it to be rough and uncomfortable, it was removed. Her course at the nursing home was one of gradual decline. She became increasingly short of breath, and anxious.

Although Mrs. Ireland knew that she was seriously ill, she was not sure just how much longer she had to live. She was approached by the social worker at Cold Springs Subacute Nursing Facility to think about joining the hospice program there. She wanted to discuss it with her daughters, but the time never seemed right.

Eventually, when Mrs. Ireland became nonverbal and was struggling to breathe, her oldest daughter, Carol, was approached by the facility social worker about the possibility of entering hospice care. Carol was initially upset by the conversation. She said that she felt that everyone had "given up" on her mother. "It is bad enough that her doctors have given up on her, now you are giving up on her too," she told the social worker. Carol explained that she did not understand why more was not being done. "I don't really understand what is going on with my mom. I never see any doctors, and the nurses here don't tell me anything." She felt that her mother was "dumped" at the nursing home by her doctors. This was 1 week prior to her death.

The last week of Mrs. Ireland's life was very difficult for everyone involved with her care. The nasal cannula was very uncomfortable, and Mrs. Ireland would often try to pull it away from her nose. Her former oncologist was eventually contacted by her daughter, Carol, who said he would do everything he could to keep her comfortable. New orders were written for morphine sulphate SL, q2h PRN, and to "keep O_2 sat above 90%." This led to a conversation as to whether or not Mrs. Ireland should be restrained, as removal of her oxygen tubing caused her O_2 sat to drop.

After approximately 2 weeks in the nursing home, Mrs. Ireland was found to have a 6-cm round stage III pressure ulcer on her coccyx. The nurse caring for Mrs. Ireland advocated for her to get a pressure-relieving mattress, and wrote a care plan for the pressure ulcer. The care plan included the following nursing actions: turn patient every 2 hours, wet to moist dressing to be changed daily, observe for signs and symptoms of infection, and administer pain medication prior to dressing changes.

On the day of her death, Mrs. Ireland was very anxious and was struggling to breathe. Although she was not verbally responsive, she gripped onto her side rails and would take short, rapid breaths. Her oxygen saturation was below 90%.

When the nurses would administer the morphine sulphate, her respiratory rate would drop substantially, and she would become less and less responsive with each dose. The nurses at the facility were upset because they felt that they were "killing her" with the morphine. None of the nurses wanted to be responsible for giving the final dose.

Literature Review

The case of Mrs. Ireland demonstrates many of the issues and problems that can serve as barriers to dying well. The literature reports the sometimes overwhelming symptom burden experienced by older adults at the end of life. Among residents of nursing homes and in assisted living facilities, pain and shortness of breath occur in more than half of patients, with 9% to 15% of family members reporting that these symptoms were "severe" or "horrible" for their family members at the end of life (Hanson et al., 2008). While nausea and anxiety tend to be reported less frequently, when they do occur, they are symptoms that tend to be highly distressing to patients (Kris & Dodd, 2004). Evidence-based strategies to manage these symptoms are well known, and need to be employed.

The essential elements of pain management are broadly addressed through guidelines established by the World Health Organization in their Cancer Pain Ladder (WHO, n.d.). The principles of the pain ladder suggest that pain would be assessed frequently, with higher levels of pain requiring different pain management strategies. More specific information related to the assessment and management of cancer pain can be found in the clinical practice guidelines available through a variety of nursing and medical associations (Piano et al., 2013; Ripamonti et al., 2012).

For Mrs. Ireland, management of the symptoms specific to her diagnosis of lung cancer is important. For patients with any type of pulmonary disease at the end of life, management of dyspnea and the anxiety associated with shortness of breath is foundational to high-quality care. It is understood that dyspnea and shortness of breath are highly intercorrelated and thus should be managed together (Kris & Dodd, 2004).

Elements of the management of shortness of breath should include supplemental humidified oxygen, opiate narcotics, and anxiolytic adjuvants (Simoff et al., 2013).

Late entry to hospice care poses a challenge to health care providers, hospice care workers, and patient family members. Family members of residents dying in nursing homes without the benefit of hospice reported an increased number of unmet needs, and more problems with quality of care than those who received hospice care (Teno et al., 2011). When hospice entry is delayed, patient family members are more likely to experience depression after the death of their loved one (Kris et al., 2006). Therefore, timely referral to hospice is important to help improve the quality of care in this patient population (Teno, Casarett, Spence, & Connor, 2012).

Despite the demonstrated value of hospice care, certain groups of patients are at increased risk of delayed entry into hospice. For patients with metastatic lung cancer, nearly half (47%) report that they have not discussed the possibility of hospice care with a provider. Among these residents with metastatic lung cancer, those who are Black, Hispanic, non-English speaking, married or living with a partner, or Medicaid beneficiaries, as well as those who had received chemotherapy, are at increased risk of delayed hospice entry (Huskamp et al., 2009). Patients with certain diagnoses, such as those with Alzheimer's disease as well as those with heart failure, are at increased risk of delayed entry into hospice (Adler, Goldfinger, Kalman, Park, & Meier, 2009).

While most older adults prefer to die at home, the majority, unfortunately, do not (National Center for Health Statistics [NCHS], 2011). Between 1989 and 2007, there was a shift away from hospitals and into homes and nursing homes as the site of death, and this trend is continuing (NCHS, 2011; Teno et al., 2013). In addition, there has been a significant increase in the percentage of patients being transferred out of hospitals with less than 3 days to live (Teno et al., 2013), making the coordination of care offered by nurses essential. Age is a major factor determining place of death, with older patients significantly more likely to die in a nursing home (NCHS, 2011). Patients who have delayed entry into hospice and who have poorly controlled pain are less likely to die in the setting of their choice (Jeurkar et al., 2012). The place of death and context of care can serve as a major barrier to the delivery of high-quality end-of-life care. Nursing homes have often been noted for their inadequate staffing levels, lack of supervision of staff, and substandard physical environment (Kayser-Jones, Schell, Lyons, Kris, Chan, & Beard, 2003). These quality-of-care issues are of concern to all residents and their families, but can be especially problematic for residents at the end of life, who have complex nursing care requirements.

For patients who are terminally ill residents of nursing homes, adequate communication is an essential component of care (Aspinal, Addington-Hall, Hughes, & Higginson, 2003; Hebert, Schulz, Copeland, & Arnold, 2009; Shield, Wetle, Teno, Miller, & Welch, 2010; Sloane et al., 2003; Thompson, McClement, Menec, & Chochinov, 2012). As exemplified in the case study, residents often feel a disconnection from their health care provider when they enter the nursing home. Thompson et al. (2012) describe family members as feeling as though they needed to "hunt down" their physicians, who were often "not being forthcoming," and Shield, Wetle, Teno, Miller, and Welch (2005) describe them as "missing in action." This poor communication is a major contributing factor to dissatisfaction with end-of-life care in nursing homes.

Solutions and Strategies

An emphasis in nursing education on how to manage the common symptoms associated with dying is important. Because it is the bedside nurse who will be responsible for responding to a sometimes rapidly changing symptom profile, nurses will need to be taught to frequently reassess their terminally ill patients. Careful forethought is necessary to consider not only which medications are needed presently, but which medications may be needed moving forward. Terminally ill residents should have orders on hand to immediately respond to any rapid changes in levels of pain, anxiety, or nausea.

Nursing homes need to recognize that these medically complex patients require substantial amounts of nursing care and attention, and should staff units in such a way that allows for sufficient time to deliver this care. The environment of the dying patient is important not only for the patient, but for the family members and friends who may visit. High-quality nursing homes are noted for their care, community, and compassion (Kayser-Jones, Chan, & Kris, 2005).

Hospice providers can be a source of tremendous comfort both to patients and their family members. Evidence suggests, however, that the benefit of hospice can be limited when patients enter hospice very close to death. Therefore, providers should talk with their patients about hospice care early in the stages of what will ultimately be terminal diseases.

The following are points to consider in the management of patient care at the end of life:

1. Poor symptom management
    - Assess symptoms frequently using standardized assessment tools.
    - Manage symptoms according to evidence-based practice protocols such as the WHO ladder for pain management.
    - Consider the possibility of sudden changes in the intensity of symptoms, particularly in patients at the end of life, and have a plan in place to manage these changes.
2. Delayed entry to hospice
    - Hospice should be a consideration whenever patients are seriously ill.
    - Practitioners should talk honestly and openly about the availability of hospice care across practice settings.
    - Practitioners should ensure advanced directives are present prior to nursing home placement or upon nursing home admission.
3. Lack of communication
    - The presence of nurse practitioners in nursing homes has been demonstrated to improve levels of communication and perceived support among nursing home patients and their families.
    - Early entry to hospice care can also ensure that patients have adequate levels of communication at the end of life.

Role and Cultural Considerations

The staff nurse in a nursing home is an important coordinator of care for patients who are terminally ill. This nurse, either an RN or, more commonly, an LVN/LPN, is the center of communication and symptom management, as well as coordinator of medical care. Nursing homes that employ nurse practitioners tend to have higher levels of patient satisfaction, and residents in homes with nurse practitioners report improved communication and levels of support.

Minority patients in nursing homes are at increased risk of poor-quality care. They are less likely to receive the benefit of hospice care, and are more likely to have poor symptom management at the end of life. In addition, minority patients are more likely to reside in nursing homes with poor levels of nurse staffing. Each of these concerns, when combined, means that minority patients and their families are less likely to have a positive end-of-life experience.

Clinical Reasoning Questions

1. It was decided that Mrs. Ireland was not a good candidate for chemotherapy, in part due to her age. Should age be a factor when determining appropriateness to treat? At what age is it no longer appropriate to treat advanced cancer in an older adult?
2. Mrs. Ireland was discharged to a subacute facility for "palliative care." What are the differences between palliative care, comfort care, and hospice care?
3. Hospice care may be delivered in many different settings. How does the setting in which hospice care is delivered affect the quality of the hospice care?
4. At the end of life, orders were written to keep O_2 saturation above 90%, as well as for sublingual morphine sulphate. How might you change these orders? What might be considered key orders for a patient to have in place at the end of life?
5. Mrs. Ireland's nurse wrote for the following items to be included in her care plan related to her pressure ulcer: turn patient every 2 hours, wet to moist dressing to be changed

daily, observe for signs and symptoms of infection, and administer pain medication prior to dressing changes. What do you think of these nursing actions?

6. None of the nurses at the facility wanted to be the one to administer the "final dose" of morphine. How common is that feeling, in your opinion? If you were an APRN coming into the setting, how might you discuss this issue with the staff nurses? Do you see this as part of your role?

References

Adler, E. D., Goldfinger, J. Z., Kalman, J., Park, M. E., & Meier, D. E. (2009). Palliative care in the treatment of advanced heart failure. *Circulation, 120*(25), 2597–2606.

Aspinal, F., Addington-Hall, J., Hughes, R., & Higginson, I. J. (2003). Using satisfaction to measure the quality of palliative care: A review of the literature. *Journal of Advanced Nursing, 42*(4), 324–339.

Hanson, L. C., Eckert, J. K., Dobbs, D., Williams, C. S., Caprio, A. J., Sloane, P. D., & Zimmerman, S. (2008). Symptom experience of dying long-term care residents. *Journal of the American Geriatrics Society, 56*(1), 91–98.

Hebert, R. S., Schulz, R., Copeland, V. C., & Arnold, R. M. (2009). Preparing family caregivers for death and bereavement: Insights from caregivers of terminally ill patients. *Journal of Pain and Symptom Management, 37*(1), 3–12.

Huskamp, H. A., Keating, N. L., Malin, J. L., Zaslavsky, A. M., Weeks, J. C., Earle, C. C., & Ayanian, J. Z. (2009). Discussions with physicians about hospice among patients with metastatic lung cancer. *Archives of Internal Medicine, 169*(10), 954–962.

Jeurkar, N., Farrington, S., Craig, T. R., Slattery, J., Harrold, J. K., Oldanie, B., & Casarett, D. J. (2012). Which hospice patients with cancer are able to die in the setting of their choice? Results of a retrospective cohort study. *Journal of Clinical Oncology: Official Journal of the American Society of Clinical Oncology, 30*(22), 2783–2787.

Kayser-Jones, J., Chan, J., & Kris, A. (2005). A model long-term care hospice unit: Care, community, and compassion. *Geriatric Nursing, 26*(1), 16–20, 64.

Kayser-Jones, J., Schell, E., Lyons, W., Kris, A. E., Chan, J., & Beard, R. L. (2003). Factors that influence end-of-life care in nursing homes: The physical environment, inadequate staffing, and lack of supervision. *The Gerontologist, 43*(Spec. No. 2), 76–84.

Kris, A. E., Cherlin, E. J., Prigerson, H., Carlson, M. D., Johnson-Hurzeler, R., Kasl, S. V., & Bradley, E. H. (2006). Length of hospice enrollment and subsequent depression in family caregivers: 13-month follow-up study. *The American Journal of Geriatric Psychiatry: Official Journal of the American Association for Geriatric Psychiatry, 14*(3), 264–269.

Kris, A. E., & Dodd, M. J. (2004). Symptom experience of adult hospitalized medical-surgical patients. *Journal of Pain and Symptom Management, 28*(5), 451–459.

National Center for Health Statistics. (2011). *Health, United States, 2010: With special feature on death and dying.* Retrieved from http://www.cdc.gov/nchs/data/hus/hus10.pdf

Piano, V., Schalkwijk, A., Burgers, J., Verhagen, S., Kress, H., Hekster, Y., . . . Vissers, K. (2013). Guidelines for neuropathic pain management in patients with cancer: A European survey and comparison. *Pain Practice: The Official Journal of World Institute of Pain, 13*(5), 349–357.

Ripamonti, C. I., Santini, D., Maranzano, E., Berti, M., Roila, F., & ESMO Guidelines Working Group. (2012). Management of cancer pain: ESMO clinical practice guidelines. *Annals of Oncology: Official Journal of the European Society for Medical Oncology/ESMO, 23*(Suppl. 7), vii139–vii154.

Shield, R. R., Wetle, T., Teno, J., Miller, S. C., & Welch, L. (2005). Physicians "missing in action": Family perspectives on physician and staffing problems in end-of-life care in the nursing home. *Journal of the American Geriatrics Society, 53*(10), 1651–1657.

Shield, R. R., Wetle, T., Teno, J., Miller, S. C., & Welch, L. C. (2010). Vigilant at the end of life: Family advocacy in the nursing home. *Journal of Palliative Medicine, 13*(5), 573–579.

Simoff, M. J., Lally, B., Slade, M. G., Goldberg, W. G., Lee, P., Michaud, G. C., . . . Chawla, M. (2013). Symptom management in patients with lung cancer: Diagnosis and management of lung cancer, 3rd ed.: American College of Chest Physicians evidence-based clinical practice guidelines. *Chest, 143*(5 Suppl), e455S–97S. doi:10.1378/chest.12-2366; 10.1378/chest.12-2366

Sloane, P. D., Zimmerman, S., Hanson, L., Mitchell, C. M., Riedel-Leo, C., & Custis-Buie, V. (2003). End-of-life care in assisted living and related residential care settings: Comparison with nursing homes. *Journal of the American Geriatrics Society, 51*(11), 1587–1594.

Teno, J. M., Casarett, D., Spence, C., & Connor, S. (2012). It is "too late" or is it? Bereaved family member perceptions of hospice referral when their family member was on hospice for seven days or less. *Journal of Pain and Symptom Management, 43*(4), 732–738.

Teno, J. M., Gozalo, P. L., Bynum, J. P., Leland, N. E., Miller, S. C., Morden, N. E., . . . Mor, V. (2013). Change in end-of-life care for Medicare beneficiaries: Site of death, place of care, and health care transitions in 2000, 2005, and 2009. *JAMA: The Journal of the American Medical Association, 309*(5), 470–477.

Teno, J. M., Gozalo, P. L., Lee, I. C., Kuo, S., Spence, C., Connor, S. R., & Casarett, D. J. (2011). Does hospice improve quality of care for persons dying from dementia? *Journal of the American Geriatrics Society, 59*(8), 1531–1536.

Thompson, G. N., McClement, S. E., Menec, V. H., & Chochinov, H. M. (2012). Understanding bereaved family members' dissatisfaction with end-of-life care in nursing homes. *Journal of Gerontological Nursing, 38*(10), 49–60.

World Health Organization. (n.d.). *WHO's cancer pain ladder for adults.* Retrieved from http://www.who.int/cancer/palliative/painladder/en

INDEX